Handbook of Practical Critical Care Medicine

Springer
*New York
Berlin
Heidelberg
Barcelona
Hong Kong
London
Milan
Paris
Singapore
Tokyo*

Handbook of Practical Critical Care Medicine

Joseph Varon, M.D., F.A.C.P.,
F.C.C.P., F.C.C.M.
Associate Professor of Medicine

Robert E. Fromm, Jr., M.D., M.P.H., F.A.C.P.,
F.C.C.P., F.C.C.M.
Associate Professor of Medicine

Baylor College of Medicine
and
The Methodist Hospital
Houston, Texas

With 30 Illustrations

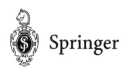 Springer

Joseph Varon, M.D.
Robert E. Fromm, Jr., M.D., M.P.H.
Baylor College of Medicine
2219 Dorrington Street
Houston, TX 77030
USA

Library of Congress Cataloging-in-Publication Data
Varon, Joseph.
    Handbook of practical critical care medicine / Joseph Varon,
  Robert E. Fromm, Jr.
        p.   cm.
    Includes bibliographical references and index.
    ISBN 0-387-95165-2 (softcover : alk. paper)
    1. Critical care medicine—Handbooks, manuals, etc.   I. Fromm,
  Robert E.   II. Title.
  RC86.8 .V364   2001
  616′.028—dc21   2001020052

Printed on acid-free paper.

Production managed by Timothy Taylor; manufacturing supervised by Joe
Quatela.
Typeset by Best-set Typesetter Ltd., Hong Kong.
Printed and bound by R.R. Donnelley and Sons, Harrisonburg, VA.
Printed in the United States of America.

9 8 7 6 5 4 3 2 1

ISBN 0-387-95165-2   SPIN 10785335

Springer-Verlag   New York Berlin Heidelberg
A member of BertelsmannSpringer Science+Business Media GmbH

To our families

Preface

Critical care medicine is a relatively new specialty. Over the past few decades, we have seen an enormous growth in the number of intensive care units (ICUs) worldwide. Medical students, residents, fellows, attending physicians, critical care nurses, pharmacists, respiratory therapists, and other health-care providers (irrespective of their ultimate field of practice) will spend several months or years of their professional lives taking care of critically ill or severely injured patients. These clinicians must have special training, experience, and competence in managing complex problems in their patients. In addition, they must interpret the data obtained by many kinds of monitoring devices, and they must integrate this information with their knowledge of the pathophysiology of disease.

This handbook was written for every practitioner engaged in critical care medicine. We have attempted to present basic and generally accepted clinical information and some important formulas as well as laboratory values and tables that we feel will be useful to the practitioner of critical care medicine. Chapter 1 provides an introduction to the ICU. Chapters 2 through 18 follow an outline format and are divided by organ system (i.e., neurologic disorders, cardiovascular disorders), as well as special topics (i.e., environmental disorders, trauma, toxicology). In addition, many of these chapters review some useful facts and formulas systematically. Finally, Chapters 19 and 20 supply lists of pharmacologic agents and dosages commonly used in the ICU and laboratory values relevant to the ICU.

It is important for the reader of this handbook to understand that critical care medicine is not a static field and that changes occur every day. Therefore, this handbook is not meant to define the standard of care but, rather, to be a general guide to current clinical practice used in critical care medicine.

Joseph Varon, M.D., F.A.C.P., F.C.C.P., F.C.C.M.
Robert E. Fromm, Jr., M.D., M.P.H., F.A.C.P., F.C.C.P., F.C.C.M.

Contents

Approach to the Intensive Care Unit

■ WELCOME TO THE ICU

What Is an ICU?

An intensive care unit (ICU) is an area of a hospital that provides aggressive therapy, using state-of-the-art technology, and both invasive and noninvasive monitoring for critically ill and high-risk patients. In these units the patient's physiological variables are reported to the practitioner on a continuous basis, so that titrated care can be provided.

As a medical student, resident physician, and attending physician, one is likely to spend several hundreds of hours in these units caring for very sick patients. Knowing the function and organization of these specialized areas will help the practitioner in understanding critical care.

Historical Development of the ICU

The origin of the ICU is controversial. In 1863, Florence Nightingale wrote, "In small country hospitals there are areas that have a recess or small room leading from the operating theater in which the patients remain until they have recovered, or at least recover from the immediate effects of the operation." This is probably the earliest description of what would become the ICU. Recovery rooms were developed at the Johns Hopkins Hospital in the 1920s. In Germany in the 1930s, the first well-organized postoperative ICU was developed. In the United States, more specialized postoperative recovery rooms were implemented in the 1940s at the Mayo Clinic. In the late 1950s, the first shock unit was established in Los Angeles. The initial surveillance unit for patients after acute myocardial infarction was started in Kansas City in 1962.

Economical Impact of the ICU

Since their initial development, there has been a rapid and remarkable growth of ICU beds in the United States. There are presently an estimated 50,000 ICU beds in the United States, and critical care consumes approximately 1.5–2% of the gross national product.

Organization of the ICU

ICUs in the United States may be open or closed. Open ICUs may be utilized by any attending physician with admitting privileges in that institution, and many subspecialists may manage the patient at the same time. These physicians do not need to be specifically trained in critical care medicine. A different system is provided in closed ICUs, in which the management of the patient on admission to the unit is provided by an ICU team and orchestrated by physicians with specialized training in critical care medicine. Although consultants may be involved in the patient's care, all orders are written by the ICU team, and all decisions are approved by this team.

ICUs may also be organized by the type of patients whom they are intended to treat. Examples include the neurosurgical ICU (NICU), pediatric ICU (PICU), cardiovascular surgery ICU (CVICU), surgical ICU (SICU), medical ICU (MICU), and coronary care unit (CCU).

Most ICUs in the United States have a medical director who, with varying degrees of authority, is responsible for bed allocation, policy making, and quality assurance and who may be, particularly in closed ICUs, the primary attending physician for patients admitted to that unit.

■ TEAM WORK

Care of the critically ill patient has evolved into a discipline that requires specialized training and skills. The physician in the ICU depends on nursing for accurate charting and assessment of the patients during the times when he or she is not at the bedside and for the provision of the full spectrum of nursing care, including psychological and social support and the administration of ordered therapies.

Complex mechanical ventilation devices need appropriate monitoring and adjustment. This expertise and other functions are provided by a professional team of respiratory therapy practitioners. The wide spectrum of the pharmacopeia used in the ICU is greatly enhanced by the assistance of our colleagues in pharmacy. Many institutions find it useful to have pharmacists with advanced training participate in rounding to help practitioners in the appropriate pharmacologic management of the critically ill. Additionally, technicians with experience in monitoring equipment may help in obtaining physiologic data and maintaining the associated equipment. Without these additional health-care professionals, optimal ICU management would not be possible.

■ THE FLOWSHEET

ICU patients by virtue of their critical illnesses present with complex pathophysiology and symptomatology. In many cases, these patients are endotracheally intubated, with mental status depression, and cannot provide historical information. The physical examination and monitoring of physiology and laboratory data must provide the information on which to base a diagnosis and initiate appropriate treatment in these cases.

The flowsheet is the repository of information necessary for the recognition and management of severe physiological derangements in critically ill patients. A well-organized flowsheet provides around-the-clock information regarding the different organ systems rather than just vital signs alone. In many institutions these flowsheets are computerized, potentially improving accessibility and allowing real-time data. These devices are complex and expensive, and, to date, no studies have proven that utilizing these electronic flowsheets decreases nursing charting time or improves care. Thus, caution in their adoption is warranted.

Major categories appropriate for an ICU flowsheet include

— Vital signs

— Neurological status

— Hemodynamic parameters

— Ventilator settings

— Respiratory parameters

— Inputs and outputs

— Laboratory data

— Medications

■ THE CRITICALLY ILL PATIENT

In general, ICU patients not only are very ill but also may have disease processes that involve a number of different organ systems. Therefore, the approach to the critically ill patient needs to be systematic and complete (see below).

Several issues need to be considered in the initial approach to the critically ill patient. The initial evaluation consists of assessment of the ABC (airway, breathing, circulation), with interventions performed as needed. An organized and efficient history and physical examination should then be conducted for all patients entering the ICU, and a series of priorities for therapeutic interventions should be established.

■ SYSTEM-ORIENTED ROUNDS

In the ICU accurate transmission of clinical information is required. It is important to be compulsive and follow every single detail. The mode of presentation during ICU rounds may vary based on institutional tradition. Nevertheless, because of multiple medical problems, systematic gathering and presentation of data are needed for proper management of these patients. We prefer presenting and writing notes in a "head-to-toe" format (see Table 1.1).

The ICU progress note is system oriented, which differs from the problem-oriented approach commonly utilized on the general medicine-surgery wards. The assessment and plan are formulated for each of the different organ systems as aids to organization, but like in the non-ICU chart, each progress note should contain a "problem list" that is addressed daily. This problem list allows the health-care provider to keep track of multiple problems simultaneously and enables a physician unfamiliar with a given case to efficiently understand its complexities if the need arises.

The art of presenting cases during rounds is perfected at the bedside over many years, but the following abbreviated guide may get the new member of the ICU team off to a good start. A "how-to" for examining an ICU patient, and a stylized ICU progress note guide are also presented. Remember that for each system reviewed a full review of data, assessment, and management plan should be provided.

When you arrive in the ICU in the morning:

1. Ask the previous night's physicians and nurses about your patients.
2. Go to the patient's room. Review the flow sheet. Then proceed by reviewing each organ system as follows:

Table 1.1. Minimum Amount of Information Necessary for Presentation During Rounds (See Text for Details)

ICU SURVIVAL GUIDE FOR PRESENTATION DURING ROUNDS

1. **Identification/Problem List**
2. **Major events during the last 24 h.**
3. **Neurological**:
   — Mental status, complaints, detailed neurological exam (if pertinent).
4. **Cardiovascular**:
   — Symptoms and physical findings, record BP, pulse variability over the past 24 h, ECG.
   — If CVP line and/or Swan-Ganz catheter in place, check CVP and hemodynamics *yourself.*
5. **Respiratory**:
   — Ventilator settings, latest ABGs, symptoms and physical findings, CXR (daily if the patient is intubated). Other calculations (e.g., compliance, minute volume, etc).
6. **Renal/Metabolic**:
   — Urine output (per hour and during the last 24 h), inputs/outputs with balance (daily, weekly), weight, electrolytes, and if done creatinine clearance. Acid-base balance interpretation.
7. **Gastrointestinal**:
   — Abdominal exam, oral intake, coffee-grounds, diarrhea. Abdominal X-rays, liver function tests, amylase, etc.
8. **Infectious Diseases**:
   — Temperature curve, WBC, cultures, current antibiotics (number of days on each drug), and antibiotic levels.
9. **Hematology**:
   — CBC, PT, PTT, TT, BT, DIC screen (if pertinent), peripheral smear. Medications altering bleeding.
10. **Nutrition**:
    — TPN, enteral feedings, rate, caloric intake, and grams of protein.
11. **Endocrine**:
    — Do you need to check TFTs or cortisol? Give total insulin needs per hour and 24 h.
12. **Psychosocial**:
    — Is the patient depressed or suicidal? Is the family aware of his or her present condition?
13. **Other**:
    — Check the endotracheal tube position (from lips or nostrils in centimeters), and check CXR position. Check all lines, transducers. Note position of the catheter, skin insertion sites.
    — All medications and drips must be known. All drips must be renewed before or during rounds.

Abbreviations: ABG, arterial blood gas; BP, blood pressure; BT, bleeding time; CBC, complete blood count; CXR, chest x-ray; CVP, central venous pressure; DIC, disseminated intravascular coagulation; ECG, electrocardiogram; PT, prothrombin time; PTT, partial thromboplastin time; TFT, thyroid function tests; TPN, total parenteral nutrition; TT, thrombin time; WBC, white blood cell count.

Identification

— Provide name, age, major diagnosis, day of entry to the hospital, and day of admission to the ICU.

Major Events Over the Last 24 Hours

— Mention (or list in the progress note) any medical event or diagnostic endeavor that was significant. For example, major thoracic surgery or cardiopulmonary arrest, computed tomography (CT) scan of the head, reintubation, or changes in mechanical ventilation.

Systems Review

Neurologic

— Mental status: Is the patient awake? If so, can you perform a mental status examination? If the patient is comatose, is he or she spontaneously breathing?
— What is the Glasgow coma scale score?
— If the patient is sedated, what is the Ramsay score, or what is the score on any other scales used at the institution for patients who are sedated?
— If pertinent (in patients with major neurological abnormalities or whose major disease process involves the central nervous system), a detailed neurological exam should be performed.
— What are the results of any neurological evaluation in the past 24 hours such as a lumbar puncture or CT scan?

Cardiovascular

— Symptoms and physical findings: It is important to specifically inquire for symptoms of dyspnea and chest pain or discomfort, among others. The physical examination should be focused on the cardiac rhythm, presence of congestive heart failure, pulmonary hypertension, pericardial effusion, and valvulopathies.
— Electrocardiogram (ECG): We recommend that a diagnostic ECG be considered in every ICU patient on a frequent basis. Many ICU patients cannot communicate chest pain or other cardiac symptomatology, so that an ECG may be the only piece of information pointing toward cardiac pathology.

— If the patient has a central venous pressure (CVP) line and/or a pulmonary artery (Swan-Ganz) catheter in place, check the CVP and hemodynamics *yourself.* Hemodynamic calculations of oxygen consumption and delivery should be noted. A detailed list of hemodynamic parameters useful in the management of critically ill patients can be found in Chapters 3 (cardiovascular) and 13 (pulmonary).

— Note the blood pressure (BP) and pulse variability over the past 24 hours.

Respiratory

— If the patient is on mechanical ventilation, the current ventilator settings need to be charted, including the ventilatory mode, tidal volume, preset respiratory rate and patient's own respiratory rate, amount of oxygen being provided (FiO_2), and whether or not the patient is receiving positive end-expiratory pressure (PEEP) and/or pressure support (PS) and their levels. When pertinent, peak flow settings and inspiration:expiration (I:E) ratio should be noted. Mechanically ventilated patients should have a daily measurement of the static and dynamic compliance, minute volume, and other parameters (see Chapters 2 and 13).

— The most recent arterial blood gases (ABGs) should be compared with previous measurements. Calculation of the alveolar-arterial oxygen gradient should be performed.

— Symptoms and physical findings should be noted, and if pertinent, sputum characteristics should be mentioned.

— Generally, a portable chest x-ray is obtained in all intubated patients daily. Attention is paid to CVP lines, endotracheal tubes, chest tubes, pericardiocentesis catheters, opacities in the lung fields (infiltrates), pneumothoraces, pneumomediastinum, and subcutaneous air.

Renal/Metabolic

— Urine output is quantified per hour and during the past 24 hours. In patients requiring intensive care for more than 2 days, it is important to keep track of their inputs, outputs, and overall daily and weekly fluid balance.

— Daily weights.

— Electrolytes are noted including magnesium, phosphorus, calcium (ionized), and if done, creatinine clearance, urine electrolytes, etc. Any changes in these values need special consideration.

— The ABGs are used for acid-base balance interpretation. The formulas most commonly used for these calculations are depicted in Chapter 14.

Gastrointestinal

— Abdominal examination: A detailed abdominal examination may uncover new pathology or allow one to assess changes in recognized problems.
— If the patient is awake and alert, mention his or her oral intake (e.g., determine whether clear liquids are well tolerated).
— The characteristics of the gastric contents or stool (e.g., coffee-grounds, diarrhea, etc.) should also be mentioned and recorded.
— Abdominal x-rays, if pertinent, are reviewed with special attention to the duration of feeding tubes, free air under the diaphragm, and bowel gas pattern.
— Liver function tests (transaminases, albumin, coagulation measurements, etc.) and pancreatic enzymes (amylase, lipase, etc.) are mentioned and recorded when pertinent, as well as their change since previous measurements.

Infectious Diseases

— Temperature curve: Changes in temperature (e.g., "fever spike" or hypothermia) should be noted as well as the interventions performed to control the temperature. Note fever character, maximum temperature (T-max), and response to antipyretics.
— The total white blood cell count (WBC) is recorded, when pertinent, with special attention to changes in the differential.
— Cultures: Culture (blood, sputum, urine, etc.) results should be checked daily with the microbiology laboratory and recorded. Those positive cultures, when mentioned, should include the antibiotic sensitivity profile when available.
— Current antibiotics: Current dosages and routes of administration as well as the number of days on each drug should be reported. If an adverse reaction occurred related to the administration of antibiotics, it should be reported.
— Antibiotic levels are drawn for many antibiotics with known pharmacokinetics to adjust their dosage (e.g., peak and trough levels for vancomycin).

— If the patient is receiving a new drug, either investigational or FDA approved, side effects and/or the observed salutary effects are reported.

Hematology

— Complete blood cell count (CBC): When presenting the results, it is important to be aware of the characteristics of the peripheral blood smear.

— Coagulation parameters: The prothrombin time (PT), partial thromboplastin time (PTT), thrombin time (TT), bleeding time (BT), and disseminated intravascular coagulation (DIC) screen (e.g., fibrinogen, fibrin split products, d-dimer, platelet count), should be addressed when pertinent.

— In this context special attention is paid to all medications that alter bleeding, both directly (e.g., heparin, desmopressin acetate) and indirectly (e.g., ticarcillin-induced thromobocytopathy, ranitidine-induced thrombocytopenia).

Nutrition

— Total parenteral nutrition (TPN): You need to state what kind of formula the patient is receiving, the total caloric intake provided by TPN with the percentage of fat and carbohydrates given. The total amount of protein is mentioned with an assessment of the anabolic or catabolic state (see Chapter 10, "Nutrition").

— Enteral feedings: These are reported similarly to TPN, with mention of any gastrointestinal intolerance (e.g. diarrhea).

— For both of the above, the nutritional needs of the patient and what percentage of these needs is actually being provided must be reported.

Endocrine

— Special attention is paid to pancreatic, adrenal, and thyroid function. If needed, a cortisol level or thyroid function tests are performed. In most situations these determinations are not appropriate in the ICU except under special circumstances (e.g., hypotension refractory to volume resuscitation in a patient with disseminated tuberculosis, Addisonian crisis), and the results are usually not available immediately.

— Insulin: The total insulin needs per hour and per 24 hours as well as the blood sugar values should be reported. The type of insulin preparation being used should be specified.

— In patients with hyperosmolal states and diabetic ketoacidosis, it is necessary to determine calculated and measured serum osmolality as well as ketones. The values for these are charted and compared with previous results.

Psychosocial

— Patients in the ICU tend to be confused and on occasion disoriented. Although these symptoms and signs are reviewed as part of the neurological examination, it is important to consider other diagnoses (e.g., depression, psychosis).
— For drug overdoses and patients with depression, specific questions need to be asked regarding the potential of new suicidal and homicidal ideations.

Other

Other parameters also must be checked daily before the morning (or evening) rounds:

— Check the endotracheal tube size and position (from the lips or nostrils in centimeters), and check its position on chest x-ray, as mentioned above.
— If the patient has a nasotracheal or orotracheal tube, a detailed ear, nose, and throat examination should be performed (because patients with nasotracheal tubes may develop severe sinusitis).
— Check all lines with their corresponding equipment (e.g., transducers must be at an adequate level). Note the position of the catheter(s) both on physical examination and on x-ray, as well as the appearance of the skin insertion site(s) (e.g., infection).
— All medications and continuous infusions and their proper concentrations and infusion rates must be known and recorded.
— At the time of "prerounding," all infusions must be renewed. TPN orders need to be written early, with changes based on the most recent laboratory findings.
— At the end of rounds every morning, it is important to keep a list of the things that need to be done that day, for example, changes in central venous lines or arterial lines, performing a lumbar puncture, etc.

■ DNR AND ETHICAL ISSUES

Ethical issues arise every day in the ICU. For example, should a particular patient be kept on mechanical ventilation when he has an underlying malignancy? Should the patient with acquired immune deficiency syndrome (AIDS) receive cardiopulmonary resuscitation (CPR) in the event of a cardiorespiratory arrest? Should the family be permitted to terminate mechanical ventilation or tube feedings?

These and similar questions are frequently asked and in reality may have no single correct answer. Patients must be allowed the opportunity to express their wishes about resuscitation. ICU physicians need to educate the patient and the family regarding prognosis. Physicians are not obliged to provide futile interventions, but communication is the key to avoiding conflicts in this arena.

Do not resuscitate (DNR) orders have become widely used in U.S. hospitals. A DNR order specifically instructs the patient's health-care provider to forego CPR if the patient undergoes cardiac or respiratory arrest. Various levels of support may be agreed upon by patients, their physicians, and family.

Different institutions have distinct categories of support. Examples include the following:

— Code A or Code I: Full support, including CPR, vasopressors, mechanical ventilation, surgery, etc.

— Code B or Code II: Full support except CPR (no endotracheal intubation or chest compressions). However, vasopressor drugs are utilized in these cases.

— Code C or Code III: Comfort care only. Depending on the policies of the institution, intravenous fluids, antibiotics, and other medications may be withheld.

A patient who is DNR may be in either of the last two groups. It is important then that a full description of a particular triage status is provided and carefully explained to the patient and/or family and discussed as needed.

As mentioned, the level of resuscitative efforts will therefore depend on the patient's wishes. When the patient cannot express his or her wishes, then these questions are asked to the closest family member or designated individual. For example, would the patient have wanted full mechanical ventilatory support for a cardiopulmonary arrest? Were provisions made for a health- care surrogate if the patient became incompetent?

Ethical problems often can be resolved by seeking consultation with a group of individuals who are experienced in dealing with these issues. In many institutions an ethics committee is available to provide consultation to practitioners and families regarding moral and ethical dilemmas.

2

The Basics of Critical Care

Critical care medicine is an integrated discipline that requires the clinician to examine a number of important basic interactions. These include the interactions among organ systems, between the patient and his or her environment, and between the patient and life support equipment. Gas exchange within the lung, for example, is dependent on the matching of ventilation and perfusion—in quantity, space, and time. Thus, neither the lungs nor the heart are solely responsible; rather, it is the cardiopulmonary interaction that determines the adequacy of gas exchange.

Critical care often entails providing advanced life support through the application of technology. Mechanical ventilation is a common example. Why is it that positive pressure ventilation and positive end-expiratory pressure (PEEP) can result in oliguria or reduction of cardiac output? Many times clinical assessments and your therapeutic plans will be directed at the interaction between the patient and technology; this represents a unique "physiology" in itself.

■ I. CARDIAC ARREST AND RESUSCITATION

Resuscitation from death is not an everyday event but is no longer a rarity. The goal of resuscitation is restoration of normal or near-normal cardiopulmonary function, without deterioration of other organ systems.

A. Etiology

The most common causes of sudden cardiac arrest are depicted in Table 2.1.

Table 2.1. Common Causes of Sudden Nontraumatic Cardiac Arrest

1. Primary Cardiac Event
    a. CAD
    b. Dysrhythmias due to
        (1) Hyperkalemia
        (2) Severe acidemia
        (3) Other electrolyte disturbances
    c. Myocarditis
    d. Tamponade
2. Secondary to a Respiratory Arrest (e.g., children)
3. Secondary to Acute Respiratory Failure
    a. Hypoxemia
    b. Hypercapnia
4. Extreme Alterations in Body Temperature
5. Drug Effects
    a. Digitalis
    b. Quinidine
    c. Tricyclic antidepressants
    d. Cocaine

   B. Pathogenesis
      1. Ventricular fibrillation (VF) or pulseless ventricular tachycardia (VT).
      2. Asystole.
      3. Pulseless electrical activity (PEA) (electromechanical dissociation). Patients arresting with PEA can have any cardiac rhythm but no effective mechanical systole (thus, blood pressure [BP] is unobtainable).
      4. Cardiogenic shock: No effective cardiac output is generated.
      5. The central nervous system (CNS) will not tolerate >6 minutes of ischemia at normothermia.
   C. Diagnosis
      1. Unexpected loss of consciousness in the unmonitored patient.
      2. Loss of palpable central arterial pulse.
      3. Respiratory arrest in a patient previously breathing spontaneously.
   D. Differential Diagnosis
      1. Syncope or vasovagal reactions
      2. Coma
      3. "Collapse"
      4. Seizures
   E. Management
      1. Cardiopulmonary Resuscitation

a. The main indications for cardiopulmonary resuscitation (CPR) in the ICU include
   (1) Cardiovascular collapse
   (2) Respiratory arrest with or without cardiac arrest
b. Mechanisms of blood flow during CPR
   (1) Direct compression of the heart between the sternum and vertebral column "squeezes" blood from the ventricles into the great vessels.
   (2) Changes in intrathoracic pressure generate gradients between the peripheral venous and arterial beds, resulting in forward flow.
   (3) During CPR, the dynamics of the chest compression process may play a major role in determining outcome of the resuscitation effort.
c. Technique
   (1) Establish an effective airway (see Chapter 15, "Special Techniques").
      (a) Assess breathing first (open airway, look, listen and feel).
      (b) If respiratory arrest has occurred, the possibility of a foreign body obstruction needs to be considered and measures taken to relieve it.
      (c) If endotracheal intubation is to be performed, the maximum interruption of ventilation should be 30 seconds.
      (d) The respiratory rate during cardiac or respiratory arrest should be 10 to 12 breaths per minute. Once spontaneous circulation has been restored, the rate should be 12 to 15 breaths per minute.
      (e) Ventilations should be performed with a tidal volume of 8 to 10 mL/kg of ideal body weight.
      (f) The highest possible concentration of oxygen (100%) should be administered to all patients receiving CPR.
   (2) Determine pulselessness (if no pulse, start CPR immediately).
   (3) Chest compressions, current advanced cardiac life support (ACLS) recommendations:
      (a) Rescuer's hand located in the lower margin of sternum.
      (b) Heel of one hand is placed on the lower half of the sternum, and the other hand

is placed on top of the hand on the sternum so that the hands are parallel.

(c) Elbows are locked in position, the arms are straightened, and the rescuer's shoulders are positioned directly over the hands, providing a straight thrust.

(d) The sternum is depressed $1\frac{1}{2}$ to 2 inches in normal-sized adults with each compression at a rate of 100/minute.

(e) Current areas of investigation and debate that have been recently been acknowledged by the American Heart Association include

    i. Mechanical versus manual CPR

    ii. High-impulse CPR

    iii. Interposed abdominal compressions

    iv. Active compression-decompression

    v. Vest CPR

(f) Determinants of efficacy of CPR:

    i. Systolic pressure of at least 60 mm Hg.

    ii. End-tidal CO_2 ($ETCO_2$): Initial $ETCO_2$ values may predict whether the patient will regain a perfusing rhythm during resuscitation.

(4) Cardiac monitoring and dysrhythmia recognition (see also Chapter 3, "Cardiovascular Disorders")

    (a) Distinguish between ventricular and supraventricular rhythms.

        i. Most rapid, wide QRS rhythms are VT.

        ii. Initiate therapy immediately (see below).

(5) Defibrillation is the major determinant of survival in cardiac arrest due to VF.

    (a) The energy requirements for different conditions vary (see below).

    (b) Electrodes should be properly placed to maximize current through the myocardium.

(6) Drug therapy during CPR may given by the following routes:

(a) Peripheral vein (antecubital or external jugular are preferred).

(b) Central venous line (subclavian or internal jugular): On occasion a long line that extends above the diaphragm can be started in the femoral vein.

(c) Endotracheal: Medications should be administered at 2 to 2.5 times the recommended intravenous (IV) dose and should be diluted in 10 mL of normal saline or distilled water. A catheter should be passed beyond the tip of the endotracheal tube, and the medication sprayed quickly followed by several quick insufflations.

(d) Intraosseous: particularly useful in pediatric patients.

(e) The different drug dosages utilized during CPR and in the immediate postresuscitation period are depicted in the appendix.

(7) The algorithm approach

(a) ABCD (see Figure 2.1).

(b) Call for defibrillator at once.

(c) If no circulation, start CPR (as above).

(d) Assess rhythm (see Figures 2.1 and 2.2).

(e) If VT/VF are present, follow the algorithm presented in Figure 2.3.

(f) If PEA is present, follow the algorithm in Figure 2.4.

(g) If asystole is present, follow the algorithm in Figure 2.5.

(h) For bradycardia follow the algorithm in Figure 2.6.

(i) For tachycardia follow the algorithms presented in Figures 2.7 to 2.10.

d. Cerebral resuscitation

(1) The best way of preserving neurologic function is obviously the early and effective restoration of cardiopulmonary function.

(2) Using standard closed-chest compressions, if circulation is not restored promptly, cerebral survival is minimal.

(3) Autoregulation of cerebral blood flow is lost after an extended periods of hypoxemia or

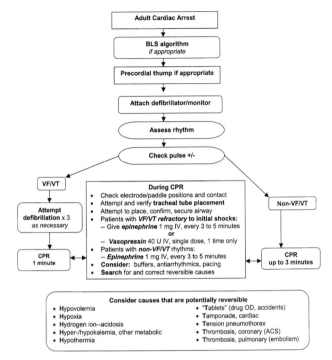

Figure 2.1. The algorithm approach.

hypercarbia. Thus, prompt correction of these variables is of extreme importance.

(4) Optimize cerebral perfusion pressure by maintaining a normal or slightly elevated mean arterial pressure and by reducing intracranial pressure if increased (see Chapter 9, "Neurologic Disorders").

(5) The use of selective calcium channe blockers (i.e., nimodipine, lidoflazine) to preserve cerebral function following a cardiac arrest is an area of controversy and is currently under investigation.

2. Predictors of poor outcome in resuscitation

a. Preterminal illness (i.e., sepsis, malignancies)

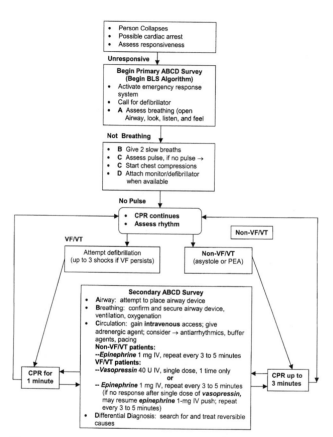

Figure 2.2. The algorithm approach.

b. Catastrophic events (i.e., massive pulmonary embolism, ruptured aneurysms, cardiogenic shock, etc).
c. Delayed performance of basic life support (BLS)/ACLS
d. Initial rhythm
   (1) Asystole or PEA: prognosis grim.
   (2) VT: good prognosis, but rarely encountered.
   (3) VF: ability to prevent deterioration to asystole is dependent on time to defibrillation.

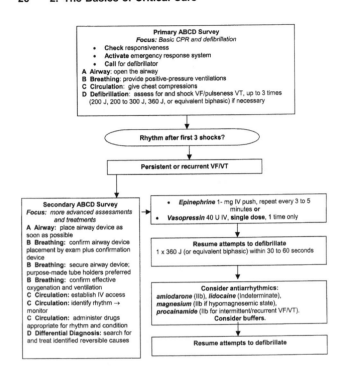

Figure 2.3. Algorithm for ventricular fibrillation (VF) and pulseless ventricular tachycardia (VT).

■ II. THE ALVEOLAR AIR EQUATION

A. Dalton's law states that the partial pressure of a mixture of gases is equal to the sum of the partial pressures of the constituent gases. Thus, the total pressure of alveolar gases must equal the sum of its constituents and, in turn, equilibrate with atmospheric pressure. We are most often concerned with the respiratory gases, O_2 and CO_2.

B. The alveolar air equation is based firmly on Dalton's law but is expressed in terms that emphasize alveolar O_2 and CO_2:

$$P_AO_2 = (P_{ATM} - P_{H2O})FiO_2 - PCO_2/RQ$$

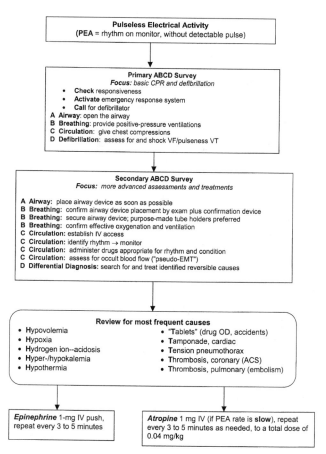

Figure 2.4. Algorithm for pulseless electrical activity (PEA) (also known as electromechanical dissociation).

P_AO_2 = partial pressure of O_2 in the alveolus under present conditions. P_{ATM} = current, local atmospheric pressure. P_{H_2O} = vapor pressure of water at body temperature and 100% relative humidity. FiO_2 = fraction of inspired O_2. PCO_2 = partial pressure of CO_2 in arterial blood. RQ = respiratory quotient.

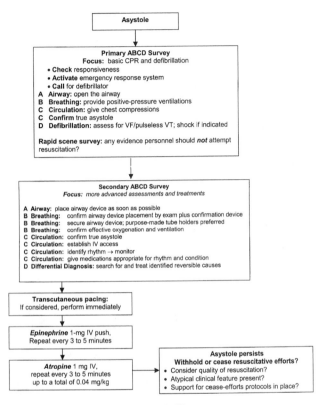

Figure 2.5. Asystole treatment algorithm.

C. Many clinical and environmental influences are immediately obvious when considering the terms of the equation:
   1. P_{ATM}: Altitude per se can clearly result in hypoxemia. A given patient's PO_2 must be considered in the context of location. A "normal" arterial PO_2 is not the same in Denver (average = 73 mm Hg) as it is a sea level (average = 95 mm Hg).
   2. FiO_2: While atmospheric air is uniformly about 21% O_2, one must ask: 21% of what? The FiO_2 on a mountain top at 11,000 feet is also 21% but there is not enough

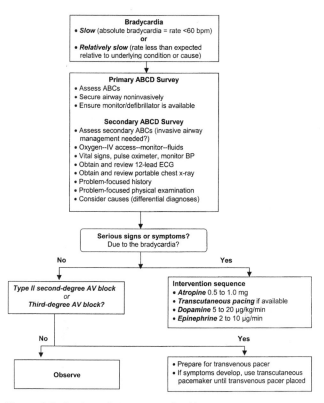

Bradycardia
• *Slow* (absolute bradycardia = rate <60 bpm)
  or
• *Relatively slow* (rate less than expected
  relative to underlying condition or cause)

Primary ABCD Survey
• Assess ABCs
• Secure airway noninvasively
• Ensure monitor/defibrillator is available

Secondary ABCD Survey
• Assess secondary ABCs (invasive airway
  management needed?)
• Oxygen--IV access--monitor--fluids
• Vital signs, pulse oximeter, monitor BP
• Obtain and review 12-lead ECG
• Obtain and review portable chest x-ray
• Problem-focused history
• Problem-focused physical examination
• Consider causes (differential diagnoses)

Serious signs or symptoms?
Due to the bradycardia?

No   **Yes**

Type II second-degree AV block
or
Third-degree AV block?

Intervention sequence
• *Atropine* 0.5 to 1.0 mg
• *Transcutaneous pacing* if available
• *Dopamine* 5 to 20 µg/kg/min
• *Epinephrine* 2 to 10 µg/min

No   **Yes**

Observe

• Prepare for transvenous pacer
• If symptoms develop, use transcutaneous
  pacemaker until transvenous pacer placed

Figure 2.6. Bradycardia treatment algorithm.

total O_2 in the rarefied air to sustain an arterial PO_2 above 60 mm Hg.

3. PCO_2: Although CO_2 coming into the alveolus does not displace O_2 (this would not obey Dalton's law), the blood PCO_2 does equilibrate with alveolar gases. Simultaneously, O_2 is taken up from the alveolus. When patients hypoventilate, not only does CO_2 accumulate, alveolar O_2 becomes depleted. Thus, elevated PCO_2 is associated with low P_AO_2 and sometimes hypoxemia. Similarly, hyperventilating patients (excess CO_2 elimination, low PCO_2, frequent replenishment of alveolar O_2) can have

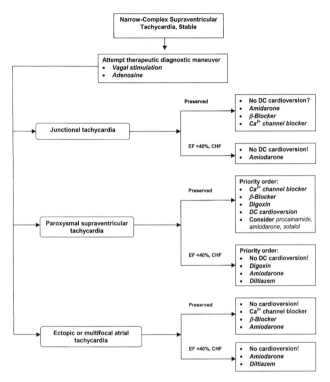

Figure 2.7. Tachycardia algorithms.

higher than normal P_AO_2 and arterial PO_2. (See Example 3 below.)

4. RQ is the ratio of CO_2 production to O_2 consumption. The ratio of alveolar gas exchange—CO_2 coming into the alveolus and O_2 leaving the alveolus—not unexpectedly, also reflects the RQ. Given a particular ratio of alveolar gas exchange, the ultimate value for P_AO_2 will also be affected by the rate of CO_2 elimination from the alveolus, i.e., alveolar ventilation.

D. The A-a Gradient

1. While the alveolar air equation predicts the partial pressure of O_2 in the alveolus (P_AO_2) under current conditions, it is not necessarily true that arterial blood will have an

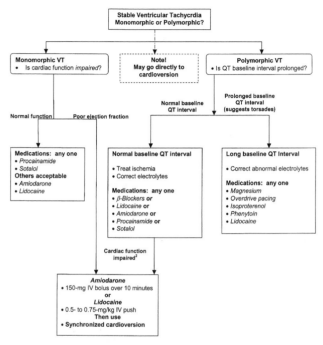

Figure 2.8. Tachycardia algorithms.

identical partial pressure of O_2 (PaO_2). We can however, measure the PaO_2 directly and compare it with the calculated value for P_AO_2. When we subtract arterial from alveolar PO_2, we obtain the A-a gradient.

Example 1: A healthy young adult breathing room air at sea level:

Arterial blood gases (ABGs): pH = 7.40, $PaCO_2 = 40$, $PaO_2 = 95$

(assume RQ = 0.8)
$P_AO_2 = (760 - 47) .21 - 40/0.8$
$P_AO_2 = 150 - 50 = 100$
A-a gradient = $P_AO_2 - PaO_2$
A-a gradient = $100 - 95 = 5$ mm Hg.

This person has an A-a gradient of 5 mm Hg, which is normal (0 to 10).

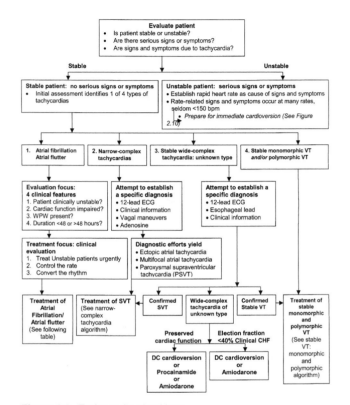

Figure 2.9. Tachycardia algorithms.

Example 2: An elderly patient in respiratory distress secondary to pulmonary edema breathing 40% O_2 (FiO_2 = 0.4):

ABGs: pH = 7.43, $PaCO_2$ = 36, PaO_2 = 70
P_AO_2 = (760 − 47) .40 − 36/0.8
P_AO_2 = 285 − 45 = 240
A-a gradient = P_AO_2 − PaO_2
A-a gradient = 240 − 70 = 170 mm Hg

This person has an A-a gradient of 170 mm Hg, which is markedly elevated.

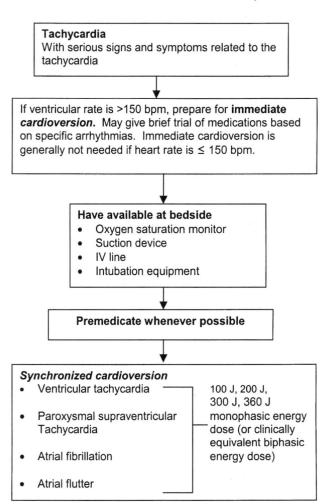

Figure 2.10. Electrical synchronized cardioversion algorithm.

2. Significance: The presence of an A-a gradient tells you that *something is wrong: gas exchange is impaired.* It does not tell you what is wrong, nor does it tell you the etiology of hypoxemia when present. A widened A-a gradient simply indicates that alveolar O_2 tension is not successfully reflected in arterial blood.

   a. Note that at a given FiO_2, P_AO_2 varies inversely as the $PaCO_2$. Thus at any A-a gradient a high $PaCO_2$ is associated with a low P_AO_2 and vice-versa. A patient who hyperventilates (low $PaCO_2$) may do so purposely to improve their P_AO_2 and thus their PaO_2.

Example 3: An emergency room patient breathing room air:

ABGs: pH = 7.50, $PaCO_2$ = 30, PaO_2 = 65

What would the patient's PaO_2 be with the same A-a gradient and a $PaCO_2$ of 40?
   Room Air:

$P_AO_2 = (760 - 47) .21 - 30/0.8 = 150 - 35 = 115$
A-a gradient = 115 − 65
A-a gradient = 50
Now, what if the PCO_2 were 40?
$P_AO_2 = (760 - 47) .21 - \mathbf{40}/0.8 = 150 - 50 = 100$
$P_AO_2 = 100$
A-a gradient = 50
Therefore PaO_2 = **50**

PaO_2 would be **50** if the patient were not hyperventilating. "Normal" ventilation ($PaCO_2$ = 40) would be associated with hypoxemia, but with hyperventilation, the patient's PO_2 is above 60. Note that it is also possible for a patient to have hypoxemia without a widened A-a gradient. There are two important examples: high altitude and alveolar hypoventilation.

Example 4: A normal adult breathing room air at altitude 11,000 feet:

A-a gradient = 0
$PaO_2 = (\mathbf{510} - 47) .21 - 40/0.8 = 47$
A-a gradient = 0
$PaO_2 = 47$

This patient has hypoxemia without an A-a gradient.

Example 5: A patient with pure alveolar hypoventilation secondary to narcotic overdose breathing room air:

$PCO_2 = 80$; A-a gradient $= 0$
$P_AO_2 = (760 - 47) .21 - 80/0.8$
$P_AO_2 = 50$
A-a gradient $= 0$
$PaO_2 = 50$

This patient has hypoxemia without an A-a gradient.

3. Summary

a. The alveolar air equation shows the relationships among atmospheric pressure, FiO_2, $PaCO_2$, and alveolar O_2 tension (P_AO_2).

b. When alveolar O_2 tension (P_AO_2) is not reflected faithfully in arterial blood (PaO_2)—i.e., a widened A-a gradient—the calculation indicates that gas exchange is impaired, but it does not tell you how or why.

c. Calculation of the A-a gradient is a useful bedside tool for evaluation of patients with respiratory distress or abnormal ABGs and to follow their progress.

d. It is possible to have hypoxemia without a widened A-a gradient. High altitude and hypoventilation (elevated $PaCO_2$) are examples.

◼ III. OXYGEN TRANSPORT

A. Oxygen Delivery: Calculations

1. Calculation of oxygen delivery ($\dot{D}O_2$) and oxygen consumption ($\dot{V}O_2$) are useful bedside techniques in the ICU.

2. $\dot{D}O_2 = CO \times CaO_2$
   Oxygen Delivery = Cardiac Output × Arterial O_2 Content

3. $CaO_2 = Hb \times SaO_2 \times K$
   Arterial O_2 Content = Hemoglobin × Arterial O_2 Saturation × a Constant*
   *We will use $1.34 \, mL \, O_2/g \, Hb$.

4. Resolving the units:
   $\dot{D}O_2 \, [mL \, O_2/min] = CO \, [mL/min] \times Hb \, [g/100 mL] \times 1.34 \, [mL \, O_2/g] \times SaO_2 \, [scalar]$

5. Normal values (70-kg man at rest)
   $\dot{D}O_2 = 5000 \, mL/min \, [CO] \times 15 \, g/100 \, mL \, [Hb] \times 1.34 \, mL \, O_2/g \, [constant] \times 1.00 \, [SaO_2]$
   $\dot{D}O_2 = 1005 \, mL \, O_2/min$

6. This value does not take into account dissolved O_2 in the plasma: $0.003 \, mL \, O_2/100 \, cc/mm \, Hg \, PaO_2$, which adds another $15 \, mL \, O_2$ of arterial O_2 content.

7. Values to remember:

Normal CaO_2 (15 g Hb, 100% SaO_2) = 20.4 mL O_2/100 cc
(20.4 vol %)
Normal $\dot{D}O_2$ (70-kg man, at rest, CO = 5000 mL/min) =
1020 mL O_2/min

B. Oxygen Transport: Concepts

Only 3 clinical variables can affect

$\dot{D}O_2$: cardiac output, hemoglobin, and oxygen saturation. Note that what looks very simple is not:

1. Cardiac output entails all of normal cardiodynamics (preload, afterload, contractility), hemodynamics, state of hydration, blood gas and electrolyte influences, the influence of mechanical ventilation and other technology, intrinsic cardiac disease, dysrhythmias, etc.

2. Hemoglobin is largely a quantitative problem (i.e., oxygen-carrying capacity), but it also includes the effects of abnormal hemoglobins, massive transfusions, pH and temperature, other causes of shift in the oxyhemoglobin dissociation curve, and hemoglobin substitutes.

3. Arterial oxygen saturation embodies the pathophysiology of acute and chronic lung disease, management of mechanical ventilation, the cardiopulmonary interaction, venous admixture, intrapulmonary or intracardiac shunting, etc.

4. If this is not complicated enough, recall that what you may be doing to support the lungs may have a detrimental effect on cardiac output (see below). Similarly, failure to correct severe blood gas abnormalities may also adversely affect cardiac function. This makes the bedside management of oxygen delivery in critically ill patients straightforward, although at times very difficult:

   a. Support oxygenation such that $PO_2 > 60$, $SaO_2 > 0.9$ on nontoxic FiO_2 (≤ 0.5).

   b. Ensure hemoglobin concentration of at least 10 g/100 cc.

   c. Optimize cardiac output (CO) under current conditions (i.e., current ventilator settings).

C. Physiologic Maintenance of Oxygen Delivery Since $\dot{D}O_2$ is dependent on only 3 variables, how does a normal person respond to abnormalities of one of the values?

1. Fall in SaO_2:

   If SaO_2 falls to 0.5, a person can achieve normal O_2 delivery by doubling CO:

   $$\dot{D}O_2 = CO \times Hb \times SaO_2$$
   $$\dot{D}O_2 = \mathbf{2}CO \times Hb \times \mathbf{1/2}SaO_2$$

   a. Therefore, in the short term, increased CO can compensate for even severe hypoxemia.

    b. Note that when $SaO_2 = 0.5$, $PaO_2 = $ **27**! This is the definition of P_{50} for normal adult hemoglobin A, namely, the PaO_2 at which hemoglobin is 50% saturated (27 mm Hg). Thus, even severe hypoxemia can be tolerated well as long as hemoglobin is normal and CO can be enhanced.

    c. In patients with chronically low SaO_2 (high altitude, chronic lung disease, cyanotic heart disease), they will also increase their hemoglobin concentration.

2. Fall in Hemoglobin:

    If hemoglobin falls dramatically, $\dot{D}O_2$ is again maintained by increasing CO.

    a. Note that SaO_2 can never increase beyond 100% and therefore cannot compensate for low hemoglobin. The ability to increase and maintain CO is an important mechanism by which anemia can be tolerated.

$$\dot{D}O_2 = CO \times Hb \times SaO_2$$
$$\dot{D}O_2 = \mathbf{2}CO \times \mathbf{1/2}Hb \times SaO_2$$

3. Fall in Cardiac Output

    What if CO falls dramatically, then how is $\dot{D}O_2$ maintained? The answer is, $\dot{D}O_2$ in totality is not maintained, but tissue $\dot{D}O_2$ is maintained by *enhanced extraction.*

    a. If fewer liters of oxygenated blood are delivered, then the tissues must extract more from *every liter that is delivered.*

    b. Normally, arterial blood is nearly 100% saturated with O_2. Venous blood returning to the heart is the same in terms of hemoglobin, and quantitatively the same as CO. Thus, it is the *venous oxygen saturation* (SvO_2) that reflects O_2 extraction. Normal $SvO_2 = .75$. Therefore, *normal extraction is about 25%.*

    c. Looking at extraction (i.e., A—V O_2 difference) is therefore a good probe (under some circumstances, such as heart failure) of the adequacy of CO: High extraction implies inadequate CO.

4. Fall in Oxygen Delivery

    Here is a general rule of thumb: A normal person can withstand a severe abnormality of any *one* of the O_2 delivery variables (CO, Hb, SaO_2) without developing lactic acidosis (lactic acidosis would indicate cellular O_2 deprivation with resultant anaerobic metabolism).

    a. Note that during cardiac arrest lactate is generated not because of hypoxemia alone but, rather, because the cardiac output is also severely compromised and unable to compensate for low PaO_2 to maintain $\dot{D}O_2$.

D. Oxygen Consumption ($\dot{V}O_2$)
   1. $\dot{D}O_2$ (oxygen delivery) is what leaves the heart both quantitatively and qualitatively. What returns to the heart should be the same quantitatively, with the same hemoglobin concentration, different *only* in terms of *oxygen saturation*.
   2. If we know the $\dot{D}O_2$ (what left the heart), and we calculate what has returned to the heart, we can then subtract to ascertain the amount consumed:

   Oxygen Consumption
   $$(\dot{V}O_2) = CO \times (CaO_2) - CO \times (C\bar{v}O_2)*$$
   what left   what returned
   the heart to   the heart

   Thus, $\dot{V}O_2 = CO(CaO_2 - C\bar{v}O_2)**$
   This is the Fick Equation
   *$C\bar{v}O_2$ is the mixed venous O_2 content.
   **$CaO_2 - C\bar{v}O_2$ is the arteriovenous O_2 content difference.
   3. CvO_2 (mixed venous O_2 content) is calculated in exactly the same way as the CaO_2 (arterial content); namely:

   $$Hb \times 1.34 \times S\bar{v}O_2$$

   ($S\bar{v}O_2$ is the mixed venous O_2 saturation).
   4. If $\dot{V}O_2$ is known, the Fick equation can be used to calculate the cardiac output:

   $$CO = \frac{\dot{V}O_2}{(CaO_2 - C\bar{v}O_2)}$$

   5. At the bedside, what do you need to calculate $\dot{V}O_2$?
      a. The patient needs a pulmonary artery (Swan-Ganz) catheter
         (1) for CO determination
         (2) to obtain a true mixed venous blood sample from the pulmonary artery ($S\bar{v}O_2$)
      b. Arterial blood gas determination (or SaO_2 determination)
      c. Hemoglobin determination
   6. Example of normal values (70-kg man at rest)

   $CaO_2 = 15$ [Hb] $\times 1.34$ [constant] $\times 1.00$ [SaO_2] $= 20.1$
   $CvO_2 = 15$ [Hb] $\times 1.34$ [constant] $\times 0.75$ [$S\bar{v}O_2$] $= 15.1$
   $CO = 5000$ mL [5 L/min]
   $VO_2 = 5000$ mL/min (20.1 mL O_2/100 mL $- 15.1$ mL O_2/100 cc
   $VO_2 = 50 (20 - 15)$
   VO_2 [normal, at rest] $= 250$ mL O_2/min

7. Bedside Application in the ICU Human life depends on oxygen. This is a good reason to assess the adequacy of DO_2 in critically ill patients. Where there is life, there is O_2 consumption.

   a. We are concerned about factors that increase resting O_2 consumption such as fever. Febrile patients increase their resting O_2 consumption by 10% to 13% °C, (approximately 7%/°F).

   b. We are also concerned when calculated O_2 consumption is less than predicted (for body surface area, temperature) such as may occur in sepsis. Many times in spite of high DO_2, patients with sepsis have low calculated $\dot{V}O_2$, lactic acidosis, oliguria, and other signs of poor parenchymal organ function.

   c. Instead of arbitrary endpoints, it is best to look for physiological endpoints. When measured O_2 consumption, the $S\bar{v}O_2$, the (A—V) O_2 content difference, and the serum lactate are all normal, then it is likely that DO_2 is adequate. Evidence that you have satisfied the body's (tissues') needs is better evidence of the adequacy of DO_2 than any arbitrary number.

   d. Make sure that you see DO_2 as an integrated variable. If you change ventilator settings (see below)— for example, raise the PEEP to enhance SaO_2—but in the process cause a fall in CO, you may not have achieved any overall benefit in terms of DO_2. Cardiac output, hemoglobin, and SaO_2 require individual attention and management.

   e. Look for opportunities to get the best results for each intervention. For example, a transfusion of packed red blood cells may increase hemoglobin and raise CO. This may be substantially better management than trying to raise CO with crystalloid IV fluids to compensate for a borderline hemoglobin and/or SaO_2.

   f. Check CO and O_2 transport variables often, and measure the response to your interventions. Note that we often record heart rate and blood pressure every hour although CO can vary over a wide range irrespective of these more traditional signs. Cardiac output is a vital sign!

   g. Current technology now provides continuous data for SaO_2, $S\bar{v}O_2$ and even CO. These can obviate the necessity of repeated blood gas determinations and facilitate frequent assessment of O_2 transport variables.

■ IV. MECHANICAL VENTILATION

Humans breathe for two reasons: to take in oxygen (oxygenation) and to eliminate carbon dioxide (ventilation). a patient's inability to perform either or both of these functions defines respiratory failure.

A. Ventilation

Normal people produce CO_2 continuously, thus, there is a constant need for CO_2 elimination. We all eliminate CO_2 by a process that entails breathing in fresh air (essentially devoid of CO_2), allowing it to equilibrate with the CO_2 dissolved in capillary blood, and then exhaling it laden with CO_2. We perform this process 10 to 14 times each minute with significant volumes of air, such that under normal conditions arterial CO_2 ($PaCO_2$) is kept nearly constant at 40 mm Hg (torr).

More precisely, we move a tidal volume (Vt) in and out at a certain frequency (f) or respiratory rate (RR). The product of rate and tidal volume is the minute ventilation (V_{min}). Thus, it is the minute ventilation that is fundamentally responsible for CO_2 elimination.

$$V_{min} = V_t \times RR$$

1. The minute ventilation can be further divided into the gases that reach the alveoli and are therefore available for exchange (the alveolar ventilation, VA) and those gases that fill the airways or that reach unperfused (see below) alveoli and therefore cannot exchange gases (the anatomical and physiological *dead space*, respectively, V_D).

2. CO_2 elimination is therefore directly proportional to the minute alveolar ventilation at any level of CO_2 production or blood PCO_2.

$$CO_2 \text{ elimination} = (V_A)_{min} \times PCO_2$$

3. Since any physiologic parameter (i.e., serum creatinine, platelet count, PCO_2) is ultimately the result of the balance between production and elimination, it follows that PCO_2 (under any conditions affecting production) can be controlled by adjusting minute ventilation.

B. Oxygenation

How people accomplish oxygenation is equally simple, but considerably different from how we accomplish ventilation. We purposely inhale an oxygen-enriched atmosphere all the way down to our alveoli to allow the oxygen to be taken up by the capillary blood—both dissolved in proportion to its partial pressure (obeying Henry's law) and in combination with hemoglobin. More precisely, the air we inspire has a certain fraction that is oxygen—that is, a certain *Fraction of inspired O_2 (FiO$_2$)*.

Although we breathe only intermittently, we need to accomplish gas exchange continuously. If there were oxygen in our alveoli only when we inhaled, then blood would pass through the lungs unoxygenated in between breaths. Thus, we need to maintain volume in our lungs even at end-exhalation. This is accomplished by maintaining a pressure gradient across the lungs between breaths. The pressure in the pleural space (outside the lungs) is negative (approximately [–] 5 cm H_2O) with respect to the atmospheric pressure present in our airways. If we subtract vectorially, there is a $0 - (-5) = +5$ cm H_2O pressure gradient across the lungs even at end-exhalation—in effect, a PEEP. Thus, oxygenation is accomplished in normal people by purposely inspiring a certain FiO$_2$ and maintaining a certain PEEP.

C. PEEP and Compliance
   1. Compliance

      The volume in the lungs is related to the transpulmonary pressure. Indeed, volume and pressure are intimately related in many systems (such as ventilator tubing, cardiac filling, resting lung volume) through the variable of *compliance* (C):

$$C = \frac{\Delta V}{\Delta P}$$

compliance is defined *as the change in volume for a given change in pressure*. Thus, in order for us to achieve a given volume change—such as a tidal volume—in our lungs, we must make a pressure change. The precise pressure necessary will be determined by the lung (and chest wall) compliance.

Mathematically, it is clear that, as compliance falls (as may occur in pulmonary edema, adult respiratory distress syndrome (ARDS), lung fibrosis, and many other conditions), one must achieve ever increasing ΔP just to achieve the same ΔV. It is often the case that a patient's inability to do the work required to increase ΔP to maintain an adequate tidal exchange (ΔV) is the ultimate cause of respiratory failure.

The fundamental role that lung compliance plays in determining the relationship between clinically significant lung volumes (e.g., tidal volume) and the pressures required to achieve them has many important clinical implications:

a. If there is no gradient of pressure ($\Delta P = 0$), then there is no volume change. When a patient develops a pneumothorax, the pressure in the pleural space equals the pressure in the airways. As a result, there is no transpulmonary pressure (ΔP) and thus no lung volume—i.e., the lung collapses—because of the lungs' intrinsic compliance (and elastance, which is defined as 1/compliance).

Pneumothorax results in no lung volume (zero ΔV), because there is no transpulmonary pressure (zero ΔP).

b. To create a volume change, we must effect a pressure change. Thus, tidal volume is determined by the ΔP generated as the chest wall expands and the diaphragm contracts. Similarly, to increase our tidal volume, we must generate a larger ΔP, or if compliance falls, we may need a larger ΔP just to achieve the same tidal volume.

c. If a person has low lung compliance (i.e., restrictive disease), then normal resting negative intrapleural pressure (ΔP) will result in lower resting lung volume (ΔV).

d. If a person has high lung compliance (i.e., emphysema with destruction of lung parenchyma), then normal resting negative intrapleural pressure will result in high resting lung volume (e.g., "barrel chest" of emphysema).

e. Since the lungs are merely populations of alveoli, these relationships among pressure, volume, and compliance apply to individual alveoli and specific lung regions as well as to whole lungs.

f. Compliance contributes to the logical connection between the requirements of gas exchange and the respiratory work:

    (1) CO_2 production demands minute ventilation.

    (2) Minute ventilation requires a certain tidal volume.

    (3) This change in volume requires a change in pressure.

    (4) How much pressure for a given volume is determined by compliance.

    (5) The amount of pressure that must be generated is a major determinant of the work of breathing.

2. PEEP

From our description of oxygenation and ventilation, it should be clear that we are clinically concerned about maintaining the adequacy of 2 important lung volumes: The tidal volume of each breath and the resting lung volume in between breaths. The pressure generated during active inspiration either by the ventilator or the patient will determine the tidal volume (mediated, of course, through compliance). But what determines the resting lung volume? The answer is the resting transpulmonary pressure. In normal people (with normal lung compliance), the vectorial difference between airway and intrapleural pressures (ΔP) determines the resting lung volume, known more precisely as the *functional residual capacity (FRC)*.

$$P_{airway} - P_{pleural} = \Delta P_{transpulmonary}$$
$$0 - (-5) = +5$$
$$\Delta P = +5 \, cm \, H_2O$$

Resting lung volume (FRC) is therefore determined by the ΔP and compliance.

$$C = \frac{\Delta V}{\Delta P}$$
$$C = \frac{FRC}{P_{transpulmonary}}$$
$$FRC = C(P_{transpulmonary})$$

Since ΔP is positive and present at end-expiration, what we are talking about is positive end-expiratory pressure (PEEP). It should also be clear that *PEEP directly determines FRC.*

We have all had the experience of inflating a balloon. It's difficult at first, then suddenly gets easier once some volume is inside. As we reach the full inflation, it may again become difficult as we reach the limits of the balloon's compliance. If we let go, the balloon recoils (elastance) and collapses.

Our alveoli, in many ways, are similar: If they start fully collapsed, they are difficult to inflate at first. Once there is some volume, it becomes easier; this point of change in compliance is referred to as *critical <u>opening</u> pressure (COP)*.

Unlike balloons, normal alveoli do not immediately lose all of their volume when pressure is released but may maintain some volume (thanks in large measure to *surfactant*) until distending pressure is critically low and then collapse. The point at which this occurs is *critical <u>closing</u> pressure (CCP)*.

If one could maintain end-expiratory pressure (i.e., PEEP) above CCP, then alveoli would not collapse; their volume would be enhanced; and, in the aggregate, *lung volume* (FRC) would be enhanced. If low lung compliance results in high CCP, then PEEP must be increased above the CCP to prevent alveolar collapse. This is precisely the rationale for PEEP in the management of acute low-compliance lung disease (e.g., ARDS).

a. Summary of the Effects of PEEP
  (1) PEEP increases FRC.
  (2) PEEP increases compliance.
  (3) PEEP reduces shunt fraction (see below) by maintaining volume for gas exchange in perfused lung units in between breaths.
  (4) PEEP increases dead space by overdistending normally compliant alveoli.
  (5) PEEP increases intrathoracic pressure, which can impede venous return into the chest or specifically restrict cardiac filling, both of which may result in reduced cardiac output.
  (6) PEEP may contribute to barotrauma because it represents the baseline (end-expiration) for all pressure changes, because it may cause overdistention of compliant lung regions, and because of the nature of the acute lung diseases in which PEEP is most frequently useful.

D. Modes of Mechanical Ventilation

Under routine conditions, when a patient develops respiratory failure and is intubated, initial mechanical ventilatory support is provided by some form of conventional *volume-cycled ventilation* (*VCV*). Volume cycled means that the endpoint for the ventilator is the delivery of a selected tidal volume, leaving the machine itself to determine what *pressure* is necessary to deliver that volume, to that patient, at that time. Recent advances in technology have made it possible to control or limit the pressure required while still having tidal volume as the endpoint (pressure-controlled ventilation).

In addition to the standard array of choices for how to deliver VCV, there are also modes that do not use quasi-physiologic parameters, such as high-frequency ventilation. These modes of mechanical ventilatory support are beyond the scope of this manual but have been reviewed in depth elsewhere.

For conventional VCV, essentially four modes are commonly used, as depicted in Table 2.2.

Table 2.2. Commonly Used Modes of Volume-Cycled Ventilation

1. Controlled Mechanical Ventilation (CMV)

2. Assisted/Controlled Mechanical Ventilation (A/C)

3. Synchronized Intermittent Mandatory Ventilation (SIMV)

4. Continuous Positive Airway Pressure (CPAP)

5. Pressure Support Ventilation (PSV) is not a separate mode but, rather, an adjunct that can be used with several other modes.

1. Controlled Mechanical Ventilation (CMV)

From our discussion above, it follows that the basic functions of ventilation and oxygenation can be accomplished by providing four basic settings: respiratory rate, tidal volume, FiO_2, and PEEP. Given these parameters, the ventilator will provide the patient with a constant minute ventilation and oxygen. These are the settings for CMV. The only gases these patients receive are from the machine breaths. These patients cannot initiate a breath, change their rate, or access any other source of fresh gases. This mode of therefore useful in a limited number of settings such as the following:

a. In the operating room when patients are fully anesthetized

b. When patients are apneic and likely to remain so

c. When patients are sedated/anesthetized and paralyzed in the intensive care unit (ICU)

It is important to note that in CMV patients absolutely cannot breathe on their own. If these patients should awaken or attempt to breathe, they can become agitated and dyspneic. It is extremely frightening to be unable to breathe and to experience essentially a chronically occluded airway. Worse yet, if these patients become detached from the ventilator, anesthetized and/or paralyzed patients will be functionally apneic and may soon experience full cardiopulmonary arrest.

2. Assisted/Controlled Mechanical Ventilation (A/C)

The settings for A/C are the same four basic ones used for CMV. There is no difference between CMV and A/C in anesthetized or apneic patients. The singular difference is that in A/C mode patients can initiate breaths. Unlike in you and me, however, the amount of effort these patients make does not determine the tidal volume. When these patients initiate a breath with sufficient force to "trigger" the ventilator, the tidal volume they receive is the one already preset to be delivered as a "controlled" breath. Moreover, the machine will use whatever pressure is required to deliver the volume, and the patients' lungs and chest must then accommodate that tidal volume. The set rate in A/C is essentially a default control rate; that is, it is the number of volume-cycled breaths the machine will deliver on its own, even if the patient is apneic. Thus the "controlled" aspect of A/C is the guaranteed minute volume delivered regardless of the patient's spontaneous efforts.

While this mode has some value in its ability to relieve dyspnea in the immediate postintubation period, it is not a good choice for prolonged mechanical support. Evidence now indicates that in accommodating "assisted" breaths, the respiratory muscles may actually be fatigued rather than "rested," as was initially intended by the design. Better choices are available for routine use.

3. Synchronized Intermittent Mandatory Ventilation (SIMV) Of currently available modes, SIMV is probably the most versatile and therefore the most widely used. What does the term mean?

  a. Mandatory ventilation represents the same guaranteed minute ventilation (respiratory rate × tidal volume) delivered by the machine as seen in CMV or A/C. Thus, if the patient becomes apneic while on SIMV, the mandatory ventilation will be provided.

  b. Intermittent ventilation is used to emphasize that the machine will deliver the desired number of breaths at intervals, leaving the patient free to breathe spontaneously in between. If for example, the set respiratory rate is 10 breaths per minute, then the machine will deliver the selected tidal volume about every 6 seconds. The patient may need or desire to breathe more often than 10 times per minute and can do so in the intervals (approximately 6 seconds) between machine breaths.

  c. *Synchronized* IMV is a relatively new refinement of the original IMV design. In the example above, the machine will cycle every 6 seconds, but it would be undesirable for the ventilator to attempt delivery of a new breath if the patient were in the process of exhaling a spontaneous breath. Without synchronization, this kind of "collision" could occur in the airways, causing very high airway pressure, a risk of barotrauma, ineffective ventilation, and enhanced (rather than relieved) dyspnea. The synchronizer looks at a "window" period when the next machine breath is due. If the patient is exhaling, the ventilator can wait to begin inspiration. If the patient initiates a breath at the time the ventilator is due to cycle, the machine breath and the spontaneous breath will merge into one synchronized breath not unlike the "triggered" breaths in A/C mode. This represents a major improvement for IMV, especially in patients with prolonged expiratory times such as those with bronchial asthma.

  d. SIMV was introduced into wide usage as a "weaning" modality. Weaning from mechanical ventilation is discussed below, but in this connection, the principle is simple. Initially, the mandatory ventilation provides the entire minute ventilation necessary to maintain the patient's PCO_2 within normal limits. As patients begin to breathe spontaneously, the mandatory ventilation is gradually reduced until they are essentially providing the entire minute ventilation (and therefore CO_2 elimination) through their own spontaneous efforts. At this point these patients no longer require mechanical ventilatory support.

  e. It should be noted here that on SIMV, as in all of the modes thus far discussed, oxygenation is still supported by the settings for PEEP and FiO_2.

4. Continuous Positive Airway Pressure (CPAP)

  CPAP is the mode in which the machine is providing only PEEP, FiO_2, and humidification (maintained in all modes) but does not deliver any mechanical breaths. In this sense, it is the mode that would result if the patient were on either SIMV or A/C and the machine respiratory rate were set at zero. Its utility is limited to essentially 2 circumstances:

  a. Patients with no ventilatory difficulty who require positive airway pressure (PEEP) to support oxygenation

  b. Patients in the final stages of weaning who are being observed while they breathe without ventilatory support.

5. Pressure Support Ventilation (PSV)

  Pressure support is not a mode of mechanical ventilation, rather it is an adjunct to other modes. All people can inhale a certain tidal volume based on their ability to create a significant negative intrapleural pressure. As noted in the description of PEEP above, the vectorial result of the *negative intrapleural pressure* is a *positive-pressure gradient across the lungs*. In simplest terms, PSV is the delivery of gas flow (during a spontaneous breath) with a defined positive pressure that one selects on the ventilator. This positive pressure is vectorially summative with the negative pressure generated by the patient's effort. The net result is that the positive pressure gradient across the lung is enhanced, and as a result, so is the spontaneous tidal volume.

No PSV:
$0 - (-10) = +10$ H$_2$O transpulmonary pressure
With PSV of + 10
$+10$ (PSV) $- (-10) = +20$ cm H$_2$O transpulmonary
pressure

The above has many implications for the use of PSV:

a. PSV only has an effect on spontaneous breaths.

b. The effect of PSV can be measured as an enhancement of *spontaneous tidal volume.*

c. In our basic description, then, PSV serves the function of ventilation.

d. PSV can facilitate the reduction of mandatory machine breaths, since it increases the effectiveness of the patient's spontaneous efforts.

e. PSV can therefore be a very useful adjunct to ventilator weaning.

f. Patients may have significant relief of dyspnea with PSV because it enhances the efficacy of their own efforts, especially in low-compliance lung disease or when the respiratory muscles are fatigued.

g. PSV can help to overcome the additional work of breathing imposed by the endotracheal tube and the ventilator circuit.

h. Although the transpulmonary pressure is enhanced by PSV, the airway pressure is limited to the pressure support selected (+10 cm H$_2$O in the example above). This can have a significant beneficial effect on hemodynamics.

i. Respiratory muscles do not benefit from "rest" defined as not contracting at all; in fact they may rapidly atrophy if not allowed to perform as they usually do. However, with acute lung disease, the work of breathing may result in fatigue. PSV should allow the respiratory muscles to perform a manageable amount of work, without the risk of atrophy on the one hand or fatigue on the other.

j. If the PSV is set at >8 to 10 cm H$_2$O, it, too, may have to be weaned gradually before mechanical ventilation is discontinued.

k. PSV can only be used in modes that allow the patient to breathe spontaneously, that is, SIMV, CPAP.

E. Initiation of Mechanical Ventilation
   1. Criteria for Initiation of Mechanical Ventilation
      a. Physical Assessment: The patient is apneic, severely tachypneic, or in respiratory distress unresponsive to therapeutic interventions and supplemental oxygen.
      b. Gas Exchange: Hypoxemia ($PO_2 < 50$) despite high-flow oxygen; hypercarbia (acute, $PCO_2 > 50$ with acidic pH).
      c. Clinical Judgment: The constellation of laboratory and physical findings may be the most compelling. A PCO_2 of 60 and a respiratory rate of 35 may be the usual baseline for some patients but may represent a dire emergency in others.
   2. Initial Ventilator Settings (See Table 2.3)

F. General Principles of Ventilator Management (See Also Table 2.4)
   1. Therapeutic Endpoints
      a. $PaCO_2$: Ventilatory parameters are adjusted to achieve a $PaCO_2$ of 35 to 45 with the pH also in the normal physiologic range of 7.35 to 7.45.
      b. PaO_2 : A $PaO_2 > 60$ that corresponds to an $SaO_2 > 0.9$ with the patient receiving nontoxic FiO_2 (≤ 0.5). If this

---

Table 2.3. Initial Ventilator Settings

1. *Mode*: Unless there is a compelling reason not to, SIMV is the most versatile mode to use.

2. *Respiratory Rate*: Generally between 8 and 12 breaths per minute adjusted according to the $PaCO_2$.

3. *Tidal Volume*: In the ICU setting, 6 to 10 mL/kg lean body weight (do not count adipose tissue or edema).

4. *FiO₂*: Many people start with 1.00 (100% O_2), but often 0.8 (80% O_2) will suffice. A phenomenon called "absorption atelectasis" occurs proportionately more with higher FiO_2. Regardless, the FiO_2 should be adjusted down as soon as possible.

5. *PEEP*: Normal people can create positive pressure in their airways with their lips, palate, and glottis. Since the endotracheal tube bypasses all of these structures, most initial setups include "physiologic" PEEP of +3 to +5 cm of H_2O.

6. *PSV*: 8 to 10 cm H_2O can usually overcome the additional work imposed by the endotracheal tube and ventilator circuit, but larger amounts may substantially reduce dyspnea. Remember, PSV only has relevance for spontaneously breathing patients.

Table 2.4. The Ventilator Principles

VENTILATOR PRINCIPLE 1: To reach a desirable clinical endpoint for the patient's $PaCO_2$, the ventilator settings you will adjust are the RESPIRATORY RATE (RR) and/or the TIDAL VOLUME (Vt) delivered by the machine.

VENTILATOR PRINCIPLE 2: To reach a desirable clinical endpoint for a patient's PaO_2, the ventilator settings you will adjust are the FRACTION OF INSPIRED O_2 (FiO_2) and/or the POSITIVE END-EXPIRATORY PRESSURE (PEEP).

VENTILATOR PRINCIPLE 3: Patients do not "buck" or "fight" the ventilator; patients buck ill-conceived ventilator settings.

is not achievable on physiologic PEEP, the PEEP can be raised in +2-cm H_2O increments to achieve this endpoint.
   (1) Note that this endpoint can be expressed as a PaO_2/FiO_2 ratio 60/0.4 = 150 (FiO_2 = 0.4 is not associated with O_2 toxicity)
   (2) PEEP will be most beneficial in acute low-compliance lung disease. Patients with markedly asymmetrical lung disease, bullous emphysema, or asthma may actually have worsening gas exchange with significant PEEP.
2. When patients are in respiratory distress, it is acceptable to change any or all of the ventilator settings at one time; during weaning the same is not true.
3. Patient Comfort
   a. Having an endotracheal tube in place is not comfortable, and because one cannot speak, frustrating as well.
   b. Patients who will be intubated for a short time should receive mild sedation with agents having no significant respiratory suppression.
   c. Patients who require high ventilator settings and will likely be intubated for several days before weaning should receive more substantial sedation.
   d. In our opinion, only a few selected patients require paralytic agents.
4. Some Simple Rules of Thumb
   a. Endotracheal tubes should be as large (diameter) as possible and cut as short as possible once position is verified.
   b. Endotracheal tubes must be carefully secured and should be out from between the patient's teeth.

    c. Suctioning is important but should be minimal or strictly prn when the patient is on >+10cm H_2O PEEP, to minimize volume loss from within the lungs.

    d. When setting up the ventilator, the peak inspiratory flow rate is best kept relatively low (≤50L/min [LPM]) but must be at least *3 times the minute ventilation* or the patient may be dyspneic.

    e. Generally, a PSV of 8 to 10cm H_2O overcomes the extra flow resistive work of the endotracheal tube, but the optimal level usually results in a spontaneous respiratory rate <25 breaths per minute and absence of accessory muscle use.

    f. Any intubated patient should have a nasogastric tube placed; this immediately empties the stomach of liquid contents and of the air that is often swallowed during respiratory distress. It can then be used for stress ulcer prophylaxis and enteral nutritional support.

G. Weaning From Mechanical Ventilation

The ultimate goal of placing patients on mechanical ventilation is to take them off of mechanical ventilation.

    1. When reducing the ventilator settings, you may change 2 settings at once, but not 2 that serve the same function: For example, you may reduce the FiO_2 and the respiratory rate at the same time, because one serves *oxygenation* and the other serves *ventilation;* you would not reduce the respiratory rate and the PSV at the same time, since both serve the minute ventilation.

    2. When beginning to wean PEEP from its peak setting, it is prudent to reduce it in 1-cm H_2O increments for the first few changes.

    3. When weaning PEEP, changes should not be made more frequently than every 3 to 4 hours; some alveoli may destabilize and collapse rapidly, others may take time; hence, whether or not the patient will tolerate the change may not be clear for 3 to 4 hours.

    4. To be successfully weaned from the ventilator and extubated (removal of the endotracheal tube), patients must meet 3 sets of criteria: gas exchange, pulmonary mechanics, and circumstantial.

        a. Gas Exchange

            (1) The FiO_2 should be ≤0.5, and the PEEP should be physiologic before active weaning is contemplated.

            (2) The $PaCO_2$ should be normal (or normal for the patient), and the pH should be in the

Table 2.5. Weaning Parameters

Tidal volume:	4–7 mL/kg
Respiratory rate:	<30 breaths/min
Negative inspiratory force:	More negative than 20 cm H_2O
Minute ventilation:	<10 L/min
Vital capacity:	>10 mL/kg

        normal range (not acidic) before parameters that serve ventilation are reduced.

    (3) In general, the desirable therapeutic endpoints outlined above should be met before the settings are reduced.

  b. Pulmonary Mechanics

    (1) Although often referred to as "weaning parameters," these are more correctly thought of as extubation criteria.

    (2) The parameters measured and desirable values are depicted in Table 2.5.

  c. Circumstantial criteria

    (1) If possible, the patient should be awake and alert for extubation.

    (2) If the patient is neurologically impaired, careful testing of the gag and cough reflexes is necessary.

    (3) Secretions should have minimized or the patient clearly demonstrated an ability to manage them.

    (4) The airway should be patent and nonedematous, and the patient should have control (voluntary or reflex) over it.

    (5) Extraneous stresses placed on respiratory requirements must be corrected, such as metabolic acidosis, anemia, fever, bronchospasm, and cardiac dysrhythmia.

    (6) Electrolyte abnormalities that compromise respiratory muscle function must be corrected, such as low values for potassium, magnesium, phosphorus, and ionized calcium.

■ V. HEMODYNAMICS

The subject of hemodynamics has 2 major components: *Cardiodynamics,* the physiology of heart function per se, and traditional *hemodynamics,* which embraces the pulmonary circulation, the systemic circulation, and the right and left sides of the heart as the functional pumps (respectively) of these circuits.

The bedside tool that is most useful for both continuous assessment of cardiac pump function and management of the hemodynamic state of the circulation is the *pulmonary artery (PA) (Swan-Ganz) catheter.* Although much useful information can be derived from the measurements and calculations made possible through the use of a PA catheter, the single most important reason to place one in a critically ill patient is to measure *cardiac* output. In the critical care unit, ensurance of the adequacy of cardiac output and its integral role in life-sustaining DO_2 is the principle rationale for placement of the catheter. Proper interpretation and manipulation of other values (e.g., the pulmonary capillary wedge pressure) depend on the cardiac output for context.

The PA catheter is *not a therapy.* It is a *monitoring device.* Like all interventions it carries an inherent risk/benefit ratio. Unless the catheter is used *actively* to assess the patient, guide management, and reassess the response to interventions, its placement is all risk and no benefit. Indeed, in recent years, the authors of this book have seldom used this device.

A. Physics and Physiology

Conceptually, the flow of any fluid through a conduit is governed by the following general principle:

Pressure = Flow × Resistance

Note that this applies to airway pressure, inspiratory flow rate, and airway resistance or, as in the present discussion, blood pressure, blood flow (cardiac output), and vascular resistance. Specifically:

MAP	=	**CO**	×	**SVR**
Mean Arterial Pressure		Cardiac Output		Systemic Vascular Resistance

or

PAP	=	**CO**	×	**PVR**
Pulmonary Artery Pressure		Cardiac Output		Pulmonary Vascular Resistance

We can solve these equations for the calculated resistances:

$$SVR = \frac{MAP \times 79.9*}{CO}$$

$$PVR = \frac{PAP \times 79.9*}{CO}$$

*79.9 is a constant that converts the units according to the resistance equation of Poiseuille.

Vascular Resistance: Conceptually, the resistance to flow of a fluid through a conduit is given by the equation of Poiseuille:

$$\text{Resistance} = \frac{8 \times \text{length} \times \text{velocity} \times \text{viscosity}}{\pi(\text{radius})^4}$$

B. Cardiodynamics

The pump function of the heart results from the interaction of 3 variables: *preload*, *afterload*, and *contractility*.

1. Preload

   In simplest terms, preload is the amount of cardiac filling during diastole. In this sense, one can think of it as the end-diastolic volume (EDV), which is either the cause or the result of end-diastolic pressure (EDP). In purest terms, the preload is the resting fiber length of the myofibrils and forms the fundamental basis for the Frank-Starling curve.

2. Afterload

   In simplest terms, afterload can be thought of as the impedance to cardiac ejection. If, for example, the diastolic blood pressure were high, the heart would have to overcome that pressure just to open the aortic valve. In truth, afterload is much more complicated than simply blood pressure. In physiological terms, afterload is *the developed wall tension* during systole and is affected by several factors. Generally speaking, anything that makes it easier for the heart to eject blood is an *afterload reducer*, and anything that makes it more difficult increases afterload.

3. Contractility

   Contractility is literally the force with which the heart contracts. Note that, given any amount of filling and a constant afterload, the amount of blood ejected by a given heart beat will depend on the force of contraction.

4. Cardiac Output

   The CO is the product of the amount of blood pumped each time the heart contracts (stroke volume, SV) times the number of contractions per minute (HR).

   $$\textbf{CO} = \textbf{HR} \times \textbf{SV}$$

   $$\textbf{SV} = \frac{\textbf{CO}}{\textbf{HR}}$$

   It is clear from the above that a person can have a CO of 5 LPM with a HR of 70 or a HR of 140. Part of the clinical assessment of the CO includes looking at the efficiency of cardiac performance. In general, better SV and lower HR represents greater efficiency.

5. Indexing

Normal adults come in all shapes and sizes. The absolute CO for a healthy 45-kg woman may be the same as the value for an NFL football player in hemorrhagic shock. How can we compare the values? The answer is to index the values to body surface area (BSA). Thus, raw values for CO in adults may vary widely, while indexed values are usually closely comparable:

a. 45-kg female: CO = 4.0 LPM, BSA = $1.387 \, m^2$

$$CI = \frac{CO}{BSA} = \frac{4.0 \, LPM}{1.387 \, m^2} = \mathbf{2.88 \, LPM/m^2}$$

b. 145-kg male: CO = 8.0 LPM, BSA = $2.77 \, m^2$

$$CI = \frac{CO}{BSA} = \frac{8.0 \, LPM}{2.774 \, m^2} = \mathbf{2.88 \, LPM/m^2}$$

Notice that in the above example a 4-LPM CO yields on excellent cardiac index (CI) for the smaller patient but would result in a value (1.44) for the larger patient consistent with a diagnosis of shock.

Any of the values calculated as part of a hemodynamic profile can be indexed: CI, stroke volume index (SVI), systemic vascular resistance index (SVRI), etc. The normal values for these indices are useful, since they are the standard for comparison of all patients, not just those of average size.

6. Basic Approach to Hemodynamic Management

Bedside pulmonary artery catheterization in the ICU is not the same procedure as diagnostic cardiac catheterization in the laboratory. The fundamental purpose in the ICU is to measure, monitor, and manage the CO as an integral part of oxygen delivery. Since many of the patients are intubated, on positive pressure ventilation (VCV), and may have multiple other problems that affect cardiac performance (even if not of cardiac origin per se), the CO must be managed to meet O_2 transport endpoints, not to make "the numbers" look like textbook normal.

a. Do not place a pulmonary artery catheter unless you are going to use it: The actual bedside methodology for catheter placement is reviewed elsewhere. The important principles to remember follow:

(1) The catheter is placed to measure CO; all of the other values and calculations are only

useful for management in the context of a known CO.

(2) Record and evaluate all of the values during placement of the catheter: central venous pressure (CVP), right atrial pressure (RA), right ventricular pressure (RV), pulmonary artery pressure (PA systolic, diastolic, and mean), and the pulmonary capillary occlusion (wedge) pressure (PCWP). All of these can be helpful in assessment, diagnosis, and, most importantly, management.

(3) Understand the clinical circumstances of the catheterization. Interpretation of the measured pressures in a patient on PEEP (see below) and positive-pressure ventilation differs markedly from interpretation of the same values in a nonintubated, spontaneously breathing patient.

b. If the CO is lower than you desire for good O_2 transport, or is acceptable but achieved inefficiently such as with low SV and a significant tachycardia, then the following interventions are recommended:

(1) Optimize the Preload: In general, the higher the filling pressure (PCWP) the higher the EDV; thus, the higher the preload. Remember, the endpoint is optimized CO as part of optimized O_2 delivery. On any Starling curve, maximal CO (or SV, or stroke work index [SWI]) is achieved at an optimal filling pressure of about 18 to 22 mm Hg. This is true only as a general rule of thumb. It does not take into account other mitigating factors such as oncotic pressure, capillary permeability, or the transmural pressure (which may be markedly different in a patient on significant PEEP) (see below).

(2) Inotropic Support: If CO is still not adequate or still achieved inefficiently, then the addition of an inotrope is justified. An inotrope enables the heart to achieve a higher function curve at the same filling pressure. A good choice for this intervention is dobutamine at between 5 and 30 µg/kg/min.

(3) Reduced Afterload: If CO is still less than desired, further enhancement may be achieved by afterload reduction. Dobutamine itself has some peripheral vasodilating properties. Amrinone is a phosphodiesterase inhibitor with

both inotropic and vasodilating properties and may work well in tandem with dobutamine. If the patient's blood pressure is frankly elevated, afterload reduction can be achieved by adequate blood pressure control with a variety of agents.

(4) Perform a Two-Dimensional Echocardiogram: If available, a bedside two-dimensional echocardiogram can further enhance your assessment.

    (a) Evaluate chamber size/ventricular volume.

    (b) Evaluate contractility/regional wall motion.

    (c) Evaluate valvular function, which may be hemodynamically important.

    (d) Estimate ejection fraction.

(5) Reevaluation: After each incremental intervention (volume loading, inotropic support, afterload reduction), reevaluate CO, oxygen transport, and the derived hemodynamic profile.

c. Transmural Pressures: In our discussion of transpulmonary pressure, we looked at the gradient across the lungs from the airways to the pleural space. An exactly analogous gradient exists across the wall of the heart between intracavitary pressure (inside the atria or ventricles) and the intrathoracic (intrapleural) pressure (ITP). Again, it is the vectorial difference across the wall of the heart that is the true transmural pressure and therefore the real determinant of ventricular volume. This concept has many important physiologic implications:

(1) A "normal" filling pressure for the right ventricle of $5\,cm\ H_2O$ (i.e., a normal CVP) is not really 5 but, rather, 10; i.e., $5\,cm\ H_2O$ filling from *within* and $-5\,cm\ H_2O$ pulling from *without*:

$$CVP - ITP = P_{transmural}$$
$$5 - (-5) = +10\,cm\,H_2O$$

(2) This is a fundamental observation of the Starling relationship: When people inhale (more negative ITP), right ventricular filling is enhanced and, as a result, so is cardiac output.

(3) Similarly, a "normal" PCWP (which serves as left ventricular filling pressure) is not the measured intracavitary pressure (normal ≈ 8 to

12 mm Hg) but, rather, the *transmural* pressure, which includes the effect of negative ITP.

(4) Note that the heart (or any of its chambers) has *compliance*. Just as transpulmonary pressure determines lung volume through compliance, so does transmural filling pressure determine ventricular volume (EDV, i.e., true *preload*).

(5) Since ventricular volume (EDV) is the *preload* and a major determinant of CO, appreciation of transmural pressures may help you in the management of CO and DO_2.

d. Spontaneously breathing patients with negative ITP make it easy to use readily measured values for CVP or PCWP. When patients are on positive-pressure ventilation (any conventional mode of VCV) and especially when they are on PEEP, ITP may no longer be negative and may even been substantially positive. Thus, instead of *enhancing* transmural filling pressures, positive (+) ITP may *reduce* transmural gradients, ventricular filling and therefore, cardiac output.

No PEEP:
$$CVP - ITP = P_{transmural}$$
$$+5 - (-5) = +10 \, cm \, H_2O$$
PEEP = +10 cm H_2O:
$$CVP - ITP = P_{transmural}$$
$$+12 - (+10) = +2 \, cm \, H_2O$$

(1) Note that even though the measured CVP (inside the vena cava) is higher (+12) in the patient on PEEP, the transmural filling pressure is substantially lower, and as a result, so is the preload (and CO).

(2) Normally, if the CVP or PCWP rises, one presumes that the RVEDV and the LVEDV also increase (respectively). This is because the normally negative ITP vectorially enhances the transmural pressures and therefore end-diastolic volumes.

(3) If positive ITP actually "squeezes" the heart from without, the measured filling *pressure* within the chambers will go *up* as the *volume* (EDV) is going *down!*

(4) A patient on high PEEP who has high measured values for CVP and PCWP may have any of the following:

(a) High end-diastolic volume, good pre-load, and therefore good CO, as would normally be predicted by elevated filling pressures.

(b) Less than expected EDVs and CO because of restricted cardiac filling secondary to increased ITP.

(c) Very small EDVs because of "squeezing" from positive ITP with resultant poor CO.

(5) *No algorithm* can tell you to what degree PEEP is affecting the measured filling pressures nor the degree to which positive airway pressure (PEEP) is transmitted to the pleural space and mediastinum. The very best indicator of adequate filling pressures (CVP and/or PCWP) is a *good CO* achieved *efficiently* with a good SV.

(6) A bedside echocardiogram maybe of value to look at chamber size (EDV) and correlate it with measured filling pressures (from the PA catheter). This will help you decide whether a given PCWP does indeed yield a good preload (EDV) and whether the CO may benefit from further volume (preload) enhancement. The findings can also help you decide whether inotropic support should be added.

C. Summary

1. The PA catheter can tell you a great deal about the patient's condition but nothing more important than the cardiac output. Its use in recent years is controversial.

2. The CO is 1 of only 3 parameters you can manipulate to optimize life-sustaining oxygen delivery.

3. The derived hemodynamic calculations and profiles may help you categorize shock states and suggest specific management (see Chapter 3, "Cardiovascular Disorders").

4. Regardless, in the ICU setting, particularly with patients on positive-pressure ventilation, all manipulations of the patient will likely have hemodynamic effects, and thus you must use the catheter as a monitoring device and update data frequently.

5. Ventilator setting changes, diuresis, IV fluids, fever, anemia, acidosis/alkalosis, electrolyte abnormalities, medications, anesthesia/analgesics—all can and *will affect cardiac performance*, CO, and as a result, DO_2.

■ VI. THE CARDIOPULMONARY INTERACTION

A. Proper gas exchange within the lungs depends on the matching of ventilation (V) and perfusion (Q_T). It is immediately obvious that both pulmonary and cardiac function are intimately involved.

B. By far the most common cause of arterial hypoxemia is mismatching of V and Q_T. If ventilation and perfusion are not matched in space, in quantity, or in time, then some mixed venous blood will pass from the right side of the heart to the left side of the heart without being oxygenated.

1. Matching in Space

   If there is a region of lung that receives blood flow but there is little or no ventilation in the same region, then mixed venous blood flowing through that area will reach the left side of the heart without picking up oxygen. A good clinical example of this problem is acute atelectasis.

2. Matching in Quantity

   Suppose a region of lung receives normal capillary blood flow but a reduced amount of ventilation. When fresh gas is present in the alveoli, the capillary blood is initially well oxygenated, but because of reduced ventilation, the O_2 tension in the alveolus falls and subsequent blood flow is poorly oxygenated until alveolar gas is replenished. This kind of V/Q_T abnormality is very common in both acute and chronic lung disease. It follows that supplemental O_2 (which allows capillary oxygen uptake to take place over a longer period of time) improves the hypoxemia which results from this V/Q_T abnormality.

3. Matching in Time

   Imagine a region of lung that only has ventilation during the inspiratory phase of respiration but no residual gas after exhalation (see discussion of PEEP above and Figure 2.1). Gas exchange would take place only during inspiration. Note that ventilation and perfusion would not be present at the same time, and mixed venous blood would be allowed to pass unoxygenated through the lungs between active inspirations. Such severe mismatch can occur in acute low-compliance lung disease such as hyalin membrane disease or ARDS.

4. Overall V/Q_T Matching

   Note that any of the scenarios above—V and Q_T not in the same place, not in equal quantities, not present together at the same time—could all be represented mathematically as a *low* V/Q_T ratio. However, such a depiction would hide the individual pathogenesis and the accompanying rationale for therapy.

5. Venous Admixture

In the examples above of mismatching of V and Q_T, note that the low V/Q_T ratio means that some venous blood is not oxygenated and is returned as such to the left side of the heart. Thus, either as the result of disproportionately high perfusion for the ventilation, perfusion that exhausts available oxygen, or blood that passes an alveolus that is only intermittently ventilated, some quantity of mixed venous blood is added to oxygenated blood with resultant decrease in the final PaO_2 or frank hypoxemia.

6. True Shunt

A true shunt occurs when there is zero ventilation and some measurable perfusion. This shunted blood never comes in contact with air and thus reaches the left side of the heart as unaltered mixed venous blood. No change in FiO_2 will improve the resultant hypoxemia, since oxygenated blood cannot saturate beyond 100% and a fixed quantity of unoxygenated blood (shunt) will be added to the final mix.

B. General Principles

1. Venous Admixture

The venous admixture will show improvement in hypoxemia with enhanced FiO_2. The component that is the result of low V/Q will be corrected, and the true shunt component will not.

2. True Shunt

A true shunt does not show any improvement of hypoxemia with enhanced FiO_2. If you increase the FiO_2 by 10% increments three times (.21 to .30 to .40 to .50) and the PO_2 increases <10 torr, you are dealing with a fixed shunt.

3. Clinical Endpoints

PO_2 > 60 torr, SaO_2 > .90 achieved a nontoxic FiO_2 (≤0.5) are acceptable. If the patient requires either higher FiO_2 or fails to reach these endpoints regardless of FiO_2, then therapy directed at shunt reduction per se should be instituted.

4. Shunt Reduction

Shunt reduction may occasionally be achieved rapidly such as by relieving atelectasis or collapse, but it often requires positive-pressure ventilation and PEEP. The rationale for this approach is the recruitment and stabilization of alveoli such that there is now measurable ventilation in perfused lung regions where previously there was none.

   a. Normal people have <5% shunt resulting from some venous blood being returned directed to the left heart (most importantly, the bronchial circulation).

   b. Patients with >15% usually require mechanical ventilation.

   c. It is interesting to note that the desirable clinical endpoints ($PO_2 > 60$, $SaO_2 > 90$ on $FiO_2 \leq .5$ and PO_2/FiO_2 ratio ≥ 150) all are achieved when Qs/Q_T is reduced to <15%.

   d. Shunt reduction is often achieved by mechanical ventilation per se, sometimes by the application of PEEP (above physiologic), but it ultimately depends on reversal of the pathologic condition (e.g., atelectasis, pulmonary edema, ARDS).

5. Shunt Equation

   In a modified form, the shunt equation can be used at the bedside to calculate the "shunt fraction" and followed during the course of management:

$$\frac{Q_s}{Q_T} = \frac{1 - SaO_2}{1 - SvO_2}$$

C. The Cardiopulmonary Interaction

   From the above it is clear that management of V/Q_T means the *management of V and the management of* Q_T. It is of paramount importance that you realize that the two are intimately and inextricably related.

   1. Cardiac Output and Hypoxemia

      As discussed previously, a typical response to low CO is enhanced peripheral extraction (and low SvO_2). If the patient has a significant quantitative shunt, it will be qualitatively enhanced by low SvO_2. Improvement in CO can thus result in improvement in PO_2 without a single "pulmonary" intervention. There are also times when a fixed shunt flow (Qs) represents a larger fraction of a low CO (Q_T), whereas the same Qs may be a less significant fraction of an improved CO. The message is: *Hypoxemia may improve significantly with enhancement of CO, and conversely, a low CO can have a serious adverse effect on oxygenation in the patient with respiratory failure and significant shunt.*

   2. Ventilators and Cardiac Output

      Patients who require shunt reduction to reach clinical endpoints are likely to be on positive-pressure ventilation and PEEP. While positive airway pressure may help recruit and stabilize alveoli, it may also significantly impede venous return to the chest, restrict cardiac diastolic filling, and thus reduce CO (see discussion above). Note that in the scheme of optimizing DO_2, raising the SaO_2 with a maneuver (e.g., raising PEEP) that results in loss of CO achieves nothing in terms of $\dot{D}O_2$:

a. $\dot{D}O_2 = \mathbf{10}\ (CO) \times 12\ (Hb) \times 1.34 \times \mathbf{0.80}\ (SaO_2) = 1286$
b. $\dot{D}O_2 = \mathbf{8}\ (CO) \times 12\ (Hb) \times 1.34 \times \mathbf{0.99}\ (SaO_2) = 1273$

$\dot{D}O_2$ is the *same* in both cases: What has been *gained in SaO_2 has been lost in CO*—perhaps secondary to the application of PEEP.

■ VII. INTEGRATED CARDIOPULMONARY MANAGEMENT PRINCIPLES

A. Practical Suggestions

Based on the acknowledged interdependence of ventilator management and hemodynamics, below are some practical suggestions:

1. Adjust the ventilator settings to reach clinical endpoints as outlined previously.
2. If the patient requires PEEP > physiological, and especially $\geq 15\ cm\ H_2O$, the patient probably should have a PA catheter placed to assist management.
3. CO (CI) should be optimized to (at least) within normal limits on the current ventilator settings.
4. Do not detach the patient from the ventilator to try to obtain "true readings." The relevant hemodynamics are those measured on the ventilator.
5. Optimize CO first by preload enhancement followed by use of inotropes or afterload-reducing agents as indicated.
6. *Reassess.* You may see that the ABGs improve with good hemodynamic management and no further escalation of ventilator support will be needed.
7. If the filling pressures are elevated or suggest *high preload with poor cardiac output* in a patient on PEEP, an echocardiogram may help define ventricular volume and ventricular function and help you to interpret the measured filling pressures.
8. PEEP (like everything else) should be increased as much as necessary and as little as possible.
9. If the patient is breathing spontaneously, you may reduce the number of IMV breaths as tolerated and maintain

V_{min} with spontaneous (usually with appropriate PSV) breaths. The fewer positive-pressure breaths, the less impedance to venous return and ventricular filling and, therefore, cardiac output.

10. There are 1440 minutes in a day. A reduction in IMV breaths from 10 to 8 spares the heart 2880 positive-pressure breaths and translates into many liters of CO and $\dot{D}O_2$.

11. Do not forget to make measurements and calculations frequently. $\dot{D}O_2$, $\dot{V}O_2$, Qs/Q_T, CO, PCWP, SV, SVR, and others can all be assessed and reassessed anytime. These are much more precise insights into why a patient is hypoxemic or hypotensive than the simple measure of PO_2 or blood pressure.

12. Patients on positive-pressure ventilation and PEEP should receive dopamine at $\leq 3\mu g/kg/min$ to enhance renal blood flow.

13. Patients with respiratory failure who are on mechanical ventilation should also receive
    a. Stress ulcer prophylaxis
    b. Nutritional support (preferably enteral)
    c. Deep venous thrombosis prophylaxis
    d. Appropriate sedation/analgesia

14. Noninvasive and/or continuous monitors such as pulse oximetry, end-tidal CO_2 monitoring, and $S\bar{v}O_2$ fiberoptic catheters can all help guide dynamic management and reduce the need for arterial and mixed venous blood gas determinations.

15. Invasive arterial and central venous lines are needed for monitoring, blood sampling, and administration of vasoactive substances, concentrated electrolytes, or emergency medications.

16. Such patients should have a daily chest x-ray to verify positions of tubes and catheters, follow lung pathology, and monitor for complications such as barotrauma, atelectasis, or ICU-acquired disease.

3

Cardiovascular Disorders

Cardiovascular disease is the number one cause of death in the United States, killing more than 900,000 patients each year. Recent advances in our understanding of the pathogenesis of some of these disorders, as well as new therapeutic techniques, have greatly improved our ability to treat these patients.

■ ISCHEMIC HEART DISEASE

I. Unstable Angina Pectoris
   A. Definition
      Angina pectoris is chest discomfort that occurs when myocardial oxygen demand exceeds supply. Unstable angina is the manifestation of coronary artery disease that falls somewhere between angina pectoris and myocardial infarction. It is characterized by
      1. Recent onset of ischemic chest pain
      2. Increase of severity, duration, or frequency or chronic anginal chest pain, or
      3. Angina pain that occurs at rest
      Recently, the term *acute coronary syndrome* has been used to describe the spectrum of acute unstable manifestations of coronary disease including unstable angina and myocardial infarction.
   B. Risk Factors
      1. Increased age
      2. Male sex
      3. Family history

        4. Smoking history
        5. Hypertension
        6. Diabetes mellitus
        7. Hyperlipidemia

C. Pathophysiology

Coronary artery atherosclerosis most commonly underlies unstable angina. Unstable atheromatous plaque with the development of thrombus is thought to cause the transformation of a stable angina picture into that of unstable angina. Up to 7% to 9% of hospitalized patients with unstable angina will develop myocardial infarction (MI). Coronary artery spasm, hemorrhage, and increased platelet aggregation have been argued to play a role in this syndrome.

D. Clinical Presentation

Substernal pain (pressure, heaviness, tightness, and/or burning) that is new in onset, prolonged, or occurring at rest is common. Shortness of breath, diaphoresis, nausea, and pain in the left arm may be present. On occasion, back and jaw pain are the cardinal features.

E. Differential Diagnosis
    1. Acute MI
    2. Acute aortic dissection
    3. Pulmonary disorders including pulmonary embolism, pleurisy, pneumothorax, and pneumonia
    4. Peptic ulcer disease, pancreatitis, esophageal reflux and spasm, cholecystitis, and biliary colic
    5. Musculoskeletal conditions, chest wall pain, costochondritis
    6. Herpes zoster

F. Diagnostic Studies
    1. Diagnosis is made primarily by history.

Physical examination is usually unraveling. However, one should look for evidence of hyperlipidemia, hypertension, and congestive heart failure as well as the presence of murmurs.

    2. Electrocardiograms (ECGs) during episodes of pain may show tangent repolarization abnormalities. Normal tracing may be present also. Chest radiographs should be obtained and may show evidence of cardiomegaly and/or pulmonary edema.

G. Treatment

A patient with unstable angina should be placed on bed rest in the intensive care unit (ICU).
    1. Pharmacotherapy

a. Nitrates

This class of agents causes relaxation of vascular muscle and venodilatation. Diastolic ventricular wall tension is reduced by decreased venous return following administration of these agents, thus decreasing myocardial oxygen consumption. Therapy may be started with sublingual nitroglycerin, 0.4 mg (1/150) q5min × 3. Topical therapy with 2% nitroglycerin ointment ($^1/_2$ to 2 inches) q6h may also be instituted. Recurrent bouts of pain should prompt institution of intravenous nitroglycerin beginning at 10 µg/min and titrated upward to the desired effect (absence of pain, systolic blood pressure no less than 90 to 100 mm Hg).

b. Beta-Adrenergic Blocking Agents

These agents reduce myocardial oxygen demand by decreasing heart rate, blood pressure, and contractility. Patients with bradycardia of <50 beats per minute, systolic blood pressure <100 mm Hg, chest x-ray evidence of pulmonary edema, second- or third-degree atrioventricular (A-V) block or a PR interval ≥0.24 seconds, and those with bronchospastic lung disease should not receive these agents. Intravenous and oral beta-blocker dosage schedules are depicted in Table 3.1.

Table 3.1. Commonly Used Beta-Blockers in Unstable Angina

Drug	Acute intravenous dose	Oral dose
Atenolol	5 mg over 5 minutes, repeat × 1 after 10 minutes.	50 mg q12h or 100 mg q24h
Metoprolol	5 mg q5 min × 3 doses	50 mg q6h; after 48h, 100 mg q12h
Labetolol	20–80 mg bolus 2-mg/min infusion titrate to effect	100 mg bid
Nadolol		40–80 mg qd
Propanolol	0.5–3 mg slow IV bolus, repeat as necessary	40–800 mg/d given bid to qid

Table 3.2. Oral Calcium-Channel Antagonists Used in Unstable Angina

Agent	Oral dose
Verapamil	240–480 mg/day
Diltiazem	180–360 mg/day

c. Calcium-Channel Antagonists

These agents decrease myocardial ischemia by coronary and peripheral vasodilatation, negative effects on contractility, and also heart rate. They are not first-line agents but may be used in refractory cases.

Oral doses of representative calcium channel antagonists are noted in Table 3.2. Because of their negative inotropic effect, these agents should not be administered in patients with congestive heart failure.

d. Aspirin

Aspirin has been shown to decrease the rate of myocardial infarction and coronary death in patients with unstable angina. Various dosing regimens ranging from 160 to 325 mg qd have been advocated. Some studies have demonstrated a 50% reduction in cardiovascular death or nonfatal MI.

e. Anticoagulants

Intravenous heparin has been a useful adjunct in unstable angina, demonstrating reduced incidence of MI and refractory angina in some studies. Intermediate and high-risk presentations are usually treated with heparin. Doses of 60 IU/kg intravenous (IV) bolus followed by 12 IU/kg/h infusion are recommended. Enoxaparin or deltaheparin are low molecular weight heparins that may be superior to unfractionated heparin dosed at 1 mg/kg bid.

f. Thrombolytic Therapy

Despite the benefits in acute myocardial infarction, thrombolytic therapy has not been shown to improve outcome in patients with unstable angina.

g. Glycoprotein IIb/IIIa Receptor Inhibitors

These agents block the receptors that lead to

platelet aggregation. Two relatively short-acting (4 to 8 hours) agents (eptifibatide, tirofiban) and one longer acting antibody (abciximab) are available. These agents are beneficial during percutaneous coronary interventions, and the shorter acting agents are approved for use in non-Q MI and unstable angina being medically managed. Decreased combined endpoints of death, infarction, and urgent intervention have been reported. These agents should be administered to high-risk patients (ST depression >1 mm, persistent or recurrent symptoms, widespread electrocardiographic [ECG] abnormalities, depressed left ventricular [LV] function, positive cardiac markers)

(1) Eptifibatide, 180-μg/kg IV bolus followed by a 2-μg/kg/min infusion. A double-bolus regimen has been shown to improve platelet inhibition in some clinical studies (180 μg/kg × 2, 10 minutes apart).

(2) Tirofiban, 0.4 μg/kg/min × 30 minutes followed by 0.1 μg/min infusion.

(3) Abciximab, 0.25-mg/kg IV bolus followed by 0.125 μg/kg/min infusion.

2. Nonpharmacologic Therapy

Persistent chest pain despite maximal therapy with nitrates, beta-blockers, aspirin, heparin, etc. may require early cardiac catheterization, with the view toward potential mechanical intervention (percutaneous transluminal coronary angioplasty (PTCA) or coronary bypass surgery). Intra-aortic balloon pump (IABP) insertion should be performed with the goal of stabilizing the patient when needed. The IABP relieves pain and may provide relative stability for evaluation before intervention.

II. Myocardial Infarction

A. Definition

Myocardial infarction (MI) is necrosis of the cardiac muscle resulting from insufficient supply of oxygenated blood.

1. Q-Wave MI

Q-wave MI presents with ST-segment elevation and the subsequent development of pathologic Q waves in the ECG.

    2. Nonacute MI

        More than 50% of acute MIs in the United States do not present with ST-segment elevation but rather have nonspecific ECG changes or even normal ECGs.

B. Pathophysiology

    1. MI is nearly universally the result of coronary artery atherosclerosis.

    2. Atherosclerotic lesions reduce and limit the flow through coronary arteries, resulting in ischemic myocardial cells.

    3. The formation of thrombi plays a significant role in acute MI, and almost all ST-segment elevation infarcts will have an occlusive thrombus in the infarct-related artery if examined early enough in the course of the MI.

    4. Occlusion of the right coronary artery (RCA) generally results in inferior/posterior MI.

    5. Occlusion of the left anterior descending artery (LAD) generally leads to anterior infarctions, while blockage of the left circumflex artery (LCA) results in lateral and/or inferior/posterior MI.

    6. Spasm of the coronary arteries may also play a role in MI. As many as 2% of all MI patients, a significantly higher percentage of those patients who are less than 35 years of age, will have angiographically normal coronary arteries, and presumably spasm is a significant pathophysiologic event.

C. Risk Factors

    Risk factors for coronary artery disease including MI are age, male sex, family history, smoking, hypertension, elevated cholesterol, and diabetes mellitus. Cocaine use has recently arisen as a risk factor for MI.

D. Clinical Presentation

    1. Patients present with chest pain (typically substernal) lasting 30 minutes or longer, which is unrelieved by rest or nitroglycerin, and pain that may radiate from left or right arm into the jaw. The pain is typically nonpleuritic and may be associated with dyspnea, diaphoresis, nausea, or vomiting.

    2. As many as 20% of all MIs are painless.

    3. "Burning" discomfort is as predictive of acute MI as pressure-type discomfort.

E. Physical Findings

    1. Skin may be cool. Diaphoresis may be evident.

2. Heart may demonstrate an apical systolic murmur, mitral regurgitation secondary to papillary muscle dysfunction. S_3 or S_4 gallop sounds may be present.

3. Advanced signs of congestive heart failure (CHF) with pulmonary edema may be present with rales auscultated in lung fields.

4. In many instances the physical examination will not reveal specific abnormalities.

F. Diagnostic Studies

1. The diagnosis of MI must be presumptive, based on history, physical examination, and ECG.

2. Electrocardiogram (see Table 3.3)

a. Q-Wave MI: The classic description of the evolution of Q-wave MI includes the following:

(1) ST-segment elevation is indicative of an area of injury (see Figure 3.1).

(2) T-wave inversion, a sign of ischemia.

(3) Q waves indicate areas of infarction. Development of Q waves may be early or may not occur for several days during the evolution of a MI.

Table 3.3. ECG Localization of Infarcts

Infarct location	ECG abnormality
Anterior	V_1-V_4
Anteroseptal	V_1-V_2
Anterolateral	I, aVL, V_4, V_5, V_6
Lateral	I and AVL
Inferior	II, III, aVF
Posterior	R > S in V_1

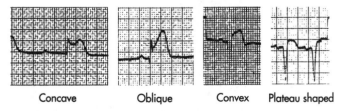

Concave   Oblique   Convex   Plateau shaped

Figure 3.1. Different types of ST elevations in acute myocardial infarction. (From Conover MB: *Understanding electrocardiography*, ed. 6, St. Louis, 1992, Mosby-Year Book.)

   b. Non Q-wave infarction: ST-segment depression and T-wave inversion may be seen.
3. Enzyme Studies

   Necrotic heart muscle cells release enzymes into the bloodstream. Classically, creatine kinase (CK, or CPK), have been used in laboratory diagnosis of MI.

   a. CK becomes elevated within 24 hours. CK is also present in the skeletal muscle and brain and thus may be released in other clinical conditions. To increase specificity, the assay of the MB isoenzyme of CK is used. This enzyme is found primarily in the myocardium.

   b. Cardiac-specific Troponin I and Troponin T are regulatory components of the contractile apparatus of the heart. These proteins are very specific for myocardial injury and are released into the blood in the hours following myocardial infarction. They are not reliably elevated until at least 10 to 12 hours after infarct onset. They remain elevated for several days and are thus quite useful in patients presenting late after infarct.

   c. Myoglobin is a cytosolic protein found in all muscle cells. It is released quickly after MI but is unfortunately not very specific for myocardial injury.

   d. CK-MB Subforms: The MB isoenzyme of CK exists in only one form in the myocardial cell. After it is released into the blood stream, enzymatically mediated cleavage of a terminal lysine residue occurs, creating 2 subforms of CK-MB. The ratio of the freshly released CK-MB to the old cleaved CK-MB is a very sensitive and specific early marker of myocardial injury.

4. Nuclear Medicine Techniques

   Thallium 201 is taken up by perfused viable cardiac myocytes and may indicate areas of infarction by the presence of "cold spots". Unfortunately, this technique may not distinguish between acute MI and previous scar. Technetium 99 (Tc^{99}) results in "hot spots" as the tracer accumulates in damaged myocardial cells.

5. Other diagnostic studies in patients with suspected MI that should be obtained include blood

counts, electrolytes, glucose, blood urea nitrogen (BUN), and creatinine and lipid profile.

G. Treatment of Acute MI

Several goals exist in the management of acute MI: Minimizing the amount of infarcted myocardium, optimizing function, and controlling the complications of acute MI.

1. Patients with suspected MI should have continuous ECG monitoring and an IV line established. They should also receive supplemental oxygen to maintain adequate oxygen saturation.

2. If the clinical condition of the patient permits, sublingual nitroglycerin (0.4 mg q5min × 3) should be given to help differentiate those patients who may be suffering from angina rather than MI.

3. Aspirin (ASA) should be given to *all* patients without contraindications (160 to 325 mg PO).

4. Thrombolytic Therapy

   a. Patients with ST-segment elevation without contraindications for thrombolytic therapy and who present within 6 to 12 hours of the onset of their symptoms should be considered for thrombolytic therapy.

   b. Patients presenting perhaps up to 24 hours may also be considered for thrombolysis, as some studies have reported improved outcomes (ISIS II trial LATE trial).

   c. Guidelines for Thrombolytic Agent Administration

      (1) Symptoms suggestive of acute MI not resolved with sublingual nitroglycerin, lasting >20 minutes and <12 hours

      (2) ST-segment elevation in 2 or more contiguous ECG leads or left bundle branch block not known to be old.

      (3) Exclusion Criteria

         (a) Bleeding diathesis

         (b) Active gastric or duodenal ulcers

         (c) Significant surgery within 3 weeks

         (d) Severe trauma within 6 months

         (e) History of cardiovascular accident (CVA) within 1 year or other central nervous system (CNS) processes or hemor-

rhage with a potential for bleeding
  (f) Severe, poorly controlled hypertension (>180/110)
  (g) Poor underlying prognosis (i.e., malignancy) where risk/benefit assessment may not favor treatment
(4) Thrombolytic Agents
  (a) Tissue plasminogen activator (rt-PA, Activase) dosage 100 mg (accelerated dosing improves patency rates without increasing complications). Give 15 mg as an IV bolus followed by 50 mg infused over 30 minutes and the remaining 35 mg infused over 60 minutes. Concomitantly administer heparin intravenously (HART trial evidence suggests unacceptable reocclusion rates if rt-PA is given without heparin). ASA should be given as well.
  (b) Streptokinase (Streptase) 1.5 million units IV over 1 hour. Because of the systemic state induced by streptokinase and high levels of fibrin split products, the need for heparin therapy with streptokinase has been questioned.
  (c) Anistreptolase anisoylated (plasminogen/streptokinase activator complex, Eminase). This drug is given as a bolus of 30 U over 5 minutes. Like streptokinase, heparin therapy is uncertain.
  (d) Reteplase: This agent is a modified rt-PA. In Gusto III reteplase had similar efficacy to rt-PA. It is given as two IV boluses of 10 U over 2 minutes 30 minutes apart. Heparin and ASA should be used.

(e) Tenecteplase (TNK): This is a modified rt-PA that is given as a single IV bolus (0.5 mg/kg). In ASSENT-II, this drug was equivalent to rt-PA in overall mortality, with fewer rates of some bleeding complications. Heparin and ASA should be used.

5. Percutaneous Transluminal Coronary Angioplasty (PTCA)

   PTCA is an excellent alternative revascularization technique where available quickly. This should be strongly considered in patients with contraindications to thrombolytic therapy. If skilled operators and facilities for rapid institution are available, the outcome of patients with primary PTCA appears equivalent to or better than that obtained with thrombolytic therapy.

6. Beta-Blockers

   Beta-blockers are useful in preventing tachydysrhythmias and in reducing myocardial oxygen consumption. Early intravenous beta-blockade followed by oral maintenance therapy reduces recurrent ischemia and infarction, even in patients receiving thrombolytic therapy. Patients without contraindications should receive these agents. (See Table 3.1.)

7. Angiotensin-Converting Enzyme (ACE) Inhibitors

   ACE inhibitors in the setting of large acute MI may have an impact on LV remodeling and improve survival in patients with LV dysfunction. These drugs should probably not be administered in the first few hours after infarction.

8. Patients should be classified clinically for prognosis as well as to determine therapy (see Tables 3.4 and 3.5).

9. Additional management of patients may be based on the hemodynamic subset in which they fall.

   a. Uncomplicated MI

      (1) In addition to the therapeutic regimens mentioned above, IV nitroglycerin should be used in pain control. Clinical studies have suggested that mortality and infarct size may be reduced by the use of nitrates.

Table 3.4. Killip Classification of Acute MI

Class I	No heart failure: Mortality < 10%.
Class II	Mild heart failure: Mortality 10%–20%.
Class III	Severe heart failure: rales > 50% of lung fields. Mortality 35%–50%.
Class IV	Cardiogenic shock: Mortality 80%.

Adapted from Killip PT: *Am J Cardiol* 1967;20:457.

Table 3.5. Hemodynamic Subsets After Acute MI

Subset	Cardiac index (L/m^2)	Wedge pressure (torr)
No pulmonary congestion or peripheral hypoperfusion.	2.7 + 0.5	12 ± 7
Isolated pulmonary congestion.	2.3 ± 0.4	23 ± 5
Isolated peripheral hypoperfusion.	1.9 ± 0.4	12 ± 5
Pulmonary congestion and hypoperfusion.	1.6 ± 0.6	27 ± 8

Adapted from Forrester GA: *Am J Cardiol* 1977;39:137.

Therapy should be started at 10 μg/min and increased until the patient is free of pain, or the systolic blood pressure falls below 100 mm Hg, or a maximal dose of approximately 200 μg/min has been achieved.

(2) Morphine sulfate in 2-mg (IV) increments as needed for pain unrelieved by nitroglycerin.

(3) Heparin 5000 SQ q8–12h or low molecular weight heparin in deep venous thrombosis (DVT) prophylaxis doses in patients without contraindications and who are not receiving full-dose heparin should be given. *Note:* Patients with anterior wall MI have a lower incidence of LV thrombosis if full heparinization is used.

(4) Strict bed rest for 24 hours followed by gradual increase in activity.

          (5) Stool softener, commonly docusate sodium (Colace) 100 mg PO qd.

          (6) A low-cholesterol, no-added salt diet should be prescribed.

b. Complicated MI (see Table 3.5)

    (1) Left Ventricular Dysfunction Manifested by Pulmonary Congestion

        (a) Decrease left ventricular end-diastolic pressure with IV nitroglycerin, consider dobutamine, diuretics, or other vasodilators (see dosages below).

    (2) Patients With Hypoperfusion Without Pulmonary Congestion

        (a) Careful IV hydration with normal saline. Pulmonary capillary wedge pressure is targeted at approximately 18 mm Hg.

        (b) Right ventricular MI accompanying inferior infarct may present in this manner. Diagnosis may be made using right-sided precordial chest ECG leads. Significant volume administration may be required for adequate LV preload.

    (3) Severe LV Dysfunction

      Pulmonary artery cannulation should be performed.

        (a) If the systolic blood pressure is >100 mm Hg, dobutamine up to 20 μg/kg/min intravenously should be started. If the patient demonstrates hypotension with systolic blood pressure (BP) <70–100 mm Hg, dopamine 2.5 to 20 μg/kg/min IV should be administered. More profound hypotension may require norepinephrine 0.5 to 30 μg/min intravenously.

        (b) Hypertensive patients should be treated with IV nitroglycerin beginning at 10 μg/min. If this is unsuccessful, sodium nitroprusside (Nipride) 0.5 μg/

kg/min should be titrated to effect. Thiocyanate accumulation is a potential problem with sodium nitroprusside. Caution should be exercised with prolonged administration and in patients with renal insufficiency.

    (c) Mechanical support with IABP may improve cardiac output and coronary perfusion while more definitive interventions are being considered.

    (d) c. Other Complications Following MI

(1) Mitral Regurgitation: This is characterized by the sudden appearance of a systolic murmur (radiating to the axilla) and worsening CHF.

    (a) Diagnostic Studies: Physical examination will demonstrate a systolic murmur and worsening pulmonary congestion. Cardiac catheterization will demonstrate giant V waves in the pulmonary wedge tracing.

    (b) Therapy: Afterload reduction (i.e., IV sodium nitroprusside) to decrease pulmonary capillary wedge pressure. Hypotensive patients may require catecholamines (i.e., dopamine and/or dobutamine).

    (c) IABP may improve coronary perfusion and ventricular emptying.

    (d) Surgical Repair

(2) Ventricular Septal Defect (VSD): VSD is an event occurring in <1% of Q-wave MIs and may occur at any point from several hours to several days after the onset of symptoms. It is most commonly seen during the first 7 days.

    (a) Diagnosis: Acute VSD results in a loud holosystolic murmur and sudden severe CHF with cardiogenic shock. Right heart catheterization with oxygen saturation measurements will exhibit an oxygen saturation step-up between the right atrium and right ventricle, and "contrast" echocardiography will many times identify the defect.

   (b) Treatment: Acute afterload reduction with IV sodium nitroprusside and IABP is required for acute VSD with subsequent surgical repair.

d. Dysrhythmias Following MI: Ninety percent of the patients suffering from acute MI will have dysrhythmias during the first 24 hours.

   (1) Sinus Bradycardia: The most commonly seen dysrhythmia in acute MI. It should be treated only when signs of diminished cardiac output are present. Atropine 0.5 to 1 mg IV q3–5min until a total dose of 0.04 mg/kg has been given. If this proves ineffective, dopamine up to 20 µg/kg/min and epinephrine 10 µg/min should be considered.

   (2) Supraventricular Dysrhythmias: Sinus tachycardia should be addressed by treating the underlying cause. Pain relief and sedation many times are all that is required. Patients with atrial fibrillation or flutter in emergent conditions may require acute cardioversion. Stable patients should be treated with calcium channel blockers, beta-blockers, etc.

   (3) Paroxysmal Supraventricular Tachycardia: This should be approached initially with vagal maneuvers and if these are unsuccessful, with adenosine 6-mg rapid IV push; if unsuccessful, adenosine 12-mg rapid IV push; followed by verapamil 2.5- to 5-mg IV push.

   (4) Ventricular Dysrhythmias: Prophylactic therapy with lidocaine does not

result in improvement of overall survival and thus *is not indicated* in patients with acute MI. In the patient showing stable ventricular tachycardia with normal LV function, lidocaine at 1- to 1.5-mg/kg IV bolus up to a total loading dose of 3 mg/kg and a continuous IV drip of lidocaine at 2 to 4 mg/min may also be used. Other choices include procainamide, administered at 20 to 30 mg/min to a maximum dose of 17 mg/kg/h. Endpoints for therapy include abolition of dysrhythmia, 50% widening of the QRS complex, and/or hypotension. A continuous infusion of 1 to 4 mg/min should be instituted. Amiodarone is another alternative given as 150 mg over 10 minutes followed by 360 mg over 6 hours and 0.5 mg/min over 18 hours. Amiodarone is a preferred agent if depressed LV function is present.

(5) Magnesium sulfate has also been demonstrated to be useful, particularly in polymorphic ventricular tachycardia: 1 to 2 g over 1 to 2 minutes, IV.

e. Conduction Disturbances Accompanying Acute MI

(1) Atrioventricular (A-V) Conduction Disturbances

(a) First-Degree A-V Block: Occurs in 4% to 14% of acute MIs.

(b) Second-Degree A-V block, Mobitz Type I: This is progressive prolongation of the PR interval with intermittent nonconduction of an atrial beat. It is commonly seen in inferior infarction and rarely progress to complete heart block.

(c) Second-Degree A-V block, Mobitz Type II: Represents 10% of all second-degree blocks during acute MI. This is commonly seen in anterior infarction and infrequently progresses to complete heart block.

(d) Third-Degree A-V Block: Occurs in 6% of patients. Mortality with inferior MI is 20% to 25%, mortality with anterior MI is even greater.

(e) Intraventricular Block: Refers to abnormalities within the three divisions of the intraventricular conduction system. These blocks may progress to higher degrees of heart block. One in 5 patients with bundle branch block in acute MI will develop second-degree or third-degree A-V block. Mortality rates are double those who do not.

(f) Complete Heart Block: Occurs frequently in MIs with right bundle branch block plus block of the anterior fascicle or posterior fascicle and less frequently, an isolated left or right bundle branch. Similarly, patients with alternating forms of bundle branch block have a high incidence of complete heart block.

(2) Therapy

  (a) Atrioventricular Block

    i. First-Degree A-V Block: no specific therapy.

    ii. Mobitz Type I Second-Degree A-V Block: Unless unusually slow ventricular rates occur, therapy is not needed. Atropine is given (as for bradycardia) followed by temporary transvenous pacemaker insertion in those patients who are symptomatic.

        iii. Mobitz Type II Second-Degree A-V Block: Particularly when associated with anterior MI, should result in placement of transvenous pacemaker.

        iv. Complete Heart Block: Temporary transvenous pacemaker (some would advocate pacemaker therapy in inferior MI for hemodynamically compromised individuals only).

        v. Intraventricular Conduction Disturbances: A transvenous pacemaker should be inserted for right bundle branch block plus either anterior fascicular, posterior fascicular, or alternating bundle branch blocks. Patients with first-degree A-V block and new onset right or left bundle branch block also should receive transvenous pacing.

III. Cardiac Pacemakers
    A. Definition

        Cardiac pacemakers are complicated devices that may be used to accelerate cardiac rate, bypass, block conduction tissue and/or disrupt dysrhythmias. Advancing technology has resulted in new modes of operation. A five-position code has been developed to describe clinical pacing mode (see Table 3.6), *The North American Society of Pacing and Electrophysiology/British Pacing Electrophysiology Group Generic Pacemaker Code.*

    B. Pacemaker Evaluation

        Rhythm strips and 12-lead ECGs can be useful in determining the mode of functioning of cardiac pacemakers placed in ICU patients. Patients should be examined for failure to sense, as indicated by inappropriate pacemaker spikes, and failure to capture, as indicated by pacemaker spikes without subse-

Table 3.6. Pacemaker Codes

Chamber paced	Chamber sensed	Response to sensing	Programmability	Antitachycardic functions
O = none	O = none	O = none	O = none	O = none
A = atrium	A = atrium	I = inhibited	S = simple programmable	P = antitachycardia
V = ventricle	V = ventricle	T = triggered	M = multiprogrammable C = communicating	S = shock
D = dual	D = dual	D = dual	R = rate modulation	D = dual

quent chamber depolarizations. More detailed information can be obtained by querying appropriately equipped pacemakers and examining pulse characteristics with appropriate devices.

IV. Congestive Heart Failure
  A. Definition
     CHF is the clinical state that occurs when the heart cannot pump sufficient oxygenated blood to meet the metabolic needs of the tissues.
  B. Etiology
     CHF may result from the failure of either the left ventricle or the right ventricle. In many instances, both pumping chambers of the heart fail. Common causes of left ventricular failure include heart disease (aortic stenosis [AS], aortic regurgitation [AR], mitral regurgitation [MR], hypertension, ischemic heart disease, cardiomyopathy, myocarditis). Common causes of right ventricular failure include pulmonary hypertension (primary and secondary), cardiomyopathy, and right ventricular infarction. Biventricular failure commonly results from left ventricular failure. Additional causes of CHF include dysrhythmias, anemia, thyrotoxicosis, medication, and arteriovenous fistulas.
  C. Clinical Manifestations
     1. Shortness of breath
     2. Orthopnea
        Increased venous return associated with a recumbent position leads to worsening shortness of breath.
     3. Paroxysmal nocturnal dyspnea
        This is the result of a number of physiologic factors including the increased venous return in patients who are recumbent.
     4. Fatigue and lethargy
     These are due to a low cardiac output.
  D. Physical Examination
     Signs of left ventricular failure on physical examination include tachycardia and tachypnea. Pulmonary venous congestion results in rales bilaterally. S_3 and S_4 gallop sounds may be heard. Patients with valvular heart disease may manifest cardiac murmurs. Signs of right heart failure include venous distension in the jugular veins, peripheral edema, ascites, and congestive hepatomegaly with hepatojugular reflux.

Table 3.7. New York Heart Association Classification of CHF

Class I.	Symptomatic with extraordinary activity.
Class II.	Symptomatic with ordinary activity.
Class III.	Symptomatic with minimum activity.
Class IV.	Symptomatic at rest.

E. Classification of CHF

Functional classification is commonly reported per the New York Heart Association criteria (see Table 3.7).

F. Chest X-Ray

Cardiomegaly with enlargement of involved heart chambers may be seen. Pulmonary vascular congestion progressing to alveolar edema.

G. Therapy

1. Correct and identify the underlying cause (i.e., treat anemia, infections, hypertension).
2. Decrease cardiac workload with bed rest.
3. Sodium restriction.
4. Preload reduction
   a. Nitrates: Venous dilatation associated with nitrates results in prompt improvement of symptoms in many patients with CHF. (See angina section in the beginning of this chapter for dosing recommendations.)
   b. Diuretic Agents
      (1) Loop-Acting Agents
         (a) Furosemide (Lasix) 10 to 240 mg IV or PO or a continuous IV infusion) induces a prompt diuresis and results in venodilatation with rapid improvement in patient symptomatology.
         (b) Bumetanide (Bumex) 0.5 to 1 mg IV or 4.5 to 2 mg PO.
         (c) Thiazides (i.e., hydrochlorothiazide 25 to 50 mg) are less potent diuretics that may be of value in mild-to-moderate CHF.
         (d) Metolazone (Zaroxolyn) may potentiate the effect of loop-acting diuretics in doses of 2.5 to 10 mg.

        (e) Morphine sulfate has traditionally been used in the management of severe pulmonary edema because of its venodilatory properties and its anxiolytic effects. This agent may depress respirations, and thus, other vasoactive substances may be preferable. If used, increments of 2 mg IV titrated to effect are recommended.

    5. Arterial Dilatation (Afterload Reduction)
        (a) ACE Inhibitors: These agents result in dilatation of the arteriolar resistant vessels and also increase venous capacity, having effects on both preload and afterload. They decrease mortality in patients with CHF. Enalaprilat is available for IV administration (1.25 mg IV over several minutes). Oral ACE inhibitors are also available.

    6. Inotropic Agents

        Intravenous infusions of dopamine and/or dobutamine have positive inotropic effects and may result in a decrease in pulmonary capillary wedge pressures, which is associated with an increase in cardiac output.

    7. Digitalis Glycosides

        These agents have limited value in the acute setting of pulmonary edema but may be useful in reducing the heart rate of patients with atrial dysrhythmias and in the long-term management of patients with CHF.

    8. Aminophylline

        Aminophylline has been used in patients with severe pulmonary edema. It is a weak diuretic and has a positive inotropic effect. The margin of safety with this agent is narrow, and its routine use is discouraged.

    9. In severe unresponsive cases or in cases where a different procedure is indicated due to erythrocytosis, phlebotomy may be used.

V. Cardiomyopathies
    A. Dilated Congestive Cardiomyopathy
        1. Etiologies
            Primary disorders of heart muscle in which dilatation of the ventricles and enlargement of the heart occurs (see Table 3.8).

Table 3.8. Etiologies of Dilated Cardiomyopathy

Idiopathic
Collagen vascular disease
Postmyocarditis
Peripartum
Familial
Toxins and nutritional deficiency
Radiation

  2. Symptoms of CHF, dysrhythmias, and pulmonary
     and systemic embolization.
  3. Physical Examination
     Signs of CHF are commonly seen. A laterally
     placed point of maximal impulse [PMI] may be
     noted along with gallop sounds.
  4. Diagnostic Studies
       a. Chest X-Ray: Cardiac enlargement may be
          seen, pulmonary congestion with interstitial
          edema, pleural effusion, etc. also may be seen.
       b. ECG: Dysrhythmias may be seen, as may
          conduction abnormalities, chamber enlarge-
          ment/hypertrophy, and nonspecific repolar-
          ization abnormalities.
       c. Echocardiography: May demonstrate a low
          ejection fraction and global hypokinesis and
          chamber enlargement.
  5. Therapy
       a. Treat the underlying cause.
       b. Management of CHF as noted above.
       c. Prevent thromboembolism.
       d. Consider low-dose beta-blockade.
       e. Consider transplantation with potential
          mechanical support as bridging maneuver
          (i.e., left ventricular assist device).
B. Restrictive Cardiomyopathy
   This is a myocardial disorder characterized by
   decreased ventricular compliance.
     1. Etiology
        Infiltrative disorders (sarcoidosis, hemochro-
        matosis, amyloidosis, etc.), radiation, endocar-
        dial fibroelastosis, endomyocardial fibrosis,
        scleroderma.
     2. Symptoms
        Right-sided CHF signs, fatigue, and weakness.
     3. Specific Diagnostic Studies
        Echocardiogram or magnetic resonance
        imaging (MRI) may help distinguish restrictive
        cardiomyopathy from constrictive pericarditis

(pericardial thickening). Cardiac catheterization and/or biopsy may be used.

4. Therapy

Control of CHF as previously noted. Special attention of volume status.

C. Hypertrophic Cardiomyopathy

Familial or sporadic disorder with marked hypertrophy of the myocardium. Focal or diffuse forms of hypertrophy may occur.

1. Symptoms: Syncope, dyspnea, chest pain, palpitations, sudden death.

2. Physical Findings

a. Crescendo-decrescendo murmur at the left sternal border, which increases with Valsalva's maneuver

b. S_4 gallop sound

3. Diagnostic Studies

Chest x-ray may be normal; ECG may show left ventricular hypertrophy, abnormal Q-waves (anterior, lateral, and inferior leads); echocardiography demonstrates ventricular hypertrophy.

4. Treatment

a. Beta-blockers (i.e., propranolol 160 to 240 mg/day).

b. Verapamil.

c. Surgical and nonsurgical myectomy should be used when optimal medical therapy has failed in appropriately selected patients. Ethanol septal infusion reduces aortic gradient and symptoms in a large proportion of cases and is rapidly becoming the therapy of choice in severely symptomatic cases.

d. Digitalis, nitrates, diuretics, and vasodilators *may worsen the clinical condition* of this subset of patients.

VI. Myocarditis

Myocarditis is an inflammatory condition of the myocardium.

A. Etiology

1. Infection

a. Viral (echovirus, adenovirus, etc.)

b. Bacterial

c. Mycoplasma

d. Mycotic

e. Rickettsial

f. Spirochetal

g. Parasitic (trichinella, *Trypanosoma cruzi*)

    2. Toxins
    3. Collagen vascular disease (scleroderma, systemic lupus erythematosus, rheumatic fever, sarcoidosis)

B. Symptoms
    1. Dyspnea
    2. Chest discomfort

C. Physical Examination
    1. Tachycardia
    2. Pericardial friction rub (in the presence of coexistent pericarditis)
    3. Evidence of CHF

D. Therapy
    1. Supportive Care
        a. Treatment of CHF
        b. Treatment of dysrhythmias as necessary
        c. Anticoagulation to prevent thromboembolism
    2. Treat the underlying cause (the use of corticosteroids and immunosuppressive therapy is not advocated, although some data support their use in selective populations with inflammatory infiltrates on endomyocardial biopsy).

VII. Pericarditis

Inflammation of the pericardium associated with many different etiologic factors.

A. Etiology (see Table 3.9)

B. Symptoms
    1. Anterior chest pain commonly radiating to arms and back, which classically increases with

Table 3.9. Etiologies of Pericarditis

1. Idiopathic

2. Infectious (tuberculosis, bacterial, viral, fungal, protozoal)

3. Collagen vascular disease

4. Drug induced

5. Trauma

6. Acute MI and post MI (Dressler's syndrome)

7. Uremia

8. Postradiation

9. Rheumatic fever

10. Neoplasms

inspiration and is relieved by sitting up or leaning forward. Palpations and tachycardia may also occur.

C. Physical Examination
1. Pericardial friction rub is best heard with the patient upright and leaning forward.
2. Tachycardia or other dysrhythmias may be auscultated.
3. If pericardial tamponade occurs, low blood pressure, narrow pulse pressure, and accentuated *pulsus paradoxus* may be seen.

D. Diagnostic Studies
1. ECG (see Figure 3.2)
   An acute MI evolutionary pattern of ECG is seen with initial ST-segment elevations with concavity upward, subsequent T-wave inversion, and finally, late resolution of the repolarization abnormalities. PR segment depression may also be seen.
2. Laboratory Evaluation
   MI should be ruled out as noted above. Other potential useful studies might include erythrocyte sedimentation rate (ESR), anti-nuclear antibodies (ANA), rheumatoid factor, viral titers, and tuberculin skin test (PPD).

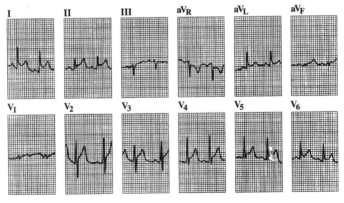

Figure 3.2. Pericarditis. Note the elevation of the ST segment as well as the depression of the PR interval. (From Hurst, JW: *Cardiovascular diagnosis: the initial examination.* St. Louis, 1993, Mosby-Year Book.)

3. Echocardiogram
   To document pericardial effusion (may not be present).

E. Treatment
1. Anti-inflammatories (i.e., indomethacin 25 to 50 mg PO q8h or salicylates 3 to 5 g/d). In severe cases, corticosteroids (i.e., prednisone 60 mg PO qd).
2. Analgesia for pain unrelieved by anti-inflammatories.
3. Observation for signs of cardiac tamponade.
4. Treatment of underlying causes.

F. Complications
1. Cardiac Tamponade
   Accumulation of pericardial fluid may impair cardiac function, mainly through thinning of diastolic filling.
   a. Symptoms: Dyspnea, orthopnea, and fatigue
   b. Physical Findings
      (1) Neck pain
      (2) Distant heart sounds
      (3) Tachycardia
      (4) Pulsus paradoxus
      (5) Hypotension and a narrow pulse pressure
   c. Diagnostic Studies
      (1) ECG: Decreased QRS amplitude and beat-to-beat changes in the R wave.
      (2) Echocardiography: Demonstrates effusions and early right ventricle diastolic collapse.
      (3) Cardiac Catheterization: Right heart catheterization will reveal equalization of diastolic pressures, which includes pericardial pressure if measured.
   d. Therapy
      (1) Pericardiocentesis (see Chapter 15, "Special Techniques"). Removal of a relatively small amount of pericardial fluid will improve diastolic filling in the ventricle and greatly improve the patient's symptomatology. A drainage catheter may also be left in place. Fluid obtained should be tested for protein, lactic dehydrogenase (LDH), cell count, Gram's stain, acid-fast

bacilli stain (AFB), culture/sensitivity, and cytology.

(2) Pericardiectomy, Pericardial Window: These surgical procedures may be performed to relieve pericardial tamponade.

VIII. Valvular Heart Disease

  A. Aortic Stenosis

    1. Etiology

      a. Rheumatic inflammation of the aortic valve

      b. Progressive stenosis secondary to congenital bicuspid valve

      c. Congenital aortic stenosis

      d. Idiopathic calcification stenosis of the aortic valve

    2. Pathophysiology

Stenosis of the aortic valve results in increased resistance to ventricular ejection and increased left ventricular pressure. Hypertrophy of the ventricle will occur. Normal aortic valve area is approximately $3\,cm^2$. Aortic valves of $<1\,cm^2$ generally produce symptoms, and those with $<0.5\,cm^2$ with pressure gradients of $\geq 50\,mm\,Hg$ are considered severe.

    3. Symptoms

      a. Syncope: Commonly with exertion and frequently associated with vasodilatation in muscle beds, leading to cerebral ischemia.

      b. Transient Dysrhythmias

      c. Angina

      d. CHF

    4. Physical Findings

      a. Slow-rising, delayed carotid upstroke with decreased amplitude

      b. Narrowing of pulse pressure

      c. Loud systolic ejection murmur heard at the base of the heart and radiating to the neck, often with a palpable thrill

    5. Diagnostic studies

      a. ECG

        (1) Left ventricular hypertrophy

        (2) Nonspecific repolarization abnormalities

      b. Chest x-ray

        (1) Pulmonary congestion in patients with CHF

(2) Aortic dilatation

(3) Calcification of the aortic valve

c. Echocardiography

(1) Hypertrophy of the left ventricular wall

(2) Visualization of the abnormal aortic valve

d. Cardiac catheterization documents severity of disease and calculation of valve area

6. Therapy

a. Judicious management for CHF and angina as they occur (see appropriate sections as above. These patients may be very "preload sensitive").

b. Valve replacement should be reserved as palliative therapy for patients who are poor surgical risks.

B. Aortic Insufficiency

1. Etiology

a. Infective endocarditis

b. Trauma with valvular rupture

c. Congenital bicuspid aortic valve

d. Rheumatic fibrosis

e. "Myxomatous" degeneration

f. Accompanying aortic dissection

2. Pathophysiology

Left ventricular pressure increases secondary to regurgitation of blood from the aorta, resulting in diastolic volume overload and subsequent decompensation.

3. Symptoms

a. Many patients remain asymptomatic for many years.

b. Symptoms during decompensation include dyspnea on exertion, syncope, chest pain, and CHF.

4. Physical Findings

a. Widening pulse pressure with bounding pulses. Rapid rise and sudden fall in arterial pressure may result in head bobbing, capillary pulsations in the nailbeds (Quincke's pulse), and "water-hammer" pulse. In addition, a murmur can be heard over the femoral arteries.

b. PMI may be displaced laterally, and S_3 gallop may be heard. A diastolic blowing decrescendo murmur occurs along the left sternal border.

   c. Austin-Flint murmur (apical diastolic rumble of low pitch secondary to aortic regurgitation, which affects the anterior mitral leaflet).

   d. Systolic apical ejection murmur may also be heard.

5. Diagnostic Studies

   a. Chest X-Ray: May show left ventricular and or aortic dilation.

   b. ECG: Left ventricle hypertrophy is usually present.

   c. Echocardiogram: Increased left ventricular dimensions and Doppler documentation of regurgitant aortic flow. Fluttering of the anterior mitral leaflet may also be seen.

   d. Cardiac Catheterization: Contrast study of the aortic root will demonstrate aortic regurgitation.

6. Therapy

   a. Medical management of CHF as noted above.

   b. Surgical therapy for patients unresponsive to medical management or with acute aortic regurgitation and left ventricular failure or with a declining ejection fraction.

C. Mitral Stenosis

1. Etiology

   a. Rheumatic fever

   b. Congenital defects

2. Pathophysiology

The normal mitral orifice is 4 to 6 cm^2 in area. An obstruction of the orifice results in impedance of flow into the left ventricle. When the orifice area approaches 1 cm^2, symptoms appear.

3. Symptoms

   a. Dyspnea, orthopnea, and paroxysmal nocturnal dyspnea (pulmonary edema may develop following exertion).

   b. Systemic embolization secondary to thrombi forming in a dilated left atrium.

   c. Dysrhythmias, particularly atrial fibrillation.

   d. Hemoptysis secondary to persistent pulmonary hypertension.

4. Physical Findings

a. Auscultation reveals an opening snap in early diastole.

b. Apical presystolic or mid-diastolic rumble.

c. Accentuated S_1, Graham-Steel murmur.

d. Pulmonary regurgitation.

5. Diagnostic Studies

    a. ECG: Right ventricle hypertrophy, right axis deviation, left atrial enlargement, atrial fibrillation

    b. Chest X-Ray

        (1) Left atrial enlargement is seen on the lateral chest and a double density on the chest x-ray.

        (2) Elevation of the left main stem bronchus and widening of the angle between the right and left main stem bronchi.

        (3) Pulmonary arterial prominence.

    c. Echocardiography: Abnormalities of the valve itself may be seen with calcification and reduction of the E-F slope of the anterior mitral leaflet during diastole.

6. Treatment

    a. Control of ventricular rate in patients with atrial fibrillation and anticoagulation to prevent thromboembolism.

    b. Management of CHF as noted above.

    c. Surgical therapy if the valve orifice is less than approximately $0.8\,cm^2$ or if symptoms persist despite optimal therapy.

    d. Balloon valvuloplasty may be of value in poor surgical candidates.

D. Mitral Regurgitation

1. Etiology

    a. Papillary muscle dysfunction or rupture of the chordae tendineae (i.e., MI)

    b. Infective endocarditis

    c. Left ventricle dilatation of any cause

    d. Mitral valvular calcification

    e. Rheumatic heart disease

    f. Mitral valve prolapse

    g. Idiopathic myxomatous degeneration of the mitral valve

    h. Atrial myxoma

2. Symptoms

    a. Dyspnea, orthopnea, and CHF of varying severity

       b. Hemoptysis
       c. Atrial fibrillation
       d. Systemic embolization

    3. Physical findings
       a. Holosystolic murmur at the apex with radiation to the base or to the left axilla
       b. Rarely, early to mid-diastolic rumble secondary to increased mitral blood flow
       c. Signs of CHF
       d. Left ventricular lift and apical thrill

    4. Diagnostic Studies
       a. ECG: Left atrial enlargement, left ventricular hypertrophy, atrial fibrillation
       b. Chest X-Ray: Left atrial enlargement, left ventricular enlargement, pulmonary congestion
       c. Echocardiography
          (1) Hyperdynamic left ventricle with enlarged left atrium
          (2) Doppler studies demonstrating regurgitant flow
          (3) Flail leaflet in patients with ruptured chordae

    5. Therapy
       a. Medical management of CHF as noted above, with particular attention to afterload reduction and control of ventricular rate.
       b. Severity of acute disease may be temporized with IABP or surgical intervention.

IX. Aortic Dissection

    A. Definition

       Although commonly called aneurysms, this disorder is more appropriately termed *aortic dissection*. This condition results when there is a tear of the aortic intima, dissection of blood into the media, and stripping away of the vessel wall from the adventitia.

    B. Etiology
       1. Hypertension (present in 90% of patients)
       2. Connective tissue disorders (i.e., Marfan's syndrome, Ehlers-Danlos syndrome)
       3. Bicuspid aortic valve
       4. Granulomatous arteritis and syphilitic aortitis
       5. Pregnancy
       6. Aortic injury

    C. Classification

       These lesions are commonly classified by their location. Type A dissections involve the proximal aorta from the aortic valve to the aortic arch, and Type B dissections arise beyond the takeoff of the left subclavian artery.

D. Symptoms
   1. Chest pain (almost always present and usually abrupt, severe, and tearing or burning)
   2. Syncope
   3. CHF
   4. Cerebrovascular accidents
E. Physical findings
   1. Hypotension or hypertension
   2. Pulse deficits
   3. Aortic regurgitation murmur
   4. Pericardial friction rub
   5. Neurologic signs
   6. Horner's Syndrome and/or hoarseness
F. Diagnostic studies
   1. Chest X-Ray
      a. Abnormal in 90% of aortic dissections
      b. Widened aortic shadow
      c. Pleural effusions
      e. Aortic calcification
   2. ECG: Frequently abnormal (90%); however, nondiagnostic.
   3. Computed tomography of the chest with or without contrast will reveal the lesion.
   4. Echocardiogram: Transthoracic and transesophageal studies may reveal the dissection.
   5. Aortogram: The "gold standard" for diagnosis.
G. Therapy
   1. Surgical
      a. Proximal dissections (Type A)
      b. Distal dissection, particularly if vital organs are compromised or persistent pain occurs despite medical management
   2. Medical
      a. Aggressive control of blood pressure. The typical regimen is administration of IV beta-blocker (traditionally, propranolol 1 mg IV q5min until evidence of beta-blockade) followed by sodium nitroprusside to maintain systolic blood pressure of approximately 100 to 120 mm Hg. Although not as well studied, the pharmacologic effects of labetalol infusion would seem to make this agent ideal for aortic dissection.
      b. Transcatheter stenting techniques have been introduced. Their role is not entirely clear at present.

X. Shock States

Shock can be defined as a state of inadequate tissue perfusion, which, unless reversed, results in progressive organ dysfunction, damage, and death. Mortality rates for shock of many causes still exceeds 50%. In early stages of shock, the patient may be relatively asymptomatic. Sympathetic discharge and other compensatory mechanisms may cause tachycardia and mild peripheral vasoconstriction in attempts to maintain blood pressure. When the state of shock worsens, organ hypoperfusion continues, and blood pressure declines; signs of organ dysfunction including restlessness and agitation, decreased urine output, and cool and clammy skin become evident.

A. Classification and etiology

A number of classification schemes for shock states have been devised. These include cardiogenic shock; myopathic (reduced systolic function, i.e., acute MI), mechanical (mitral regurgitation, ventricular septal defect), extracardiac obstructive shock (i.e., pericardial tamponade, massive pulmonary embolus, or severe pulmonary hypertension); oligemic shock (i.e., hemorrhage or fluid depletion); and distributive shock (i.e., septic shock, anaphylaxis, neurogenic shock, etc.).

B. Diagnostic Evaluation

1. Physical Examination

Tachycardia, hypotension, and evidence of hypoperfusion (i.e., altered mental status, decreased urine output, cool and clammy skin) are generally present. Other manifestations may be seen on physical examination, dependent upon the etiology of the shock state.

2. Laboratory Evaluation

a. ECG: Useful for identifying dysrhythmias and acute MI.

b. Chest X-Ray: Pneumothorax, abnormal cardiac silhouette, and pulmonary edema.

c. Hematology and Chemistry: CBC, BUN, creatinine, electrolytes, glucose, liver function tests (LFTs) and arterial blood gases should be obtained in the evaluation of any patient with shock.

3. Monitoring

a. Foley Catheter: Patients in shock without contraindication should receive catheter insertion for the monitoring of urine output.

     b. Arterial Line: For direct intra-arterial pressure determination and to allow easy vascular access for laboratory and arterial blood gas monitoring.

     c. Central Venous Pressure Monitoring Catheter or PA Catheter: These are commonly employed. Many patients can be managed without pulmonary artery cannulation, and the PA catheter is being used less frequently.

C. Therapy

Primary treatment goals include restoring oxygen transport and organ perfusion (i.e., urine output $1/2$ to $1\,mL/kg/h$ and the absence of lactic acidosis).

1. Airway, breathing and circulation (ABCs), as in all critically ill patients.

2. Supportive Measures

     a. Two large-bore IV catheters for those patients requiring volume resuscitation. For patients in whom fluid status is normal or elevated, a central IV line for administration of medication will usually be required. For those patients not volume overloaded, the initial management of hypotension and shock is volume administration. Volume challenges of 250 cc to 1 L at a time should be rapidly administered with reassessment of the patient's clinical condition.

     b. Supplemental oxygen appropriate for the patient's clinical status.

     c. Those patients not responding to volume administration should receive beta-receptor stimulants. Dopamine is commonly used in hypotensive patients because of its positive inotropic effects at lower doses and its vasoconstrictor effect. Initial doses are usually $5\,\mu g/kg/min$.

     d. Mechanical support of the circulation may be necessary in patients with refractory cardiogenic shock and amenable lesions.

     e. Additional interventions and therapeutic goals for management of shock must be based on specific etiologies.

XI. Infective Endocarditis

A. Definition

Infection of the endocardial structures of the heart.

B. Etiology
1. *Streptococcus viridans:* Streptococci is the most common organism isolated, excluding prostatic valve or right-sided endocarditis.
2. *Staphylococcus aureus:* The most frequent organism isolated in right-sided endocarditis.
3. *Staphylococcus epidermidis*
4. Others
    a. Gonococci
    b. Other bacteria
    c. Fungi
C. Risk Factors
A. number of disorders and behaviors are risk factors for the development of endocarditis. These include the following:
1. Valvular abnormalities
    a. Rheumatic valvulitis
    b. Bicuspid aortic valve
    c. Aortic stenosis or insufficiency
    d. Mitral stenosis, prolapse, or insufficiency
    e. Mechanical heart valves
    f. Previous endocarditis
2. IV drug abuse
3. Marfan's syndrome
4. Instrumentation
D. Diagnosis
1. History and Physical Examination
    Careful history for underlying risk factors should be elicited.
2. Physical Examination
    a. Fever: Generally present but may not be noted in elderly or immunocompromised patients.
    b. Cardiac Murmurs: Are usually present but may not be detected, particularly in right-sided endocarditis.
    c. Peripheral Manifestations: These include painless erythematous papules and macules of the soles and palms (Janeway lesions) and painful erythematous subcutaneous papules (Osler's nodes), as well as petechia and splinter hemorrhages of the nail beds.
3. Laboratory Evaluation
    a. Blood Cultures: Before antibiotic therapy, positive cultures are quite common (85% to 95%). Reasons for negative cultures include

prior antibiotic therapy, slow-growing or very fastidious organisms, or improper collection.
  b. Nonspecific Laboratory Findings
    (1) Includes decreased hemoglobin/hematocrit.
    (2) Elevated, decreased, or normal white blood cell count with a left shift, hematuria on urinalysis, and an elevated sedimentation rate. Rheumatoid factor may be positive in half of the cases by 6 weeks, and assays of teichoic acid antibodies have been advocated for *Staphylococcus aureus* endocarditis.
  c. Echocardiography: Transthoracic and transesophageal echocardiography may reveal valvular damage, impairments of left ventricular function, and valvular vegetations. Transesophageal echocardiography enhances sensitivity. Some patients will not demonstrate abnormal echocardiographic studies.
E. Major Complications
  1. CHF secondary to valvular destruction, dysrhythmias, or myocarditis
  2. Embolization
  3. Cardiac dysrhythmias
  4. Myocarditis and pericarditis
F. Therapy
  1. Antibiotics appropriate for the clinical setting. For a valve endocarditis, penicillin G IV (12 to 24 million U/d) and gentamicin (dosed by body weight and renal function) are commonly advocated. For IV drug addicts, penicillinase-resistant penicillin or vancomycin plus gentamicin are advocated.
  2. Surgical therapy for endocarditis should occur if severe heart failure or valvular obstruction is present or if uncontrolled infection exists. Relative indications for cardiac surgery include two or more embolic events, unusually large vegetations, extension of the infection to other intracardiac structures, or in the case of prosthetic valve endocarditis, periprosthetic leak.

XII. Dysrhythmias (See Also Chapter 2, "The Basics of Critical Care")

A. Supraventricular Dysrhythmias

A group of dysrhythmias whose site of origin and pathway is not confined to the ventricles.

1. Paroxysmal   Supraventricular   Tachycardia (PSVT)

PSVT commonly originates through a re-entrant mechanism in the AV node. Characterized by abrupt onset and termination. PSVT may occur in young patients without other evidence of cardiac disease, as well as patients with acute MI, Wolf-Parkinson-White Syndrome, or other structural heart diseases.

a. ECG Characteristics: Regular tachycardia of 150 to 220 beats per minute. Atrial activity (P waves) may or may not been seen, depending upon the rate and relationship between atrial and ventricular depolarization. QRS complex is frequently narrow. However, a wide QRS complex may be seen.

(1) Symptoms

(a) Palpitations

(b) May produce hypotension during acute MI or may precipitate CHF.

(2) Therapy

(a) ABC's.

(b) For patients demonstrating clinical instability (i.e., cardiogenic shock, ischemic chest pain, or CHF), synchronized DC countershock should be used.

(c) Treatment of the stable patient should begin with a vagal maneuver. Valsalva or carotid sinus massage following exclusion of carotid disease may abort the dysrhythmia.

(d) Adenosine should be administered to those patients who do not respond to vagal maneuvers, 6-mg rapid IV bolus. A second bolus of 12 mg rapid IV may be given. Methylxanthines (i.e., theophylline, aminophylline, caffeine) are competitive antagonists, and dipyridamole enhances the pharmacologic effect of adenosine.

(e) Verapamil 5 to 10 mg over 5 minutes (may repeat dose in 20 to 30 minutes if ineffective) may be used if adenosine is ineffective in patients with narrow complex PSVT. Pretreatment with a slow injection of 10 mL of 10% calcium chloride may decrease the common hypotensive effects of this drug. Patients with wide-complex tachycardia that cannot be confidently diagnosed as supraventricular should not receive verapamil. Nor should patients with depressed ejection fraction. Digoxin or amiodarone as noted above for stable ventricular tachycardia should be considered.

(f) Additional considerations include digoxin, beta-blockers, pace termination, and synchronized cardioversion for patients with preserved ejection fraction.

B. Atrial Fibrillation

Atrial fibrillation is characterized by chaotic atrial activity without an organized atrial rhythm. This dysrhythmia may accompany coronary artery disease, mitral and aortic valvular disease, thyrotoxicosis, peri- and myocarditis, alcoholic heart disease, and MI without evidence of other organic cardiac disease.

1. Electrocardiogram

Irregular, chaotic atrial activity without an organized rhythmic pattern. Conductive QRS complexes will have an irregularly irregular pattern. However, atrial ventricular block with emergence of a lower pacemaker site may result in irregular ventricular response.

2. Other Diagnostic Studies
   a. Thyroid function tests
   b. Echocardiography
3. Therapy
   a. In unstable patients, as in PSVT, DC cardioversion is indicated.
   b. Digoxin Loading: Digoxin has been the traditional therapy for new-onset atrial fibrillation. Administer an 0.5-mg IV loading dose followed by 0.25 mg q3–4h until the ventricular rate is controlled. For patients with impaired ejection fraction, this remains a good choice.
   c. Alternatives for rapid rate control include
      (1) Diltiazem 20 to 25 mg IV over 2 minutes with continuous infusion of 5 to 15 mg/h.
      (2) Beta-blockers (i.e., propranolol 0.5 mg IV slowly followed by boluses of 1 mg q5min to a total of 0.1 mg/kg). Atenolol 5 mg IV slowly ×2. Metoprolol 5 mg slow IV q5min × 3.
      (3) Amiodarone in a dose of 150 mg over 10 minutes followed by 360 mg over 6 hours and 0.5 mg/min is a good choice, particularly with depressed ejection fraction.
   d. Anticoagulation is advisable pre- and post-cardioversion, particularly in patients with mitral valve disease or a history of embolic phenomenon. Patients with a duration of atrial fibrillation >48 hours should not be converted acutely if avoidable, because of embolization risk. 3–4 weeks of anticoagulation precardioversion is recommended, with at least 4 weeks of anticoagulation postcardioversion suggested.
C. Atrial Flutter
   Atrial flutter is characterized by a rapid regular atrial rate of 280 to 340 beats per minute, generally associated with varying degrees of AV block. This dysrhythmia may occur with coronary artery disease, including MI, thyrotoxicosis, pulmonary embolism, and mitral valve disease.
   1. ECG: Atrial depolarization classically has a "sawtooth" pattern with varying AV conduction block. Vagal maneuvers may slow the ventricular

response rate, making atrial flutter waves more readily apparent.
  2. Therapy
     a. As for atrial fibrillation. In patients who are compromised, cardioversion with DC countershock is indicated.
     b. Commonly responds to the pharmacologic interventions previously denoted for atrial fibrillation. In addition, atrial pacing may also terminate atrial flutter.

D. Multifocal Atrial Tachycardia
   In multifocal atrial tachycardia, a chaotic irregular atrial activity is seen, with rates between 100 and 180 and varying p-wave morphology (3 consecutive different p-wave morphologies). This disorder commonly accompanies chronic obstructive pulmonary disease, theophylline toxicity, hypoxemia, and/or other metabolic disturbances.
   1. ECG (See Figure 3.3)
      Varying P-to-P intervals and beat-to-beat variability in P-wave morphology.
   2. Therapy
      a. Treat the underlying cause. Rate may be controlled, if necessary, with diltiazem or amiodarone. In the absence of depressed ejection fraction, beta-blockers may be used. In addition, IV magnesium has been advocated by some authorities.

E. Bradycardias and AV Conduction Blocks
   These are characterized by a low intrinsic rate from the sinus node or blockade of sinus impulses between the AV node, which result in slow ventricular rates.
   1. Etiology
      a. Vagotonia
      b. Ischemic heart disease

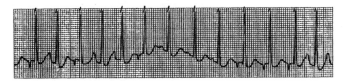

Figure 3.3. Multifocal atrial tachycardia. (From Conover MB: *Understanding electrocardiography*, ed. 6, St. Louis, 1992, Mosby-Year Book.)

       c. Cardiomyopathies

       d. Drugs

       e. Degenerative diseases of the AV conduction system

   2. Treatment

      Patients who are symptomatic due to low ventricular response rate may be treated with the following:

       a. Initially with atropine 0.5 to 1.0 mg IV, repeated every 3 to 5 minutes with a total dose of 0.04 mg/kg.

       b. Transcutaneous pacing when available may be employed.

       c. Pharmacologic therapy may include dopamine 5- to 20-µg/kg/min IV infusion or epinephrine 2- to 10-µg/min IV infusion titrated to heart rate. Patients requiring transcutaneous pacers for high degrees of AV block should receive consideration for urgent transvenous pacemaker placement.

  F. Ventricular Tachycardia

    Ventricular tachycardia is defined as 3 or more consecutive beats of ventricular origin. Common rates are between 100 and 200 beats per minute. The differentiation of ventricular and supraventricular dysrhythmia with conduction may be difficult. A good rule of thumb is that wide-complex QRS tachycardia should be considered ventricular tachycardia until proven otherwise.

    1. Monomorphic ventricular tachycardia (a single QRS morphology) should be treated as noted in Chapter 3, "The Basics of Critical Care."

    2. Polymorphic ventricular tachycardia or "torsade de pointes" may be caused by agents frequently used in the treatment of monomorphic ventricular tachycardia. Electrolyte disturbances including hypokalemia, hypomagnesemia, and the presence of cardiac and psychotropic medications should be sought. Unstable patients should receive electrical therapy as previously outlined. Stable patients may respond to overdrive pacing, IV magnesium, and correction of underlying causes.

XIII. Hypertensive Crises

    Hypertensive crises are potentially life-threatening situations that are the result of elevated blood pressure. Manifestations include hypertension with end-organ dys-

Table 3.10. End-Organ Dysfunction in Hypertensive Emergencies

Hypertensive encephalopathy
Acute aortic dissection
Acute myocardial infarction
Acute cerebral vascular accident
Acute hypertensive renal injury
Acute congestive heart failure

Table 3.11. Intravenous Antihypertensive Medications

Nitroprusside	0.5–10 μg/kg/min
Labetolol	20-mg bolus, 2 mg/min (max 300 mg/day)
Nicardipine	5 mg/h to 15 mg/h
Fenoldopam	0.1–2 μg/kg/min
Nitroglycerin	5 μg/min (increase by 5–10 μg q3–5 min as needed)
Diazoxide	25–150 mg IV over 5 min or infusion of 30 mg/min to effect

function (see Table 3.10). Rarely occur with blood pressures <130 mm Hg diastolic.

A. Treatment
   1. Blood pressure should be promptly reduced. Many authorities recommend reductions of approximately 15% in the first hour with gradual reduction to diastolic BP of 100 to 110 mm Hg or a reduction of 25% of initial reading.
   2. Reductions in BP may result in ischemia, and thus, these patients must be carefully followed. Parenteral therapy with short-acting agents are initially recommended (see Table 3.11).
   3. Patients receiving parenteral therapy commonly need continuous arterial pressure monitoring.
       a. Cyanide poisoning may occur with prolonged IV administration of sodium nitroprusside to renal failure patients. Consider this if such patients develop CNS depression, seizures, lactic acidosis, or cardiovascular instability.
           (1) May occur with infusion rate >2 μg/kg/min.
           (2) Infusion rates of >10 μg/kg/min should not be continued for prolonged periods of time because of this hazard.
           (3) If cyanide intoxication suspected, discontinue infusion, and treat as described in Chapter 16.

4. Oral therapy with clonidine (Catapress) (0.1 mg PO q20min) or a host of other agents may be used in less severe cases of hypertension in the ICU patient.

XIV. USEFUL FACTS AND FORMULAS

A. **Pressure = Flow × Resistance** This is true in the airways as well as in the cardiovascular system. For example:

Mean arterial pressure
= cardiac output × systemic vascular resistance.
Mean pulmonary arterial pressure
= cardiac output × pulmonary vascular resistance.

The unmeasured resistance term is usually calculated by solving the equations:

systemic vascular resistance

$$= \frac{\text{mean arterial pressure}}{\text{cardiac output}}$$

B. The Primary Determinants of Cardiovascular Performance
1. Heart rate
2. Preload
3. Afterload
4. Contractility

C. Other Principles and Conversion Factors

Fluid flow:

$$\text{Fluid flow} = \frac{(\text{pressure difference})(\text{radius})^4}{(\text{vessel length})(\text{fluid viscosity})^8}$$

Conversion to mm Hg

Pressure in mm Hg = Pressure in cm H_2O/1.36

LaPlace's law:

$$\text{Wall tension} = \text{distending pressure} \times \frac{\text{vessel radius}}{\text{wall thickness}}$$

Ohm's law:

$$\text{Current (I)} = \frac{\text{electromotive force (E)}}{\text{resistance (R)}}$$

Poiseuilles' law:

$$Q = v\pi r^2$$

where Q = rate of blood flow (mm/sec); πr^2 = cross-sectional area (cm^2); v = velocity of blood flow.

Vascular capacitance:

Vascular compliance (capacitance)

$$= \frac{\text{increase in volume}}{\text{increase in pressure}}$$

Vascular distensibility:

Vascular distensibility

$$= \frac{\text{increase in volume}}{\text{increase in pressure} \times \text{original volume}}$$

D. Direct measurements of the heart rate are relatively easy. Preload, afterload, and contractility are more difficult to assess clinically. In assessment of cardiovascular performance, the following hemodynamic measurements are commonly measured or calculated:

1. *Arteriovenous Oxygen Content Difference (avDO₂)*

   This is the difference between the arterial oxygen content (CaO₂) and the venous oxygen content (CvO₂).

2. *Body Surface Area (BSA)*

   Calculated from height and weight, BSA is generally used to index measured and derived values according to the size of the patient.

3. *Cardiac Index (CI)*

   Calculated as cardiac output/BSA, CI is the prime determinant of hemodynamic function.

4. *Left Ventricular Stroke Work Index (LVSWI)*

   LVSWI is the product of the stroke index (SI) and (mean arterial pressure [MAP]—pulmonary artery occlusion pressure [PAOP]), and a unit correction factor of 0.0136. The LVSWI measures the work of the left ventricle (LV) as it ejects into the aorta.

5. *Mean Arterial Pressure (MAP)*

   The MAP is estimated as one third of pulse pressure plus the diastolic blood pressure.

6. *Oxygen Consumption ($\dot{V}O_2$)*

   Calculated as $C(a–v)O_2$ H CO H 10, it is the amount of oxygen extracted in mL/min by the tissue from the arterial blood.

7. *Oxygen Delivery ($\dot{D}O_2$)*

   Calculated as (CaO_2) H CO H 10, it is the total oxygen delivered by the cardiorespiratory systems.

8. *Pulmonary Vascular Resistance Index (PVRI)*

   Calculated as (MAP – PAOP)/CI, it measures the resistance in the pulmonary vasculature.

9. *Right Ventricular Stroke Work Index (RVSWI)*

   RVSWI is the product of the SI and (mean pulmonary artery pressure [MPAP]—central venous pressure [CVP]), and a unit correction factor of 0.0136. It measures the work of the right ventricle as it ejects into the pulmonary artery.

10. *Stroke Index (SI)*

    Calculated as CI/heart rate, SI is the average volume of blood ejected by the ventricle with each beat.

11. *Systemic Vascular Resistance Index (SVRI)*

    Calculated as (MAP – CVP)/CI, SVRI is the customary measure of the resistance in the systemic circuit.

12. *Venous Admixture (Qva/Q_T)*

    Calculated as $(C\bar{c}O_2 – CaO_2)/(C\bar{c}O_2 – C\bar{v}O_2)$, it represents the fraction of cardiac output not oxygenated in an idealized lung.

E. Cardiac Output Formulas

Output of left ventricle

$$= \frac{O_2 \text{ consumption (mL/min)}}{[AO_2]–[\dot{V}O_2]}$$

It may also be measured by thermodilution techniques:

$$Q = V(Tb – Ti)K \Big/ \int Tb(t)dt$$

where $\dot{Q}$ = cardiac output; V = volume of injectate; Tb = blood temperature; Ti = injectate temperature; K = a constant including the density factor and catheter characteristics; $\int Tb(t)dt$ = area under the blood-temperature-time curve.

The same principle is applicable for the pulmonary blood flow:

$$\dot{Q} = B/(C\bar{v} - Ca)$$

where Q = pulmonary blood flow; B = rate of loss of the indicator of alveolar gas; Cv = concentration of the indicator in the venous blood; Ca = concentration of the indicator in the arterial blood.

$$\dot{Q} = \dot{V}/(CaO_2 - C\bar{v}O_2)$$

where $\dot{Q}$ = total pulmonary blood flow; $\dot{V}O_2$ = oxygen uptake; CaO_2 = arterial oxygen concentration; $C\dot{V}O_2$ = mixed venous oxygen concentration.

F. Other Cardiovascular Performance Formulas/Tables

Alveolar-arterial O_2 difference or "A-a gradient"
= Alveolar pO_2 – arterial pO_2
Normal < 10 torr (10 mm Hg)

Alveolar pO_2 at sea level (PAO_2)
= $(FiO_2 \times 713) - 1.2 \times PaCO_2$

Arterial blood O_2 content (CaO_2)
= $(PaO_2 \times .003) + (1.34 \times$ Hb in g $\times$ arterial blood Hb O_2 sat %)
Normal = 18–20 mL/dL

Arteriovenous oxygen difference ($avDO_2$)
= $(CaO_2) - (C\bar{v}O_2)$
Normal = 4–5 mL/dL

Cardiac index (CI) = cardiac output/body surface area
Normal = 3.0–3.4 L/min-m^2

Ejection Fraction (EF)

$$= \frac{\text{end-diastolic volume} - \text{end-systolic volume}}{\text{end-diastolic volume}}$$

$$= \%$$

Mean arterial (or pulmonary) pressure
= DBP + 1/3 (SBP-DBP)

Mean pulmonary arterial pressure
= DPAP + 1/3 (SPAP-DPAP)

O_2 delivery index (DO_2I) = $CaO_2 \times$ cardiac index $\times$ 10
Normal = 500–600 mL/min-m^2

O_2 consumption index ($\dot{V}O_2I$)
   = Arteriovenous O_2 difference × cardiac index × 10
Normal = 120–160 mL/min^2

O_2 extraction (O_2 Ext)
   = (arteriovenous O_2 difference/arterial blood O_2
      content) × 100
Normal = 20% to 30%

Pulmonary vascular resistance index (PVRI)
   = 79.92 (Mean PAP − $\overline{\text{PAOP}}$)/CI
Normal = 255 to 285 dyne-sec/cm^5·m^2

Shunt % = (Q_s/Q_T)

$$Q_s/Q_T(\%) = \frac{CcO_2 - CaO_2}{C_cO_2 - C\overline{v}O_2}$$

CcO_2 = Hb in g × 1.34 + (Alveolar pO_2 × .003)
Normal < 10%
Considerable disease = 20% to 29%
Life-threatening > 30%

Stroke volume (SV)
   = (end-diastolic volume) − (end-systolic volume)

Systemic vascular resistance index (SVRI)
   = 79.92 (MAP − CVP/CI)
Normal = 1970–230 dyne-sec/cm^5·m^2

Venous blood O_2 content ($C\overline{v}O_2$)
   = (PvO_2 × .003) + (1.34 × Hb in g × venous blood
      Hb O_2 sat %)
Normal = 13 to 16 mL/dL

Normal hemodynamic parameters are depicted in
Tables 3.12 to 3.14 below:

Table 3.12. Normal Hemodynamic Parameters, Adult

Parameter	Equation	Normal Range
Arterial Blood Pressure (BP)	Systolic (SBP)	90–140 mm Hg
	Diastolic (DBP)	60–90 mm Hg
Mean Arterial Pressure (MAP)	[SBP + (2 × DBP)]/3	70–105 mm Hg
Right Atrial Pressure (RAP)		2–6 mm Hg
Right Ventricular Pressure (RVP)	Systolic (RVSP)	15–25 mm Hg
	Diastolic (RVDP)	0–8 mm Hg
Pulmonary Artery Pressure (PAP)	Systolic (PASP)	15–25 mm Hg
	Diastolic (PADP)	8–15 mm Hg
Mean Pulmonary Artery Pressure (MPAP)	[PASP + (2 × PADP)]/3	10–20 mm Hg
Pulmonary Artery Wedge Pressure (PAWP)		6–12 mm Hg
Left Atrial Pressure (LAP)		6–12 mm Hg
Cardiac Output (CO)	HR × SV/1000	4.0–8.0 L/min
Cardiac Index (CI)	CO/BSA	2.5–4.0 L/min/m^2
Stroke Volume (SV)	CO/HR × 1000	60–100 mL/beat
Stroke Volume Index (SVI)	CI/HR × 1000	33–47 mL/m^2/beat
Systemic Vascular Resistance (SVR)	80 × (MAP − RAP)/CO	800–1200 dynes-sec/cm^5
Systemic Vascular Resistance Index (SVRI)	80 × (MAP − RAP)/CI	1970–2390 dynes·sec/cm^5/m^2
Pulmonary Vascular Resistance (PVR)	80 × (MPAP − PAWP)/CO	<250 dynes-sec/cm^5
Pulmonary Vascular Resistance Index (PVRI)	80 × (MPAP − PAWP)/CI	255–285 dynes-sec/cm^5/m^2

Table 3.13. Hemodynamic Parameters, Adult

Parameter	Equation	Normal Range
Left Ventricular Stroke Work (LVSW)	SV × (MAP − PAWP) × 0.0136	58–104 g-m/beat
Left Ventricular Stroke Work Index (LVSWI)	SVI × (MAP − PAWP) × 0.0136	50–62 g-m/m²/beat
Right Ventricular Stroke Work (RVSW)	SV × (MPAP − RAP) × 0.0136	8–16 g-m/beat
Right Ventricular Stroke Work Index (RVSWI)	SV × (MPAP − RAP) × 0.0136	5–10 g-m/m²/beat
Coronary Artery Perfusion Pressure (CPP)	Diastolic BP-PAWP	60–80 mm Hg
Right Ventricular End-Diastolic Volume (RVEDV)	SV/EF	100–160 mL
Right Ventricular End-Systolic Volume (RVESV)	EDV-SV	50–100 mL
Right Ventricular Ejection Fraction (RVEF)	SV/EDV	40%–60%

Table 3.14. Oxygenation Parameters, Adult

Partial Pressure of Arterial Oxygen (PaO_2)		80–100 mm Hg
Partial Pressure of Arterial CO_2 ($PaCO_2$)		35–45 mm Hg
Bicarbonate (HCO_3)		22–28 mEq/L
pH		7.38–7.42
Arterial Oxygen Saturation (SaO_2)		95%–100%
Mixed Venous Saturation ($S\bar{v}O_2$)		60%–80%
Arterial Oxygen Content (CaO_2)	$(0.0138 \times Hb \times SaO_2) + 0.0031 \times PaO_2$	17–20 mL/dL
Venous Oxygen Content ($C\bar{v}O_2$)	$(0.0138 \times Hb \times S\bar{v}O_2) + 0.0031 \times P\bar{v}O_2$	12–15 mL/dL
A-V Oxygen Content (CaO_2)	$CaO_2 - C\bar{v}O_2$	4–6 mL/dL
Oxygen Delivery ($\dot{D}O_2$)	$CaO_2 \times CO \times 10$	950–1150 mL/dL
Oxygen Delivery Index ($\dot{D}O_2I$)	$CaO_2 \times CI \times 10$	500–600 mL/min/m^2
Oxygen Consumption ($\dot{V}O_2$)	$(C(a-v)O_2) \times CO \times 10$	200–250 mL/min
Oxygen Consumption Index ($\dot{V}O_2I$)	$(C(a-v)O_2) \times CI \times 10$	120–160 mL/min/m^2
Oxygen Extraction Ration (O_2ER)	$[(CaO_2 - CvO_2)/CaO_2] \times 100$	22%–30%
Oxygen Extraction Index (O_2EI)	$(SaO_2 - SvO_2)/SaO_2 \times 100$	25%–25%

4

Endocrinologic Disorders

■ I. ADRENAL INSUFFICIENCY

A. Definition

Adrenal insufficiency is a deficiency of glucocorticoid production, which can result from adrenal gland failure (primary adrenal insufficiency) or failure of hypothalamic-pituitary secretion of corticotropin-releasing hormone (CRH) or adrenocortical trophic hormone (ACTH) (secondary adrenal insufficiency).

B. Pathophysiology

1. Glucocorticoid synthesis is regulated by the hypothalamic-pituitary-adrenal (HPA) axis (hypothalamus secretes CRH, which stimulates the pituitary to release ACTH, which increases release of cortisol by the adrenal cortex).
2. Cortisol is a negative feedback on further CRH and ACTH production.
3. Mineralocorticoid production is regulated primarily by the renin-angiotensin system, blood pressure, and extracellular potassium level.
4. Catecholamines are synthesized by the adrenal cortex and medulla.
5. The adrenal cortex is composed of the zona glomerulosa (aldosterone synthesis), zona fasciculata (glucocorticoid synthesis), and zona reticularis (androgen and glucocorticoid synthesis).
6. Primary adrenal insufficiency usually results in loss of both glucocorticoid and mineralocorticoid secretion.
7. Patients with secondary adrenal insufficiency maintain normal secretion of the mineralocorticoids.

C. Etiology
    1. Infection (acquired immune deficiency syndrome [AIDS], tuberculosis [TB], cytomegalovirus, meningococcemia, fungus, pseudomonas septicemia)
    2. Adrenal hemorrhage (coagulopathies, anticoagulant therapy, sepsis, trauma, pregnancy)
    3. Withdrawal of exogenous steroids or HPA axis suppression from recent (up to 1 year prior) treatment with exogenous corticosteroids
    4. Drugs that interfere with adrenal steroid synthesis (ketoconazole, etomidate, aminoglutethimide)
    5. Tumor destruction
    6. Adrenal infarction (arteritis, thrombosis)
    7. Autoimmune disorders (sarcoidosis, amyloidosis)

D. Clinical Manifestations
    1. Weakness
    2. Weight loss
    3. Anorexia
    4. Hyperpigmentation (only in primary adrenal insufficiency with ACTH production)
    5. Circulatory collapse
    6. Gastrointestinal disturbances (nausea/vomiting, abdominal pain, diarrhea, constipation)
    7. Dehydration
    8. Fever
    9. May have only vague symptoms (malaise, arthralgias)

E. Associated Laboratory Abnormalities
    1. Increased potassium and calcium
    2. Decreased sodium and chloride
    3. Decreased glucose
    4. Metabolic acidosis
    5. Increased blood, urea, nitrogen/creatinine (BUN/Cr) ratio
    6. Normocytic, normochromic anemia, neutropenia, lymphocytosis, eosinophilia

F. Diagnostic Evaluation
    1. Physical examination
        a. Hypotension
        b. Hyperpigmentation (not in acute or secondary adrenal insufficiency)
        c. Females may have loss of axillary hair
    2. Laboratory Evaluation
        a. Measurement of a single plasma cortisol level usually does not allow reliable appraisal of pituitary and adrenal function; however, in stressed, critically ill patients, it is sufficient to rule out or to suggest the diagnosis of adrenal insufficiency (a serum cortisol

level ≥20 μg/dL indicates adequate adrenal glucocorticoid secretion following stress, ACTH, or CRH).

b. If the patient is hemodynamically unstable and adrenal insufficiency is suspected, a random cortisol level should be drawn and treatment with hydrocortisone (see "Therapy" section below) should be initiated immediately.

c. If the patient is hemodynamically stable and adrenal insufficiency is suspected, a random cortisol level may be measured and the patient treated with dexamethasone (stress dose of 2 to 10 mg IV q6h) until the result is available; then, if the cortisol level is <20 μg/dL, a screening synthetic ACTH stimulation test may be performed:

   (1) Measure baseline cortisol level.

   (2) Give cosyntropin (synthetic ACTH) 0.25 mg IV.

   (3) Measure cortisol level again after 60 minutes.

   (4) An increase of <7 μg/dL is suggestive of primary adrenal insufficiency if the basal cortisol level is <20 μg/dL.

   (5) If diagnosis of adrenal insufficiency is confirmed by plasma cortisol <20 μg/dL, further testing (3-day ACTH infusion test) may be required to establish the exact etiology, *but* this should *only* be done when the patient is out of the intensive care unit (ICU).

d. Diagnostic imaging may help determine the etiology (bilaterally enlarged adrenal glands by computed tomography (CT) scan suggest adrenal hemorrhage, neoplastic disease, TB, or fungal infection whereas small adrenal glands suggest autoimmune disease or lack of ACTH).

e. High ACTH levels associated with low cortisol levels or failure of the adrenal gland to respond to prolonged ACTH stimulation are consistent with primary adrenal insufficiency.

f. Measurement of plasma renin (PRA) and aldosterone (ALDO) levels may help distinguish primary from secondary adrenal insufficiency (PRA/ALDO ratios are high in primary adrenal insufficiency and low in secondary adrenal insufficiency).

g. Patients with primary adrenal insufficiency have decreased 24-hour urinary cortisol, 17-OHCS, and 17-KS, and increased ACTH (assessment of these substances, impractical in most ICU situations, should not be undertaken before or in lieu of treatment).

G. Therapy
   1. Treat patients with circulatory collapse and suspected adrenal insufficiency immediately (draw random cortisol level if possible first, but do not wait to treat).
   2. Administer hydrocortisone 100 mg IV q8h for 24 hours; if the patient shows a good clinical response (or cortisol level confirms diagnosis), the dosage may be tapered gradually and eventually changed to oral.
   3. Provide adequate volume replacement with D5NS, until hypotension, dehydration, and hypoglycemia are corrected.
   4. Identify and treat any precipitating factors (infections, hemorrhage).

H. Complications
   1. Short-term corticosteroid therapy is safe.
   2. When there is a question of adrenal insufficiency during an emergency, short-term supplemental corticosteroids should be given until adrenal integrity can be assessed.
   3. It is of the utmost importance to treat patients in these situations, because adrenal crises will progress to death if untreated.

■ II. DIABETES INSIPIDUS

A. Definitions
   1. Diabetes insipidus is a disorder of fluid homeostasis resulting from inadequate vasopressin or antidiuretic hormone (ADH) secretion or action.
   2. Neurogenic diabetes insipidus may be caused by a lack of production of ADH precursor molecule by the hypothalamus or inadequate secretion of ADH by the posterior pituitary.
   3. Nephrogenic diabetes insipidus is caused by unresponsiveness of renal tubules to ADH.
   4. Both types of diabetes insipidus result in excretion of large volumes of hypotonic fluid.

B. Etiology
   See Table 4.1.

C. Clinical Manifestations
   1. Polyuria: Urine volume usually >30 mL/kg/d
   2. Neurologic manifestations: Seizures, profound central nervous system (CNS) dysfunction
   3. Dehydration

Table 4.1. Causes of Diabetes Insipidus

1. Neurogenic diabetes insipidus (ADH deficiency)
   a. Head trauma*
   b. Postoperative (secondary to neurosurgical procedures)*
   c. Neoplasms of the brain or pituitary fossa*
   d. Postanoxic/ischemic injury*
   e. Vascular injury (subarachnoid hemorrhage)*
   f. Meningoencephalitis*
   g. Infiltrative hypothalamic disorders (sarcoidosis, histiocytosis)
   h. Familial (autosomal dominant)
   i. Idiopathic

2. Nephrogenic diabetes insipidus (ADH resistance)
   a. Pharmacologic causes (lithium, amphotericin B)*
   b. Postobstructive*
   c. Metabolic disturbances (hypercalcemia, hypokalemia)*
   d. Pyelonephritis
   e. Polycystic kidney disease
   f. Sickle cell disease and trait
   g. Infiltrative diseases (sarcoidosis, amyloidosis)
   h. Familial (X-linked recessive)

3. Diabetes insipidus of pregnancy (secondary to ADH degradation by vasopressinase produced by the placenta)—a rare form of diabetes insipidus and even less commonly seen in the ICU

---

* A cause likely to be seen in critically ill patients.

    4. Polydipsia: Not likely to occur in the critically ill patient with limited access to water

  D. Evaluation of Polyuria
    1. History
      a. Review clinical history for evidence of recent trauma, neurosurgical procedure, pharmacologic causes.
      b. Rule out excess water administration.
      c. Rule out solute load.
    2. Laboratory Evaluation
      a. Decreased urine specific gravity (≤ 1.010)
      b. Inappropriately dilute urine ($\leq 300\,mOsm/kg\ H_2O$)
      c. Electrolytes: Hypernatremia, hypercalcemia, hypokalemia
      d. Increased plasma osmolality ($>300\,mOsm/kg\ H_2O$)
    3. Differential Diagnosis
      a. Diabetes insipidus
      b. Solute diuresis (glucose, mannitol, urea, IV contrast media, sodium diuresis secondary to diuretic or dopamine administration)
      c. Primary polydipsia

E. Diagnostic Approach
  1. First exclude solute diuresis as etiology (check urine glucose, osmolality, and specific gravity).
  2. If the patient has hypernatremia and either an inappropriately low plasma ADH level or an inappropriately low urine osmolality, the diagnosis of diabetes insipidus is made (further testing is needed only to distinguish the type of diabetes insipidus):
      a. Administer a therapeutic trial of 1 μg DDAVP (desmopressin) subcutaneously.
      b. If urine osmolality increases ≥50%, the diagnosis of neurogenic diabetes insipidus is confirmed and therapy can be instituted.
      c. If urine osmolality does not increase in response to DDAVP, renal resistance to ADH is suggested and nephrogenic causes of diabetes insipidus should be addressed.
  3. If the plasma sodium is <145 mEq/L, and the patient is hemodynamically stable, a water-deprivation test may be initiated (to stimulate secretion of ADH and to determine if the patient will respond appropriately to ADH):
      a. Fluid restriction should be continued until plasma osmolality is ≥295 mOsm/kg or sodium level is ≥145 mEq/L (attempt to decrease fluid intake to ≤1 to 2 L/d and follow serial urine output, osmolality, and plasma sodium).
      b. If plasma sodium ≥145 mEq/L while urine osmolality remains ≤300 mOsm/kg, DDAVP may be given (as above) to distinguish between neurogenic and nephrogenic diabetes insipidus.
      c. If plasma sodium ≥145 mEq/L and urine osmolality ≤300 mOsm/kg, secondary diabetes insipidus is suggested (nondiagnostic).
      d. If the patient tolerated the fluid restriction well, it may be continued on the suspicion that the cause is excessive water administration.
      e. If the patient develops thirst or evidence of hypovolemia before polyuria resolves, DDAVP therapy may be started with close monitoring of water balance until further testing can be performed safely (testing of plasma ADH levels may be needed when the patient is out of the critical care setting) to distinguish between partial neurogenic diabetes insipidus and nephrogenic diabetes insipidus.

F. Therapy
  1. Neurogenic Diabetes Insipidus

    a. Desmopressin or DDAVP (vasopressin analog desamino-D-arginine-8-vasopressin) is preferred because it can be administered easily (parenterally, intranasally, or directly onto the buccal mucosa); it has a relatively long duration of action; and this preparation does not have vasoconstrictor or intestinal motility effects (note that others have advocated use of aqueous vasopressin in critically ill patients because of the shorter duration of action allowing for flexibility as the patient's status changes). (See Table 4.2.)

    b. Regardless of initial sodium levels, avoid excess water administration and development of iatrogenic syndrome of inappropriate antidiuretic hormone (SIADH), especially after neurosurgical procedures, which may have short duration of diabetes insipidus.

    c. Patients with trauma or postoperative related diabetes insipidus should have therapy withheld every 3 to 5 days for assessment of potential resolution of diabetes insipidus.

    d. Many patients with neurogenic diabetes insipidus will require long-term hormone replacement.

2. Incomplete Neurogenic Diabetes Insipidus

    a. The preferred agent in critically ill patients is DDAVP.

    b. Other options include medications that augment ADH action in the kidney or increase ADH release:

        (1) Chlorpropamide (Diabinese) 100 to 500 mg qd (concern is hypoglycemia).

        (2) Clofibrate (Atromid-S) 500 mg q6h (associated with increased risk of gallstones).

        (3) Carbamazepine (Tegretol) 200 to 600 mg qd.

3. Nephrogenic Diabetes Insipidus

    a. Discontinue all medications that could be causative, if possible.

Table 4.2. Replacement Therapy for Diabetes Insipidus

Agent	Dose	Route	Duration
Desmopressin (DDAVP)	1–4 μg 5–40 μg	Subcutaneous, intravenous, intranasal	12–24 h 8–20 h
Aqueous vasopressin	5–10 U	Subcutaneous, intramuscular	2–8 h
Vasopressin tannate in oil	2.5–5.0 U	Intramuscular	24–72 h

b. During critical illness, these patients will require fluid administration titrated against urine outputs and plasma sodium levels.

c. These patients frequently respond well to chronic therapy with thiazide diuretics, which cause volume contraction and subsequent increased proximal tubule water and sodium reabsorption, decreased water delivery to the distal nephron, and ultimately decreased urine output.

4. Diabetes Insipidus of Pregnancy

a. Due to the unique pathophysiology, this form of diabetes insipidus will not respond well to treatment with vasopressin (aqueous or in oil), but responds well to DDAVP, which is resistant to vasopressinase action.

■ III. SYNDROME OF INAPPROPRIATE ANTIDIURETIC HORMONE SECRETION (SIADH)

A. Definition

SIADH is a state of euvolemic hyponatremia caused by excessive excretion of ADH.

B. Pathophysiology

1. ADH secretion is independent of normal osmotic or hemodynamic stimuli.

2. Excess ADH may be secreted ectopically or by the posterior pituitary.

3. Normal controls of sodium balance are maintained; high sodium intake increases urinary sodium excretion, and low sodium intake reduces urinary sodium excretion, resulting in maintenance of extracellular volume within normal limits.

4. Free water cannot be excreted normally; persistent ADH secretion causes water retention, hyponatremia, and progressive expansion of intracellular and extracellular fluids.

5. Expanded extracellular fluid (ECF) stimulates natriuresis with an isotonic loss of ECF, bringing the extracellular compartment back to its baseline volume.

6. The intracellular compartment remains expanded.

C. Etiology

1. Postoperative (surgical stress, anesthetic agents, positive pressure ventilation)

2. CNS disorders (head trauma, neoplasm, meningitis, encephalitis, brain abscess, hydrocephalus, intracranial hemorrhage)

3. Pulmonary diseases (pneumonia, TB, bronchiectasis, chronic obstructive pulmonary disease [COPD], status asthmaticus)
4. Drug-induced (vasopressin, DDAVP, chlorpropamide, carbamazepine, clofibrate, oxytocin, thiazide diuretics, vincristine, vinblastine, cyclophosphamide, phenothiazines, tricyclic antidepressants, narcotics, nicotine, monoamine oxidase inhibitors)
5. Ectopic ADH production by tumors (carcinoma of lung, duodenum, pancreas, thymoma, lymphoma, hepatoma, carcinoid tumors, Ewing's sarcoma)
6. Stress or pain
7. Nausea
8. Acute psychosis
9. Endocrinologic disorders (myxedema, ACTH deficiency, panhypopituitarism)

D. Clinical Manifestations
1. Mental status changes may be present (confusion or lethargy).
2. Seizures or coma may occur, especially if the hyponatremia is severe or of rapid onset.

E. Diagnostic Evaluation
1. Physical Examination
   a. Evaluate for evidence of euvolemia.
   b. Edema may be absent.
2. Laboratory Evaluation
   a. Serum sodium ≤130 mEq/L
   b. Urine osmolality >200 mOsm/kg (most reliable diagnostic test)
   c. Urinary sodium usually >30 mEq/L (due to increased atrial natriuretic hormone or suppressed aldosterone)
   d. Plasma osmolality <280 mOsm/kg
   e. Normal or decreased BUN, normal creatinine
   f. Decreased uric acid
   g. Normal thyroid, adrenal, and cardiac function

F. Differential Diagnosis
1. Factitious hyponatremia (substantial elevations of serum proteins or lipids, osmotically induced shifts of water into the intravascular space)
2. Hypovolemic hyponatremia (gastrointestinal losses, renal dysfunction, diuretics, aldosterone deficiency)
3. Hypervolemic hyponatremia (congestive heart failure, nephrotic syndrome, cirrhosis)
4. Hypothyroidism
5. Adrenal insufficiency

G. Therapy
   1. Therapy must be individualized.
   2. Treat the underlying disease (antibiotics for TB, evacuate subdural hematoma).
   3. Restrict fluids to 500 to 800cc/d (difficult in the ICU, at least attempt to decrease free water intake).
   4. It is important to distinguish acute onset (<2 to 3 days) *versus* chronic hyponatremia and to determine the presence or absence of neurological symptoms.
   5. Acute hyponatremia with symptoms may be treated with isotonic or hypertonic (3%) saline combined with a loop diuretic (furosemide is usually added to diminish the ability of the renal tubules to concentrate urine and therefore increase free water excretion) aimed at increasing the serum sodium by ≤ 1 mEq/L/h (maximum safe increase of 10 to 12 mEq/L/d).
   6. Although infusion of isotonic saline alone would seem to be reasonable, since isotonic saline is hypertonic relative to the patient's plasma, the patient with SIADH can excrete the infused sodium in a more concentrated form than it was given (the net effect can be further retention of free water and exacerbation of hyponatremia).
   7. Hypertonic saline (3%) should be given slowly (1 to 2 mL/kg/h) until the sodium is at a "safe" asymptomatic level (usually 120 to 125 mEq/L); monitor serum sodium levels every 1 to 2 hours when using hypertonic saline to avoid dangerously rapid correction, which can result in neurologic sequelae or death.
   8. In chronic hyponatremia with minimal symptomatology, the sodium should be corrected more slowly at approximately 0.5 mEq/L/h to avoid central pontine myelinolysis, which can result from aggressive sodium replacement and can result in permanent neurological impairment or death.
   9. Fluid balances should be measured every 4 to 8 hours until the serum sodium level is >125 mEq/L or is corrected halfway to normal.
   10. Demeclocycline 300 to 600 mg PO bid may be useful in patients with chronic SIADH (it causes nephrogenic diabetes insipidus and counteracts the effects of the high ADH levels).

H. Precautions Regarding Therapy
   1. It is never necessary to rapidly raise the serum sodium to normal or even to a preconceived "safe" level if that requires an increase of >10 to 12 mEq/L/d.
   2. Water moves freely across the blood-brain barrier in response to osmotic gradients; therefore, even small

increases in plasma osmolality will reduce brain edema to some extent.

3. Brain water can never increase by more than 10%, due to constraints imposed by the skull; a 5% to 10% increase in sodium concentration (6 to 12 mEq/L) can be expected to virtually eliminate cerebral edema, and clinical experience has shown this to be effective in symptomatic patients.

■ IV. DIABETIC KETOACIDOSIS AND HYPEROSMOLAR NONKETOTIC COMA

A. Definitions
   1. Diabetic ketoacidosis (DKA) and hyperosmolar nonketotic coma (HNKC) are hyperglycemic states in patients with diabetes mellitus characterized by insulin deficiency and relative excess of glucagon and other counterregulatory hormones.
   2. DKA is also characterized by ketosis.

B. Pathophysiology
   1. Insulin deficiency leads to
      a. Increased glucagon, which causes excessive hepatic glucose production (gluconeogenesis/glycogenolysis)
      b. Decreased glucose clearance from peripheral tissues
      c. Development of hyperglycemia causing an osmotic diuresis (loss of Na^+/H_2O), hypovolemia, and decreased glomerular filtration rate (GFR)
      d. Increased muscle proteolysis and decreased protein synthesis leading to loss of nitrogen and electrolytes from intracellular fluid (ICF) to ECF to urine.
   2. In DKA, insulin deficiency also leads to
      a. Increased cortisol, epinephrine, and growth hormone, which stimulate excessive adipose tissue lipolysis and free fatty acid delivery to liver and subsequent ketogenesis and hyperketonemia (beta-hydroxybutyrate and acetoacetate) in DKA
      b. Development of an anion gap metabolic acidosis (secondary to ketoacids, which neutralize the bicarbonate buffering system) and loss of K^+, Na^+, which buffer urinary excretion of ketoacids
   3. In HNKC, insulin levels may be sufficient to prevent lipolysis and ketogenesis.

C. Etiology
   1. Common precipitating events include
      a. Infection

b. Acute stress (myocardial infarction, stroke, trauma)
c. Discontinuation of insulin
d. Discontinuation of parenteral nutrition
e. Use of some medications (glucocorticoids, diphenyl-hydantoin, propranolol)

2. Rarely, nondiabetics may develop HNKC.
   a. Iatrogenic (hypertonic intravenous hyperalimentation, hyperosmolar peritoneal dialysis)
   b. Severe fluid losses in burned patients
   c. Feeding infants hypertonic oral formulas

D. Diagnostic Evaluation
   1. History
      a. DKA develops in patients of all ages (75% of DKA patients are adults) with insulin-dependent diabetes mellitus (IDDM) and infrequently with non-insulin-dependent diabetes mellitus (NIDDM) in the setting of coexisting severe medical problems.
      b. HNKC patients are typically elderly with a history of NIDDM.
      c. Duration of symptoms averages 12 days in HNKC and 3 days in DKA.
      d. Gastrointestinal symptoms are common (abdominal pain $\approx$ 50%, nausea or vomiting $\approx$ 75%).
      e. Seizures are common in HNKC.
   2. Physical Examination
      a. Altered mental status (severely depressed sensorium in HNKC, associated with osmolalities of 340 to 350 mOsm/kg)
      b. Dehydrated (dry mucous membranes, orthostatic hypotension, tachycardia)
      c. Patients with DKA may also have
         (1) Fruity breath
         (2) Hyperventilation (Kussmaul respirations)
         (3) Abdominal tenderness
   3. Laboratory Evaluation
      a. Table 4.3 lists the common diagnostic laboratory findings in DKA and HNKC.
      b. DKA may also be associated with
         (1) Low serum Na^+ (if corrected for hyperglycemia, may be normal or slightly elevated).
         (2) Normal to slightly elevated serum K^+ (note total body K^+ depleted).
         (3) Leukocytosis (with neutrophilia) may occur secondary to stress or dehydration instead of infection.
         (4) Serum amylase is often elevated (even without pancreatitis).

Table 4.3. Laboratory Values in DKA and HNKC

Lab Test	DKA	HNKC
Blood glucose (mg/dL)	200–2000	Usually > 600
Blood ketones*	Present	Absent
Arterial pH	<7.4	Normal[†]
Anion gap	Elevated (usually > 18)	Normal or elevated
Osmolality	Slightly elevated	Elevated
Urine dipstick	Glucose and ketones	Glucose

* Beta-hydroxybutyrate/acetoacetate.
[†] May be low if hypovolemia causes poor tissue perfusion.

E. Management
1. Initial Evaluation
   a. Rule out infection as precipitant
      (1) Complete blood count (CBC), urine analysis (UA), chest x-ray, appropriate cultures
      (2) Altered mental status: Consider lumbar puncture to rule out meningitis
      (3) Abdominal pain: Consider appendicitis, diverticulitis, pelvic inflammatory disease
   b. R/O myocardial infarction (electrocardiogram) in older patients or those with long-standing DM (even without complaint of chest pain)
2. Institute insulin therapy: 0.1 U/kg regular insulin IV bolus, and begin infusion of regular insulin at rate of 0.1 U/kg/h. (If IV access unobtainable, may use 0.1 U/kg IM q1h.)
   a. Expect blood glucose to decrease by ~75 mg/dL/h on this regimen.
   b. Follow blood glucose q1h.
   c. If blood glucose levels do not begin to decrease after 4 hours of insulin therapy, increase insulin dosage every hour until blood glucose begins to decrease (doses of >100 U/hour have occasionally been required in a rare, extraordinarily insulin-resistant patient).
   d. Continue infusion until blood glucose level is 250 to 300 mg/dL and serum ketones are negative (or positive only in undiluted serum) or urine ketones are "small or moderate"; anion gap should also be decreasing to near normal range unless additional cause of persistent metabolic acidosis exists.
   e. Lower insulin infusion to 2 U/h, and change IVF to D_5 0.45% Normal Saline (NS) or D_5NS (add K^+ if appropriate), aiming for blood glucose levels 150 to 200 until patient can eat and drink.

    f. Give regular insulin dose (5 to 10 U SQ) *before* stopping continuous infusion (because half-life of insulin via infusion is only 6 to 8 minutes) to avoid recurrence of hyperglycemia and ketosis.

3. Immediately begin volume repletion.

    a. Restore circulating volume (isotonic fluid: NS or Lactated Ringer's [LR]).

       (1) First liter IV over the first 30 minutes.

       (2) Second liter IV over the next hour.

       (3) Then reassess volume status and continue as clinical situation warrants.

       (4) If the patient presents in shock:

          (a) May use colloid for volume expansion

          (b) May require 2 to 3 L (or more) over first 1 to 2 hours

    b. Replace intracellular and total body fluid losses.

       (1) Patients typically lose water and sodium at around 100 mL H_2O/kg and 7 mEq Na^+/kg, so 0.45% NS is a good choice at this stage.

       (2) Gradual replacement is appropriate (150 to 300 cc/h × 12 to 24 h).

       (3) Patients are continuing to have excessive urinary losses via osmotic diuresis while hyperglycemia persists.

       (4) Fluid balance should be followed every 1 to 2 hours, and positive fluid balance should be maintained (adjust rate of IV replacement as needed).

       (5) The average patient in DKA requires 5 to 7 L positive balance during treatment.

       (6) When the patient's blood glucose level is ≤250 mg/dL, intravascular fluid (IVF) should contain 5% dextrose.

4. Monitor patient.

    a. CBC, Na^+/K^+/Cl^-/HCO_3^-/Cr, UA, chest x-ray, electrocardiogram (ECG), and appropriate cultures on admission.

    b. Follow vital signs.

    c. Record cumulative patient intake and output every hour.

    d. Check blood glucose q1h while the patient is on continuous insulin infusion and q4h after changing to SQ insulin.

    e. Check serum potassium 2 hours after insulin treatment started and q2–4h thereafter.

    f. Check serum electrolytes (Na^+/HCO_3^-/Cl^-), and determine the anion gap q4–6h.

g. Check the serum ketone level q4h.
h. Check arterial blood gases (ABGs) on admission, and repeat as clinical situation warrants.
i. Check serum phosphate, magnesium, and ionized calcium levels on admission. If low, replace.
j. Check urine dipstick q1h for presence of glucose/ketones until they are negative/small.

5. K^+ Supplementation
   a. Serum K^+ level decreases as soon as insulin action begins.
   b. K^+ administration should begin when serum $K^+ \leq$ 5.0 mEq/L and urine output is documented.
   c. Goal of K^+ supplementation at this point is to keep serum $K^+ \geq$ 3.5 mEq/L to help prevent cardiac arrhythmias.
   d. Patients typically have average total K^+ deficit of ~5 mEq/kg (but it can be much greater).
   e. Total K^+ repletion can be completed gradually (after DKA is resolved).
   f. If admission K^+ is <3.5, immediately add 40 mEq KCl to each liter of IVF (KCl usually used initially; if phosphate is low, may use KPhos).
   g. Use IV K^+ until DKA is reversed and patient can take potassium orally.

6. Metabolic Acidosis
   a. Insulin inhibits lipolysis and ketogenesis.
   b. Fluid replacement restores perfusion.
   c. Bicarbonate administration has not been shown to accelerate resolution of acidosis and is generally not advisable. The exception is in severe hyperkalemia with characteristic ECG changes, i.e., widened QRS or peaked T waves.
      (1) If needed, use 50 to 100 mEq $NaHCO_3$ in 500 to 1000 cc 0.45% saline over 1 to 2 hours.
      (2) The main risk of bicarbonate therapy is the induction of severe hypokalemia as potassium enters cell in exchange for hydrogen ions.

7. Phosphate Supplementation
   a. Phosphate depletion in DKA averages ~1.0 mmol/kg.
   b. Prospective randomized studies showed no beneficial effect of phosphate treatment on recovery from DKA.
   c. Frequently, phosphate levels plummet to ~1.5 mg/dL with insulin treatment.
   d. IV replacement is usually not essential.
   e. However, if phosphorus levels are ≤1.0 mg/dL, then replacement is generally given (potassium phosphate

IV is usually the best choice with concomitant hypokalemia), since severe hypophosphatemia may cause respiratory failure.

8. Magnesium Supplementation
   a. Mild magnesium depletion occurs in DKA and also falls with insulin treatment.
   b. Typically does not need parenteral supplementation.
   c. If the patient develops ventricular irritability with hypomagnesemia, magnesium sulfate 1 to 2 g IV may be given.

F. Complications
   Cerebral edema may develop; its therapy is not clear, but mannitol may be helpful.

■ V. MYXEDEMA

A. Definition and Epidemiology
   1. Myxedema is severe thyroid hormone deficiency, which can lead to a decreased level of consciousness, even coma.
   2. It has a reported fatality rate as high as 80%.
   3. Actual coma associated with severe hypothyroidism is rare (only about 200 cases reported in the literature).
   4. The incidence of myxedema is 3 times higher in females than males; elderly females seem most susceptible to myxedema coma.

B. Pathophysiology
   1. Thyroid hormone is essential for normal metabolism of all cells
   2. Thyroid-stimulating hormone (TSH) secreted by the pituitary (under regulation of the hypothalamus) stimulates the thyroid to secrete thyroxine (T_4) and smaller amounts of triiodothyronine (T_3), which is the active form of thyroid hormone.
   3. Most T_3 is produced in the peripheral tissues by monodeiodination of circulating T_4.
   4. T_3 and T_4 circulate bound to serum proteins; the free T_3 and T_4 are metabolically active.
   5. T_3 feeds back on the pituitary gland to inhibit production of TSH.
   6. In myxedema coma, the cause of coma is multifactorial (decreased cerebral perfusion associated with low cardiac output from bradycardia and reduced stroke volume, decreased circulating levels of thyroid hormones resulting in decreased mental responsiveness).

7. Hypothermia may result from decreased T_3 or T_4, leading to reduced metabolic rate in addition to an inability to shiver.

8. Hypoventilation (alveolar) is secondary to respiratory center depression (exacerbated by use of analgesics, sedatives, and anesthesia), defective respiratory muscle function, and occasionally airway obstruction (enlarged tongue).

9. Hyponatremia often accompanies myxedema and may have associated hypochloremia (may contribute to altered mental status).

10. Decreased plasma volume and intense peripheral vasoconstriction are typical.

C. Etiology

1. Occasionally, myxedema may be the result of chronic, severe primary thyroid failure; patients with classic signs and symptoms lapse into stupor, coma, and death.

2. Myxedema may be precipitated in patients with moderate or unrecognized hypothyroidism by a superimposed acute illness (infection) or following administration of narcotics or sedatives.

3. See Table 4.4.

D. Risk Factors

1. Infection
2. Surgery
3. Anesthesia
4. Myocardial infarction
5. Sedating drugs
6. Cerebrovascular accidents

Table 4.4. Causes of Hypothyroidism

1. Autoimmune thyroid disease (Hashimoto's thyroiditis)

2. Thyroid ablation (radioactive iodine or surgical)

3. Surgical thyroid resection

4. Pituitary disease (secondary hypothyroidism)

5. Hypothalamic disease (tertiary hypothyroidism)

6. Chemical agents (antithyroid drugs, e.g., lithium, organic goitrogens, iodine-containing drugs, e.g., amiodarone)

7. Congenital thyroid agenesis

8. Iodine deficiency or excess

9. Thyroid hormone resistance

       7. Bleeding
       8. Cold exposure
       9. Trauma
     10. Hyponatremia

E. Symptoms
    1. Decreased mental acuity
    2. Hoarseness
    3. Increased somnolence
    4. Cold intolerance
    5. Dry skin
    6. Brittle hair

F. Diagnostic Evaluation
    1. History
       a. Usually, the patient has a long history of gradual deterioration.
       b. Gradual weight gain or inability to lose weight.
       c. May have been noncompliant with thyroid replacement therapy.
       d. May have history of Graves' disease or other thyroid dysfunction.
    2. Physical Examination
       a. Hypothermia (core or rectal temperature <35°C)
       b. Bradycardia
       c. Hypoventilation (slow respiratory rate, shallow breaths)
       d. Hypotension
       e. Physical features consistent with long-standing hypothyroidism
          (1) Thick and doughy-appearing skin (may have orange or yellow tint)
          (2) Facial and general puffiness, periorbital edema
          (3) Large tongue
          (4) Alopecia, loss of lateral aspects of eyebrows
       f. Palpable thyroid (present in <50%) or thyroidectomy scar
       g. Cardiac examination may be consistent with pericardial effusion (e.g., muffled heart tones, cardiomegaly)
       h. Neurologic examination rarely reveals focal findings
          (1) Altered level of consciousness
          (2) Delayed relaxation phase of deep tendon reflexes may be present but difficult to detect
          (3) Disorders of muscular function (paralytic ileus, urinary retention, atonic bowel with fecal impaction)
    3. Laboratory Evaluation

   a. Confirmation of diagnosis relies on thyroid function tests to document hypothyroidism (measure TSH, T_4, free T_4, reverse T_3, T_3RU) (see Table 4.5).
      (1) TSH level is elevated in primary hypothyroidism.
      (2) In secondary and tertiary hypothyroidism, TSH is not elevated, and diagnosis will rely on other laboratory parameters and clinical judgment.
   b. Serum cortisol level should be drawn initially to evaluate for concomitant adrenal insufficiency.
   c. CBC, UA, blood, and urine cultures should be sent.
   d. Serum cholesterol is usually elevated.
   e. Chest x-ray may reveal signs of pleural or pericardial effusion or of infection.
   f. ECG is often abnormal (sinus bradycardia, small voltage QRS complexes, prolonged Q-T intervals, isoelectric T-wave changes, supraventricular tachycardia).
   g. ABG may reveal hypoxemia, hypercarbia, and respiratory acidosis.
   h. Serum glucose or sodium may be low.
   i. Normochromic, normocytic anemia is typical.

G. Differential Diagnosis
   1. Other causes of altered mental status (e.g., stroke, electrolyte disturbances such as hyponatremia)
   2. Sepsis
   3. Hypothermia (especially with associated anemia)
   4. Hypopituitarism
   5. Hypoglycemia
   6. Renal failure

H. Therapy
   1. Initiate thyroid hormone replacement upon suspicion (awaiting confirmation of the diagnosis may be too late).
      a. Intravenous administration of replacement hormone is necessary due to unreliable gastrointestinal absorption in the myxedematous state.
      b. We prefer T_3 and T_4 combination therapy (T_3 20-μg IV bolus followed by 10μg q8h with T_4 200μg IV followed by 100μg IV q24h) for 1 to 2 days, followed by T_4 alone.
      c. T_3 for IV administration recently became available in the United States, so many authors recommend treatment with IV T_3 alone.
      d. Peripheral conversion of $T_4 \rightarrow T_3$ requires the presence of some T_3 for enzyme activity.

Table 4.5. Thyroid Function Tests in Thyroid Disorders

Test	Hypothyroid	High T_4 Syndrome	Hyperthyroid	Low T_3 Syndrome	Low T_3/T_4 Syndrome
TSH	High*	Nl/low	Low	Low to sl ←	Low to sl ←
Total T_4	Low	High	High	Nl	Low
Total T_3	Low to low Nl	Low/Nl/high	High	Low	Low
Reverse T_3	Nl/low	Nl/high	High	High	High
Free T_4	Low	Nl/high	High	Nl	Nl
T_3RU	Low	Nl/low	High	Nl/high	High

Abbreviations: Nl, normal; sl, slight.
* Exceptions: TSH is low in hypothyroidism of secondary and tertiary causes.

e. An advantage of IV T_3 includes a more rapid onset of action than T_4; also, peripheral conversion of T_4 is not required for activity.

f. T_3 is more arrhythmogenic than T_4, and careful cardiac monitoring is essential, especially since the risk of coronary artery disease is high in these patients.

g. If IV T_3 is not immediately available, IV T_4 (as above) may be given with oral T_3 (25 µg q12h) until the patient can be treated with oral T_4 alone.

h. Previously, T_4 alone was frequently used (200- to 500-µg IV bolus followed by 50 to 100 µg IV q24h).

i. Controversy exists regarding the best therapeutic regimen, and controlled trials will probably never be performed because the disease is so rare.

j. Monitor T_3 and T_4 levels after 5 days, and adjust doses accordingly if the patient remains unconscious.

2. Metabolic Support

a. Hypothermia is best treated with passive rewarming (active rewarming can cause peripheral vasodilatation and worsening of shock). (See Chapter 5.)

b. Hyponatremia generally responds well to free water restriction.

c. Hypoglycemia should be treated with IV dextrose.

d. Seizures may be treated with standard anticonvulsant drugs.

e. Identify and treat precipitating causes (e.g., infection, stroke, myocardial infarction, narcotics, gastrointestinal bleeding).

3. Supportive Care

a. Respiratory support with mechanical ventilation may be required.

b. Hypotension should be treated aggressively with IV fluids (avoid free water) and vasopressor therapy (dopamine is preferable over norepinephrine, as it may better maintain coronary blood flow and renal/mesenteric blood flow).

c. Hypotension is poorly responsive to vasopressors until thyroid hormone replacement is initiated.

d. Hydrocortisone (100 mg IV q8h) should be given until initial cortisol level is available (if this indicates a normal stress response to the acute medical illness, this therapy may be stopped) or for 3 to 7 days followed by a rapid taper in the absence of hypothalamic-pituitary-adrenal disease; this therapy may be life-saving in patients with secondary/tertiary hypothyroidism.

    e. Monitor for presence of arrhythmias (decrease dosage of thyroid hormone replacement if arrhythmias occur); hypothyroidism is associated with a high incidence of coronary artery disease, and these patients should be monitored for evidence of myocardial ischemia exacerbated by increased myocardial oxygen consumption with T_3/T_4 treatment.

    f. Avoid sedatives.

I. Complications

    1. Euthyroid patients tolerate short-term administration of thyroid hormone well.

    2. Delay of treatment in a myxedematous patient can make the difference between survival and death.

    3. This treatment regimen should *not* routinely be instituted in hypothyroid patients without clinical evidence of myxedema coma because of potential cardiac complications (myocardial infarction, arrhythmias).

    4. Severe hypothermia ($<32°C$) is thought to have prognostic significance.

■ VI. THYROTOXIC CRISIS

A. Definitions

    1. *Thyrotoxic crisis*, or *thyroid storm*, is a life-threatening complication of hyperthyroidism characterized by a severe, sudden exacerbation of thyrotoxicosis.

    2. The general term *thyrotoxicosis* refers to the clinical and biochemical manifestations of excess thyroid hormone at the tissue level.

    3. *True hyperthyroidism* refers to disorders of thyroid glandular hyperfunction with increased synthesis and secretion of thyroid hormone.

    4. There are states of thyrotoxicosis without true hyperthyroidism (e.g., factitious ingestion of thyroid hormone, chronic thyroiditis with transient thyrotoxicosis, ectopic thyroid hormone production, subacute thyroiditis) that are associated with decreased thyroidal synthesis of new hormone; these states are rare in the critically ill patient with the possible exception of T_4 or T_3 overdose (see Table 4.6).

B. Pathophysiology

    1. The actual mechanisms by which a patient with thyrotoxicosis decompensates into thyroid crisis are poorly understood.

Table 4.6. Thyrotoxicosis: Etiologies and Differentiation by RAIU

RAIU High	RAIU Low	RAIU Low or High
TSH excess (e.g., pituitary tumors)	Destructive thyroid disease (e.g., subacute thyroiditis, postpartum thyroiditis)	Iodine-induced thyrotoxicosis (e.g., food or medication such as radiocontrast dye or amiodarone)
Abnormal thyroid stimulators (e.g., thyroid-stimulating antibodies—Graves's disease)	Ectopic thyroid tissue (e.g., metastatic follicular carcinoma)	
Thyroid autonomy (e.g., toxic multinodular goiter or toxic adenoma)	Exogenous sources (e.g., medication or food)	

Abbreviation: RAIU, 24-hour radioactive iodine uptake study.

2. A crisis develops most often after a stressful precipitating event (e.g., trauma, infection, DKA, surgical emergency, parturition, or myocardial infarction).
3. Whatever the cause, the resulting syndrome resembles that of prolonged, severe beta-adrenergic agonist overload.
4. Catecholamine levels appear to be normal despite the hypermetabolic state.

C. Etiology
    1. Undiagnosed hyperthyroidism (most commonly Graves's disease or toxic multinodular goiter) in a patient with major stress.
    2. Other etiologies of thyrotoxicosis may be distinguished by a 24-hour radioactive iodine uptake study when the patient is stable (see Table 4.6).
    3. Inadequate therapy in a hyperthyroid patient.

D. Symptoms
    1. Abnormal mental states (agitation, confusion, psychosis).
    2. Fever (T > 38.3°C) is almost always present.
    3. Heat intolerance, diaphoresis.
    4. Palpitations (sinus tachycardia and atrial fibrillation are the most common dysrhythmias).
    5. Gastrointestinal disturbances (diarrhea, nausea, vomiting, abdominal pain).
    6. Muscle wasting and weakness.
    7. Dyspnea.

E. Diagnostic Evaluation
   1. History
      a. Marked and rapid recent weight loss may warn of impending storm.
      b. Unexplained fever in a thyrotoxic patient may precede a storm.
      c. A precipitating event may be evident.
   2. Physical Examination
      a. Goiter (palpate cautiously, since vigorous massage may cause release of more hormone into the circulation)
      b. Tachycardia—may have tachydysrhythmias
      c. Hyperthermia
      d. Mental status changes
      e. Tremor
      f. Warm, moist skin
      g. Ophthalmic signs of hyperthyroidism (proptosis, lid lag, lid retraction)
      h. Signs of congestive heart failure (high-output failure or cardiomyopathy)
   3. Laboratory Evaluation
      a. Confirmation of the diagnosis relies on thyroid studies (see Tables 4.5 and 4.6).
         (1) Elevated T_4
         (2) Elevated T_3
         (3) Decreased TSH
      b. Routine studies include CBC, electrolytes, urinalysis, chest x-ray, and ECG.
      c. Evaluate for infection as indicated by history and physical examination.
      d. Associated laboratory abnormalities.
         (1) Hypercalcemia
         (2) Hypokalemia
         (3) Hyperglycemia
         (4) Hypocholesterolemia
         (5) Mild microcytic anemia
         (6) Lymphocytosis
         (7) Granulocytopenia
         (8) Hyperbilirubinemia
         (9) Elevated alkaline phosphatase
F. Differential Diagnosis
   1. Hypermetabolic states (sepsis, pheochromocytoma, Cushing's syndrome)
   2. Thyrotoxicosis without crisis/storm
G. Therapy
   Do **not** wait for lab values to begin treatment; diagnosis is made on clinical suspicion, and treatment should be initiated immediately.

1. Supportive Measures
   a. IV fluids for volume replacement.
   b. Acetaminophen for hyperthermia. Avoid aspirin, since it displaces T_4 from thyroid-binding globulin, thereby increasing the level of free T_4.
   c. Cooling blankets.
2. Inhibition of Thyroid Hormone Synthesis
   a. Propylthiouracil (PTU) (200 to 300 mg oral or via nasogastric tube q6h)
   b. Methimazole (20 to 25 mg oral or via nasogastric tube q4h)
3. Inhibition of Thyroid Hormone Release With Iodide Therapy (beginning 1 hour after PTU therapy)
   a. Sodium iodide (1 g IV q8h)
   b. Potassium iodide and iodine—Lugol's solution (10 drops q8h orally)
4. Inhibition of Peripheral Beta-Adrenergic Activity
   a. Most beta-blockers also block peripheral conversion of T_4 to T_3.
   b. Propranolol (Inderal) 0.5 to 1.0 mg/min IV to total dose of 2 to 10 mg IV q3–4h; may treat with 20 to 40 mg PO q6h after initial control with IV administration. An occasional patient has required up to 2 g/d PO due to variability of hepatic metabolism in thyrotoxic individuals.
   c. Esmolol (Brevibloc) 0.5- to 1.0-mg/kg bolus followed by infusion with 50 μg/kg/min; if inadequate effect within 5 minutes, repeat bolus and increase infusion to 100 μg/kg/min; can repeat procedure, to 200 to 300 μg/kg/min.
   d. Titrate beta-blockade to achieve heart rate ≤80 beats per minute.
   e. If the patient has a history of reactive airway disease, use caution and a short-acting cardioselective agent such as esmolol.
   f. Caution is also required in patients with CHF. Controlling the heart rate may be of benefit; however, these agents are negative inotropes and may worsen low-output failure.
   g. If beta-blockers are contraindicated, other sympatholytic drugs (reserpine, a depleter of catecholamines, or guanethidine, an inhibitor of catecholamine release) may be useful as second-line agents.
5. Inhibition of Peripheral Conversion of T_4 to T_3
   a. PTU (see above dosages).
   b. Beta-blockade (see above).
   c. Dexamethasone 1 to 2 mg IV or PO q6h.

6. Definitive therapy may require surgery or radioactive iodine therapy after etiology determined by RAIU.
7. Diagnose and treat underlying precipitating disorders (i.e., infection, other major stresses).

■ VII. SICK EUTHYROID SYNDROME

A. Definitions
   1. Sick euthyroid syndrome is characterized by thyroid hormone alterations associated with acute nonthyroidal illness.
   2. Two syndromes are described:
      a. Low T_3 syndrome
      b. Low T_3/T_4 syndrome
   3. These syndromes are thought to represent euthyroid states by many; however, specific tissues may actually be hypothyroid.
B. Review of Normal Thyroid Hormone Physiology
   1. Thyrotropin-releasing hormone (TRH) is released from the hypothalamus into the blood stream.
   2. TRH stimulates synthesis and release of thyrotropin (TSH) from the pituitary gland.
   3. TSH stimulates the thyroid gland to produce and secrete thyroxine (T_4) and smaller amounts of triiodothyronine (T_3).
   4. The thyroid gland secretes predominantly T_4 (80%), with smaller amounts of T_3 (20%).
   5. The remainder of T_3 (the physiologically active form of thyroid hormone) is produced in extrathyroidal tissues (primarily, the liver and kidneys) by monodeiodination of circulating T_4.
   6. T_3 and T_4 circulate bound to serum proteins; the free T_3 and T_4 are metabolically active.
   7. T_3 feeds back on the pituitary gland to inhibit production of TSH.
   8. Some of the circulating T_4 is metabolized to the inactive product reverse T_3.
   9. Both T_3 and reverse T_3 are rapidly cleared from the serum by further deiodination.
   10. Thyroid hormone activity begins with binding of T_3 to receptors on cell nuclei.
   11. Postbinding effects of T_3 are needed for normal cellular function.

12. The T_3 resin-uptake test is commonly performed to give an approximation of binding proteins (primarily thyroxine-binding globulin).

C. Pathophysiology
   1. In acute nonthyroidal illness, peripheral thyroid hormone metabolism is altered.
   2. The exact mechanism of decreased T_3 production is unknown.

D. Etiology
   1. Systemic illness (sepsis, cardiac or respiratory failure, neoplastic processes, stroke)
   2. Surgery
   3. Caloric deprivation
   4. Drug-induced (glucocorticoids, iodides, amiodarone, propylthiouracil)

E. Symptoms
   No specific symptoms are associated with the thyroidal hormone alterations.

F. Laboratory Evaluation
   1. Serum T_3 is low (see Table 4.5).
   2. Serum T_4 is low or normal.
   3. Reverse T_3 is elevated (usually this is the most useful discriminator between the sick euthyroid syndrome and hypothyroidism).
   4. Serum TSH is normal.

G. Therapy
   1. Attempts should be made to distinguish sick euthyroid syndrome from hypothyroidism.
   2. Currently, there is no proven benefit in using thyroid hormone to treat patients with sick euthyroid syndrome.
   3. Indeed, some researchers believe that the sick euthyroid state may be protective by conserving energy under stress.

■ VIII. HYPOGLYCEMIA

A. Definition
   Hypoglycemia is defined by plasma glucose <40 to 50 mg/dL. This definition does not include the presence of associated symptoms, since critically ill patients may not reliably demonstrate classic symptomatology.

B. Pathophysiology
   1. Clinical situations that result in increased insulin, inability of the liver to generate glucose from its glycogen stores, or

problems with the counterregulatory system may lead to hypoglycemia.

2. Insulin suppresses hepatic glucose production and stimulates glucose utilization by peripheral tissues such as muscle.

3. Insulin secretion lowers plasma glucose concentration.

4. In response to onset of hypoglycemia, the major counterregulatory hormones glucagon and epinephrine increase and cause an acceleration of glycogenolysis.

5. Catecholamines are glucose counterregulatory hormones but do not play essential roles as long as secretion of glucagon is initiated; however, in the presence of glucagon deficiency (long-standing diabetes mellitus or patients with total pancreatectomy), catecholamines become major counterregulatory hormones.

6. Patients treated with nonselective beta-adrenergic-blocking agents may have severe impairment of counterregulation mechanisms.

7. Patients with long-standing DM (10 to 15 years) may lose the ability to secrete epinephrine in response to hypoglycemia (becoming virtually defenseless against even moderate degrees of hyperinsulinemia).

C. Etiology
   See Table 4.7.

D. Symptoms
   1. Adrenergic activation
      a. Palpitations
      b. Tremor
      c. Diaphoresis
      d. Pallor
      e. Anxiety
   2. Neuroglycopenia
      a. Fatigue
      b. Faintness
      c. Dizziness
      d. Hunger
      e. Inappropriate behavior
      f. Visual symptoms
      g. Focal neurologic symptoms
      h. Seizures
      i. Coma

E. Diagnostic Evaluation
   1. History
      a. Check for history of DM.
         (1) Recent insulin or oral hypoglycemic therapy?
         (2) If DM is long-standing, the patient may also have glucagon deficiency and therefore be at

Table 4.7. Causes of Hypoglycemia

1. Hyperinsulin states
   a. Exogenous insulin administration*
   b. Endogenous insulin excess (e.g., insulinomas)

2. Ethanol-induced (after ingestion in otherwise healthy patients or chronic alcoholics)*

3. Drug-induced (e.g., sulfonylureas, quinine, propranolol, pentamidine)*

4. System disorders*
   a. Hepatic disease (e.g., cirrhosis, fulminant viral hepatitis)
   b. Renal disease (e.g., chronic renal disease associated with liver disease, CHF, sepsis)
   c. Sepsis (e.g., gram-negative sepsis, empyema of gallbladder)
   d. AIDS

5. Extensive thermal burns*

6. Total parenteral nutrition*

7. Insulin treatment of hyperkalemia*

8. Factitious (insulin injection or sulfonylurea ingestion)*

9. Endocrine causes (hypopituitarism, hypoadrenalism, hypothyroidism)

10. Autoimmune causes (insulin antireceptor antibodies, anti-insulin autoantibodies)

11. Starvation (severe caloric restriction)

12. Alimentary—following gastric surgery (e.g., gastrectomy)

13. Idiopathic (functional)—typically postprandial; this is a diagnosis of exclusion and is usually not seen in the critically ill patient

* Causes likely to be seen in the critically ill.

higher risk for hypoglycemia, since the counter-regulatory mechanisms may also be ineffective.
    b. Check for history of alcohol ingestion.
2. Physical Examination
    a. Tachycardia
    b. Pupillary dilation
    c. Cold, moist skin
    d. Changes in body temperature (hypothermia, hyperthermia)
    e. Between hypoglycemic episodes, the examination may be normal.
3. Laboratory Evaluation
    a. Plasma glucose level <40 to 50 mg/dL. Whole blood glucose is usually about 15% less than the corresponding plasma glucose level.

    b. The patient may have changes in blood counts.
        (1) Acute lymphocytosis is followed later by neutrophilia.
        (2) May have increased hemoglobin, total red blood cell (RBC) count, or packed RBC volume.
    c. ECG changes (ST depression, flat T waves, QT-interval prolongation)
    d. Electroencephalogram (EEG) changes (diminished frequency of alpha waves, increased delta waves).
    e. Artifactual hypoglycemia must be ruled out, especially if laboratory results indicate hypoglycemia with no apparent cause.
        (1) Samples in serum separator tubes left at room temperature for extended periods of time (blood glucose levels may decrease by 10 to 20 mg/dL/h due to ongoing blood cell metabolism).
        (2) Patients with increased numbers of blood cells (polycythemia vera, leukemia, leukemoid reactions) may have low measured plasma glucose levels secondary to increased metabolism.
        (3) These problems may be avoided by collecting blood in tubes containing oxalate and fluoride (gray tubes), since the fluoride acts as a glycolytic enzyme poison.
4. Diagnostic Approach
    a. Measure simultaneous blood glucose and plasma insulin levels during an episode of hypoglycemia. The best way to demonstrate insulin secretion inappropriate to the prevailing blood glucose concentration.
        (1) Relative hyperinsulinemia can be demonstrated by the simultaneous determination of blood glucose and plasma insulin levels after an overnight fast or during a 24- to 72-hour fast.
        (2) Diagnosis of hyperinsulinism can further be supported by elevated levels of plasma C-peptide and proinsulin concentrations.
        (3) Insulinomas can be localized by ultrasonography, CT scanning, magnetic resonance imaging (MRI), arteriography, and transhepatic percutaneous venous sampling, and intraoperative high-frequency sonography.
    b. Factitious hypoglycemia resulting from administration of insulin or sulfonylurea agents is typically characterized by inappropriately high plasma insulin levels (similar to insulinomas).

(1) C-peptide levels remain low in insulin-induced factitious hypoglycemia; the presence of insulin antibodies in patients who have no reason to take insulin injections also suggests this etiology.

(2) C-peptide levels are elevated in sulfonylurea-induced factitious hypoglycemia (similar to insulinomas); screening for plasma or urine sulfonylureas may confirm the diagnosis.

c. In spontaneous hypoglycemia, alcohol ingestion should be ruled out as a cause (alcohol levels may not be helpful, since hypoglycemia may not occur for as long as 36 hours after ingestion).

d. Associated systemic disorders must be ruled out as appropriate for each patient (evaluate for liver, renal, or endocrine dysfunction, or sepsis).

F. Therapy

1. If the patient is comatose, glucose should be administered intravenously (25 to 50 cc of 50% dextrose followed by infusion of 10% dextrose) until persistent or mild hyperglycemia is present.

2. Treatment with dextrose should cause resolution of symptoms rapidly unless organic changes have occurred in the brain.

3. Some patients may require additional IV boluses of 50% dextrose with continuous infusion of 10% dextrose.

4. In drug-induced hypoglycemia (especially secondary to chlorpropamide), prolonged treatment with IV dextrose may be required to keep the blood glucose levels in the 200-mg/dL range; if this does not maintain the blood glucose level >200 mg/dL, one of the following should be added:

a. 100 mg hydrocortisone and 1 mg glucagon per liter of 10% dextrose. Continue until blood glucose levels are maintained >200 mg/dL.

b. An additional infusion of 300 mg diazoxide in 5% dextrose given over a 30-minute period and repeated every 4 hours. Continue until blood glucose levels are maintained >200 mg/dL.

c. When the blood glucose levels rise, the hydrocortisone, glucagon, and diazoxide are stopped, and the rate of infusion of 10% dextrose is decreased.

d. Persistent hyperglycemia maintained on 5% dextrose is a sign to discontinue the infusion gradually over a 24-hour period.

5. Insulin-induced hypoglycemia in diabetic patients may be effectively treated with 0.5 to 1.0 mg glucagon IV, IM, or SQ; the patient should also ingest 20 to 40 g of carbohydrate, since the glucagon effect lasts only 1 to 1.5 hours.
6. Insulinomas may be surgically cured with resection.
7. Medical management of insulinomas is indicated for malignant insulinoma, patients with major contraindications to surgery, and rare patients in whom surgery fails.
   a. Diazoxide (3 to 8 mg/kg/d PO in 2 to 3 divided doses) is the drug of choice (it inhibits insulin secretion).
   b. Thiazide diuretics, diphenylhydantoin, propranolol, or calcium channel blockers may also be useful.
   c. Combination chemotherapy with streptozotocin and 5-fluorouracil has been reported to achieve partial or complete remission in 60% of patients with malignant insulinomas.
8. Treat the underlying cause if it is related to systemic disorders.

G. Complications
   Prompt recognition and treatment of hypoglycemia is required to prevent long-term neurologic sequelae or death.

■ IX. PHEOCHROMOCYTOMA

A. Definition and Epidemiology
   1. Catecholamine-producing tumor of the adrenergic system (chromaffin cells); ~90% are adrenomedullary.
   2. Nonadrenal tumors (~10%) arising from the sympathetic nervous system are designated extra-adrenal pheochromocytomas or functioning paragangliomas and most commonly occur in the abdomen, chest, and neck.
   3. Pheochromocytomas are rare (occur in only 1 to 2/100,000 adults).

B. Pathophysiology
   Symptoms are secondary to catecholamines secreted by the tumor:
   1. Alpha$_1$-adrenergic stimulation results in vasoconstriction.
   2. Alpha$_2$-adrenergic stimulation results in decreased insulin secretion.
   3. Beta$_1$-adrenergic stimulation results in cardiac inotropy/chronotropy.
   4. Beta$_2$-adrenergic stimulation results in bronchodilation and vasodilation.

5. Dopa$_1$-receptor stimulation results in renal and mesenteric vasodilation.
6. Excessive levels of catecholamines are toxic to the myocardium and cardiomyopathy may result.
7. Symptoms may be episodic in nature; paroxysms may last from less than 1 minute to several hours and may occur only once every few months or as frequently as multiple times per day.

C. Symptoms
  1. Hypertension (paroxysmal or persistent)
  2. Headache
  3. Pallor
  4. Hyperhidrosis
  5. Anxiety
  6. Tachycardia
  7. Palpitations
  8. Angina
  9. Hyperglycemia
  10. Weight loss
  11. Paresthesias (2° vasoconstriction)
  12. Visual disturbances (2° hypertensive retinopathy)
  13. Dilated pupils

D. Diagnostic Evaluation
  1. History
    a. Check for the presence of the above symptoms.
    b. A pressor response to histamine, glucagon, droperidol, tyramine, metoclopramide, saralasin, tricyclic antidepressants, or phenothiazides suggests the possibility of a pheochromocytoma.
  2. Physical Examination
    a. May be normal if performed during a symptom-free time interval.
    b. During a paroxysm, may exhibit above symptoms.
  3. Laboratory Evaluation
    a. Plasma or urinary catecholamine levels or urinary catecholamine metabolite (VMA or metanephrine) levels.
    b. Rarely, suppression tests (clonidine) or provocative tests (glucagon) are needed.
    c. Measurement of plasma and urinary catecholamines are interfered with by the following:
      (1) Stimulation of endogenous catecholamines (e.g., surgery, stroke)
      (2) Administration of exogenous catecholamines
      (3) Various drugs (alpha$_2$-agonists, methyldopa, converting enzyme inhibitors, monoamine

oxidase inhibitors, phenothiazines, tricyclic antidepressants)
4. Tumors may be localized by a variety of scanning techniques (CT, MRI, or venous blood sampling for catecholamines).
5. Arteriography is generally avoided because it can precipitate hypertensive crisis.

E. Differential Diagnosis
   1. Malignant hypertension
   2. Thyrotoxic crisis
   3. Hypertensive response (to stress, surgery, anesthesia)
   4. Cushing's syndrome

F. Therapy
   1. Surgical excision is the definitive treatment.
   2. Preoperative management is important in determining surgical outcome.
   3. Preoperative goals:
      a. Control blood pressure
      b. Provide adequate intravascular volume
      c. Treat tachyarrhythmias
      d. Treat heart failure
      e. Treat glucose intolerance
   4. Alpha-adrenergic blockade is the basis of hypertensive therapy, and patients are generally treated 1 to 2 weeks before surgery with phenoxybenzamine (or labetalol or prazosin) that is tapered to produce a 10- to 15-mm Hg orthostatic blood pressure decrease; 1 to 2 weeks of pretreatment allows for intravascular volume repletion (diminished by excess endogenous catecholamines).
   5. Tachycardia may occur from unopposed beta-adrenergic receptor activation, and if the heart rate is >110 beats per minute, a beta-blocker should be added; beta-blockers should *not* be used before institution of alpha-adrenergic blockade. Elimination of vasodilatory effects of beta-receptors results in unopposed alpha-adrenergic vasoconstriction and may provoke hypertensive crisis, and the negative inotropic effects of beta-blockers may precipitate heart failure in the face of hypertension.
   6. Reflex tachycardia is less with prazosin or labetalol.
   7. Alpha-methylparatyrosine (an inhibitor of tyrosine hydroxylase, the rate-limiting enzyme in catecholamine production) may be used in patients who cannot tolerate alpha-adrenergic blockade (postural hypotension) and can be especially useful in patients with cardiomyopathy. Indeed, phenoxybenzamine and alpha-

methylparatyrosine in combination result in less tachy-cardia and less postoperative hypotension.

8. Arrhythmias are treated with standard antiarrhythmic agents (e.g., lidocaine).

9. Blood should be available for transfusion in the perioperative period, since pheochromocytomas are vascular tumors and bleeding is frequent.

10. Diuretics should be used sparingly, since intravascular volume is already constricted by catecholamines; conversely, overadministration of fluids can worsen heart failure.

11. Perioperatively, drugs that cause catecholamine release or potentiate catecholamine action are to be avoided (e.g., morphine can cause histamine-induced catecholamine release).

12. Postoperatively, patients need cardiovascular and metabolic monitoring.

13. Hypoglycemia may occur following tumor removal (loss of catecholamine-induced hyperglycemia).

14. Pain is best treated with meperidine, and benzodiazepines are useful for sedation.

15. Recurrent hypertension should suggest the possibility of residual tumor.

5

Environmental Disorders

■ I. BURNS

It is estimated that 2 million people are burned annually in the United States. Although most of these burns are minor, approximately 3% to 5% of burn injuries are life-threatening.

A. Pathophysiology
1. Partial-thickness burns involve heat damage to the epidermis or a portion of the dermis. The dermis contains sensory nerve endings, vascular supply, hair follicles, and sweat glands.
2. Full-thickness burns involve injury to tissue deep to the sweat glands and hair follicles. The presence of thrombosed blood vessels or charring is characteristic of full-thickness burns. However, final determination of burn depth may not be possible for several days following the injury.
3. Shock may develop due to transudation and sequestration of fluid in the burned areas and elsewhere in the body. Cardiac output may drop in major burns, due to myocardial dysfunction.

B. Predisposition
1. Burn injury is the second leading cause of death among children under age 12 years.
2. Children are more likely to suffer burns than are adults because of their greater vulnerability to accidents due to inability to recognize or react to hazardous situations. Half of all victims of hot water burns are children under age 5 years.

C. Clinical Presentation
1. Partial-Thickness Burns
    a. First-degree burn involves only the epidermis; there is blanching erythema but no bulla formation.
    b. Second-degree burn involves a portion of the dermis and produces edema and fluid exudation. Bulla formation is characteristic. These develop quickly after burn injury. Consider infection if bulla appear 18 hours or later after a burn occurs.
2. Full-Thickness Burns
    a. Third-Degree Burn. Surface is dry and inelastic. Skin surface may become white or gray. This burn will not regenerate from unburned edges.
    b. Fourth-Degree Burn: Extends beyond the depth of the skin to involve underlying muscle, tendons, vascular structures, periosteum, or bone.
3. Survival depends on the extent and depth of the burn, the age of the patient, and associated injuries.
4. Vascular effects in burned skin are immediate vasoconstriction followed by increased capillary permeability and plasma extravasation. Burned skin also permits increased insensible water loss.

D. Complications
1. Coagulation necrosis at the burn site produces an advantageous setting for bacterial growth. Infection is one of the most important causes of death in severe burn injury.
2. Gastric dilatation and adynamic ileus occur in major burns.
3. Acute hemolysis may occur due to heat damage of red blood cells.
4. Acute renal failure may occur as a result of shock.
5. Hypertension may be present in burn victims, especially children.
6. Multiorgan failure is the leading cause of death in patients with burns.
7. Manipulation of burn wounds has been shown to result in bacteremia in 20% of cases.

E. Treatment
1. Evaluate airway (see smoke inhalation, below), and perform endotracheal intubation if indicated by upper airway edema or deterioration of arterial blood gases. Endotracheal intubation is appropriate for any patients with acute burn injury who display respiratory distress.
2. Establish intravenous access.
3. Evaluate burned areas under sterile technique.

4. Assess for presence of other injuries, especially with burns associated with explosions.
5. Insert nasogastric tube (to treat ileus) and urinary catheter to monitor urine output.
6. Obtain baseline laboratory values: complete blood count (CBC), electrolytes, serum urea nitrogen (BUN), creatinine, glucose, arterial blood gases, and carboxyhemoglobin level.
7. Estimate extent of burned area.
    a. Rule of nines for body surface area (BSA)
        (1) Adults: arms 9% each; legs 18% each; head 9%; trunk 18% anterior, 18% posterior; genitalia 1%
        (2) Children: arms 9% each; legs 16% each; head 13%; trunk 18% anterior, 18% posterior; genitalia 1%
        (3) Infants: arms 9% each; legs 14% each; head 18%; trunk 18% anterior, 18% posterior; genitalia 1%
    b. Lund and Browder chart
        (1) More accurate in children
8. Classify severity of burn.
    a. Major burns
        (1) Partial-thickness burns >20% BSA in children or the elderly or 25% BSA in adults
        (2) Full thickness burns >10% BSA
        (3) Burns involving the face, hands, feet, or perineum that may produce functional or cosmetic impairment
        (4) Caustic chemical burns
        (5) High-voltage electrical injury (see below)
        (6) Burns complicated by inhalation injury (see below) or major trauma
    b. Moderate burns
        (1) Partial thickness burns of 10% to 20% BSA in children or the elderly or 15% to 25% BSA in adults
        (2) Full-thickness burns <10% BSA
9. Fluid resuscitation.
    a. Within the first 24 hours, administer isotonic balanced crystalloid solution according to the recommended formula:
        (1) Multiple formulas for fluid administration exist, which recommend 1 to 4 mL/kg/% burn to be administered within the first 24 hours.
        (2) One recommendation (the Parkland formula) is to administer 4 mL of crystalloid solution per

kilogram per percent BSA in the first 24 hours of treatment. Administer half this quantity within first the 8 hours following the burn, one fourth during the second 8 hours, and the remaining one fourth in the last 8 hours.

b. May administer colloid-containing solution as needed after 24 hours, at least 12.5 g of albumin for every liter of crystalloid administered.

c. Monitor urine output. The patient should have at least 50 mL/h in the adult (or 1 mL/kg ideal body weight) and 1 mL/kg/h in the child.

d. Inhalation injury may significantly increase fluid requirements.

10. Topical care

a. Initially, cover burned areas with dry sterile sheets.

b. Clean burned areas with water and mild soap (Dial or Ivory), and remove particulate matter from burn.

c. Debride any overtly necrotic skin.

d. Apply topical agents, such as silver sulfadiazine or mafenide acetate.

e. Apply biologic dressings and synthetic skin substitutes to achieve temporary wound closure.

11. Nutrition

a. Early enteral feeding may attenuate the hypermetabolic response by preserving the intestinal mucosal barrier.

b. High-protein diets appear preferable to conventional diets.

12. Escharotomy

a. Circumferential burns producing a constricting eschar may result in respiratory (thorax) or circulatory (extremities) impairment.

b. Escharotomy may be necessary:

(1) Chest: diminished respiratory excursion, hypoxemia, diminished tidal volume.

(2) Extremities: diminished pulse and deterioration of circulation distal to the burn.

c. Fasciotomy may be necessary with high-voltage electrical burns or with associated crush injury.

■ II. DECOMPRESSION ILLNESS AND AIR EMBOLISM

The occurrence of decompression illness has paralleled the increased popularity of sport diving and may also occur in commercial divers and tunnel workers.

A. Pathophysiology
   1. Decompression illness occurs when gas dissolved in body fluids separates to form bubbles as ambient pressure decreases. Nitrogen accumulates in tissue during a dive, the amount being dependent on the dive's depth and duration. When a diver ascends too rapidly and ambient pressure decreases, there is insufficient time for nitrogen to equilibrate, and gas bubbles form in tissue and the venous circulation. Symptoms of decompression illness then occur.
   2. Flying shortly after diving increases the risk of decompression illness, as decreased ambient pressure at high altitude promotes gas bubble formation.

B. Predisposition
   1. Patients who are older or obese have a higher incidence of decompression illness.
   2. Prior joint injury predisposes to development of decompression illness in that joint.
   3. Air embolism tends to occur more frequently in less experienced divers.

C. Clinical Presentation
   1. Decompression Illness
      a. The vast majority of patients exhibit symptoms immediately following diving, though the onset may be delayed 12 to 36 hours.
      b. The clinical manifestations of decompression sickness (DCS) can be divided into two major groups:
         (1) Type I DCS: pain only, usually involving the joints.
         (2) Type II DCS: involvement of the central nervous system (CNS). This type accounts for 10% to 25% of instances in the United States.
      c. The most frequent presentation (two thirds to three quarters of cases) involves joint pain.
         (1) Knees, shoulders, and elbows are most commonly involved.
         (2) There may be slight tenderness or edema, but the severity of pain is out of proportion to objective clinical findings.
      d. Cutaneous decompression illness produces pruritus, erythematous eruption, or mottling.
      e. Pulmonary involvement.
         (1) Symptoms include pleuritic substernal chest pain, dyspnea, and cough.
         (2) Physical examination is usually unremarkable.
      f. Circulatory collapse and death may result from serious decompression illness.

g. Spinal cord decompression illness produces back pain, paresthesias, weakness, or paralysis due to obstruction of epidural vertebral veins.

h. Cerebral decompression illness may present with headache, confusion, hallucinations, delirium, seizures, visual disturbance, or cranial nerve involvement (especially, for unknown reasons, cranial nerve VIII, producing vomiting, vertigo, tinnitus, and nystagmus).

2. Air Embolism

a. Cerebral air embolism is an important cause of death in divers.

b. Focal neurologic deficit occurring within 15 to 20 minutes of ascent is the most common presentation. Consider air embolism if immediate loss of consciousness occurs upon ascent.

c. Mediastinal emphysema, subcutaneous emphysema, or pneumothorax may be associated with cerebral air embolism.

d. Coronary embolization can produce acute myocardial infarction or cardiac arrest.

D. Complications

1. Persistent neurologic defect may result from CNS decompression illness.

2. Osteonecrosis may be a late consequence of bone involvement, but this is less commonly seen now than previously.

E. Treatment

1. For air embolism, maintain patient in left lateral decubitus Trendelenburg position.

2. Apply 100% oxygen by mask.

3. Administer normal saline intravenously as required.

4. Treat seizures and cardiac dysrhythmias in standard fashion.

5. Treatment of all patients with decompression illness and air embolism is with recompression in a hyperbaric chamber. Recompression may be beneficial for decompression illness even if treatment is delayed several days. Major complications of hyperbaric oxygen therapy:

a. Barotrauma (e.g., pneumothorax, sinus trauma)

b. Oxygen toxicity

c. Psychiatric (e.g., claustrophobia)

6. For the location of the closest hyperbaric chamber, contact the Diving Accident Network of Duke University at (919) 694-2948 or (919) 684-5514.

■ III. NEAR-DROWNING

Drowning acounts for 6000 to 8000 deaths each year in the United States. Children under age 4 comprise 40% of these fatalities. The peak incidence is during warm-weather months. Drowning is defined as suffocation in a liquid medium. Near-drowning is defined as at least temporary survival from such submersion.

A. Pathophysiology

1. Near-drowning may be accompanied by aspiration of fluids or may be primarily the consequence of asphyxia due to laryngospasm. Aspiration of large quantities of sea water produces hypovolemia and concentration of extracellular electrolytes, whereas substantial fresh water aspiration produces acute hypervolemia with dilution of extracellular electrolytes.

   Although the early medical literature emphasized pathophysiologic differences between fresh and salt water drowning, aspiration of significant quantities of fluid required to produce the hemodilution or electrolyte changes described does not occur in most human survivors. At least 85% of survivors of drowning are thought to aspirate <22 mL of water per kilogram of body weight.

2. The adverse respiratory effects of near-drowning include the following:

   a. Intrapulmonary shunting
   b. Ventilation-perfusion mismatch
   c. Decreased compliance
   d. Intra-alveolar influx of fluid due to capillary-alveolar leak
   e. Hypoxemia resulting from all of the above

3. Hypothermia associated with immersion may predispose patients to cardiac dysrhythmias and exhaustion.

B. Predisposition

1. Age distribution peaks of near-drowning victims.

   a. Children <4 years.
   b. Males aged 14 to 24 years.

2. Alcohol intoxication is related to a large proportion of adult drownings.

C. Clinical Presentation

1. Respiratory findings usually predominate and include shortness of breath, air hunger, and tachypnea.

   a. Auscultatory findings may include rales, rhonchi, or wheezes.
   b. Respiratory deterioration may occur insidiously.

    2. Changes in mental status may be due to cerebral hypoxemia or head injury.

    3. Cardiac dysrhythmias (premature beats, bradycardia, atrial fibrillation, asystole, ventricular fibrillation) result from hypoxemia or hypothermia.

    4. Consider the presence of hypothermia or trauma, especially cervical spine injury in appropriate settings.

D. Complications

    1. Cerebral end-organ damage due to hypoxemia mediated through cerebral edema and increased intracerebral pressure.

    2. Renal failure may be produced by acute tubular necrosis, hemoglobinuria, or myoglobinuria.

    3. Bronchial hyperreactivity may follow near-drowning.

    4. Hypoglycemia is common.

E. Admission Criteria

    1. Need for assisted ventilation

    2. Coma or obtundation

    3. Cardiac arrest or dysrhythmias

    4. Hypothermia

F. Treatment

    1. Clear airway, and ensure adequate respirations.

       a. Apply 100% oxygen by mask to patients with spontaneous respirations.

       b. Perform endotracheal intubation and mechanical ventilation in apnea and as directed by hypoxemia or hypercarbia or for protection of airway in coma.

       c. Initiate positive end-expiratory pressure (PEEP) at 3 to 5cm H_2O in mechanically ventilated patients. Increase as required to maintain arterial O_2 saturation (SaO_2) $\geq 90\%$.

       d. Monitor arterial saturation in all patients.

       e. Administer bronchodilators in standard fashion in patients with bronchoconstriction.

    2. Treat cardiac dysrhythmias as indicated. Obtain an electrocardiogrm (ECG) on all patients with near-drowning.

    3. Monitor body temperature, and treat hypothermia if present (see below).

    4. Obtain chest radiograph at presentation and repeat as indicated.

    5. If circulatory shock is present, monitor with a Swan-Ganz catheter.

    6. Consider bronchoscopy in patients who have aspirated particulate matter or contaminated water.

G. Prognosis
  1. Classification of the victim's neurological status allows systematic assessment of prognosis.
      a. Category A: awake, fully conscious
      b. Category B: stuporous but arousable
      c. Category C: comatose
  2. Eighty percent of near-drowning victims recover without sequelae, 2% to 9% survive with brain damage, and 12% die.

■ IV. ELECTRICAL INJURIES

Approximately 3% of burn injuries that require hospital admission are the result of electrical injury. Of these, approximately 40% are fatal.

A. Pathophysiology
  1. Injuries are classified as high voltage (>1000 volts) or low voltage (<1000 volts). High voltage are generally more severe injuries, but the degree of injury also depends on tissue resistance and type of current.
  2. Lightning produces current with many millions of volts, but exposure may be extremely brief.
  3. Electrical energy causes injury through release of heat within tissues.
  4. The severity of tissue damage is directly related to duration of contact.

B. Predisposition
  1. There is a high incidence of electrical injury among children <6 years; most are related to injury by electrical outlets and cords.
  2. Two thirds of injuries among adults (mostly males) involve electrical and construction workers.

C. Clinical Presentation
  1. Wounds occurring at sites where electricity enters and exits the body are typically small areas of full-thickness burn. There may be considerable underlying tissue damage that is poorly reflected by the extent of visible skin damage.
  2. Musculoskeletal injury results from tetanic contraction of skeletal muscle during exposure. Fractures or dislocations may occur. Heat injury may produce bony or periosteal destruction.

3. Electrical injury may produce vascular endothelial disruption, hemorrhage, arterial or venous thrombosis, or peripheral ischemia.
4. Cardiac dysrhythmias are a frequent cause of immediate death. Dysrhythmias may continue to appear within 24 hours of injury.
   a. Sinus tachycardia, supraventricular tachycardia, ventricular tachycardia, atrial fibrillation, atrioventricular (A–V) block, and intraventricular conduction delay may occur.
   b. Myocardial injury resulting from high-voltage injury is uncommon but may occur.
   c. The most common ECG alterations are nonspecific ST-T-wave changes and sinus tachycardia.
5. Gastrointestinal tract injuries include intestinal perforation and stress ulcer formation with gastrointestinal hemorrhage.
6. Signs of CNS injury include coma, confusion, disorientation, and seizures. Central respiratory center depression may occur.

D. Complications
   1. Renal failure may result from rhabdomyolysis.
   2. Delayed or long-term motor paralysis may be caused by injury to the central or peripheral nervous system. Other long-term neural deficits include personality changes, memory or concentration impairment, and depression.
   3. Cataracts may develop 6 to 12 months following electrical injury to the head. Other ophthalmic sequelae include corneal ulceration and retinal or optic nerve damage.

E. Admission Criteria
   ICU admission criteria include
   1. Thermal injury ≥20% BSA
   2. Suspicion of inhalation injury
   3. History of loss of consciousness
   4. Cardiac dysrhythmias
   5. Cardiopulmonary arrest
   6. Rhabdomyolysis

F. Treatment
   1. Clear the airway, and support respiration if necessary.
   2. Administer intravenous fluids as required to maintain a urine output of at least 50 to 100 mL/h or 1 mL/kg ideal body weight/h. Traditional burn formulas for fluid replacement are not applicable to electrical burns.
   3. Monitor the cardiac rhythm.

4. Obtain CBC, electrolytes, BUN, creatinine, prothrombin time (PT), partial thromboplastin time (PTT), myoglobin, creatine kinase (CK), urinalysis, 12-lead ECG.
5. If myoglobinuria appears, treat with mannitol and sodium bicarbonate (see Chapter 14, "Renal and Fluid-Electrolyte Disorders").
6. Obtain surgical consultation for debridement of deep tissue as necessary. Technetium scanning may identify areas of muscular injury.
7. Observe for development of sepsis, especially with *Pseudomonas* or *Clostridium* spp. (in instances of myonecrosis). Antibiotics should be given prophylactically, as should tetanus prophylaxis.

■ V. HEAT EXHAUSTION AND HEAT STROKE

Approximately 4000 deaths due to heat-related illness occur annually in the United States. Mortality rate of heat stroke may be 30% to 80%. Heat exhaustion and heat stroke do not represent distinct pathophysiologic entities but rather constitute heat-induced illnesses of varying severity.

A. Pathophysiology

Radiation of heat from the body accounts for approximately 65% of cooling, provided that the air temperature is lower than body temperature. This mechanism becomes less effective as ambient temperature approaches 35°C. Sweating with the ensuing evaporation produces in approximately 30% of cooling. As ambient temperature rises, this becomes the primary method of cooling. When air temperature exceeds body temperature, heat gain by radiation is possible. As relative humidity rises, evaporative heat loss diminishes. Heat illness is exacerbated by excessive fluid loss and electrolyte depletion.

Physiologic responses to increased body heat:
1. Cutaneous vasodilatation
2. Increased cardiac output to maintain blood pressure
3. Splanchnic vasoconstriction
4. Increased sweat volume

B. Predisposition
1. Neonates, who have poor thermoregulatory capability
2. The elderly, especially those with cardiac disease
3. Obese individuals
4. Underlying illnesses: congestive heart failure, coronary artery disease, hyperthyroidism, dermatologic disorders, major burns

      5. Medications and drugs: beta-adrenergic blockers, phe-
      nothiazines, lithium, cyclic antidepressants, antihistamines,
      amphetamines, cocaine, phencyclidine

C. Clinical Presentation
   1. Heat Exhaustion
      a. Temperature elevation, but temperature is generally
         <39°C.
      b. Symptoms: nausea, vomiting, headache, light-headed-
         ness, malaise, muscular cramping.
      c. Diaphoresis, tachycardia, hypotension, or orthostatic
         hypotension.
      d. Mental status is unimpaired.
   2. Heat Stroke
      a. Temperature is generally >40.5°C.
      b. Signs: tachypnea (respiratory rate as high as 60/min),
         tachycardia, hypotension.
      c. Dry, hot skin is classic, but not necessary to make the
         diagnosis. Lack of sweating may be a late finding, and
         diaphoretic skin is seen in about half of cases.
      d. Major diagnostic point: CNS dysfunction (confu-
         sion, bizarre behavior, delirium, obtundation, coma,
         seizures). Ataxia may result from cerebellar involve-
         ment. Most CNS deficits are reversible with treat-
         ment but may become fixed.

D. Complications
   1. Heat Stroke
      a. Muscular injury causing rhabdomyolysis.
      b. Hypoglycemia.
      c. Hypocalcemia (does not usually require specific
         treatment).
      d. Renal failure resulting from acute tubular necrosis
         or rhabdomyolysis (see Chapter 14, "Renal and
         Fluid-Electrolyte Disorders").
      e. Hepatocellular injury producing elevation of liver
         enzymes.
      f. Disseminated intravascular coagulation (DIC) may
         occur 1 to 3 days following onset of heat stroke.
      g. Adult respiratory distress syndrome (see Chapter 13,
         "Pulmonary Disorders").
      h. Neurologic: ataxia, dementia, cerebral edema, brain
         death.

E. Treatment
   1. Heat Exhaustion
      a. Place patient in a cool environment.
      b. Fluid replacement with normal saline or half-normal
         saline; amount to be guided by vital signs. Invasive

cardiovascular monitoring may be required, especially in older patients.

2. Heat Stroke

    a. Maintain airway and breathing. Administer intravenous fluids as directed by vital signs.

    b. Maintain continuous core temperature monitoring with rectal or esophageal probe.

    c. Initiate immediate vigorous cooling by one or more of the following measures:

        (1) Evaporative technique: Spray patient with warm water (15°C) and cool with fan. This method prevents cutaneous vasoconstriction and does not induce shivering. Requires low-humidity environment.

        (2) Ice packs to neck, axilla, and groin. Produces cooling in area of major vessels and is useful as an adjunct to other techniques.

        (3) Ice water bath: May cause cutaneous vasoconstriction. It is also difficult to monitor an immersed patient.

        (4) Iced gastric lavage.

        (5) Cool (6 to 10°C) peritoneal lavage.

        (6) Intermittent positive-pressure breathing (IPPB) with cold inhaled air.

        (7) Cardiopulmonary bypass (this method produces the most rapid cooling).

    d. Do not administer antipyretics (e.g., salicylates or acetaminophen).

    e. Administer D5%/half normal saline to replace fluid loss.

    f. Monitor central venous pressure, urine output, and urine for myoglobin.

    g. Follow oxygen saturation and chest radiograph to determine the development of pulmonary complications, coagulation studies for DIC, liver enzymes, creatine kinase, BUN, creatinine.

    h. May require paralysis and mechanical ventilation (especially if associated with amphetamine use).

    i. If shivering occurs with cooling, may administer chlorpromazine (25 to 50 mg IV). However, this must be done with care, as chlorpromazine may produce cardiac dysrhythmias, hypotension, or a neuroleptic malignant syndrome, which in itself produces hyperthermia.

    j. Dantrolene may be used, 1 mg/kg IV (may be increased to as high as 10 mg/kg). The mechanism appears to involve calcium-release inhibition in skeletal muscle. Muscular weakness may be produced. Further research into the use of this agent in heat stroke is required.

■ VI. HYPOTHERMIA

Normal core temperature is 36 to 37.5°C. Thermoregulation is controlled in the hypothalamus. Shivering is initiated in the anterior hypothalamus and is the body's most effective method to raise temperature.

Hypothermia may be divided into mild (body temperature 33 to 35°C), moderate (27 to 32°C), and severe (<27°C) forms. It is seen in a variety of circumstances.

Primary (accidental) hypothermia is caused by exposure to low environmental temperature. Secondary hypothermia occurs when heat conservation mechanisms are abnormal due to underlying disease. Induced hypothermia has been used as a therapeutic measure in certain neurosurgical and cardiovascular surgical procedures.

A. Pathophysiology

In secondary hypothermia, there may be interference with the hypothalamic temperature regulating center, or an inability to shiver, redistribute blood flow or move from a cold environment.

B. Predisposition

1. Infants and the elderly are most susceptible.
   a. Infants: large surface area to mass ratio, inability to protect selves from cool environment
   b. Elderly: decreased sensory temperature appreciation, deficient centrally mediated response to cold, failure to shiver, limited ability to vasoconstrict peripheral vessels

2. Drug use and intoxication:
   a. Agents that depress the level of consciousness (especially ethanol) are often related to exposure-related hypothermia.
   b. Barbiturates depress core temperature by central effect.
   c. Phenothiazines inhibit response to cold by alpha-adrenergic blocking activity and by direct suppression of the thermoregulatory center.

3. Preexisting illness: see Table 5.1.

C. Clinical Presentation

1. Initial sympathetic response (producing peripheral vasoconstriction and tachycardia) causes transient elevation of blood pressure and cardiac output.

Table 5.1. Illness Predisposing to Hypothermia

Pathologic Reduction of Metabolic Rate
   Hypothyroidism
   Hypopituitarism
   Hypoadrenalism

Alteration of Hypothalamic Function
   Anorexia nervosa
   Hypothalamic tumors
   Head trauma
   Cerebrovascular accident
   Wernicke's encephalopathy
   Sarcoidosis (involving the hypothalamus)

Other Mechanisms
   Hypoglycemia
   Spinal cord transection
   Extensive body surface burns
   Exfoliative erythrodermas
   Sepsis
   Severe protein malnutrition

      a. Increased renal perfusion produces increased urine production ("cold diuresis"), which may lead to hypovolemia, hemoconcentration, and increased blood viscosity.

      b. Response is ablated below 30°C.

  2. Clouding of sensorium regularly occurs at 30 to 32°C.

  3. Mild hypothermia: Tachypnea, tachycardia, shivering, amnesia, ataxia, dysarthria.

  4. Moderate hypothermia: Decreased level of consciousness, mydriasis, atrial fibrillation, bradycardia.

  5. Severe hypothermia: Absent reflexes and response to pain, coma, hypotension.

  6. Cardiac complications:

      a. Dysrhythmias: atrial fibrillation is common.

      b. Patients are increasingly susceptible to ventricular fibrillation with diminishing temperature. Below 28°C, even minor procedures, such as moving or repositioning the patient, may initiate ventricular fibrillation.

      c. Ventricular fibrillation is resistant to pharmacologic treatment or electrical defibrillation until temperature has increased.

      d. Susceptibility to ventricular dysrhythmias may persist for several days, even after normal body temperature has been restored.

      e. ECG changes include PR, QT, and QRS prolongation and J-point elevation ("Osborn wave").

D. Complications
   1. Morbidity and mortality are related to the degree and duration of hypothermia and to appropriate therapy.
   2. Bronchorrhea and depressed cough reflexes lead to bronchopneumonia and aspiration pneumonitis.
   3. Punctate hemorrhages may occur in the gastrointestinal tract, but significant bleeding is rare.
   4. Pancreatitis is common.
   5. Fatal disseminated intravascular coagulation may occur.

E. Treatment
   1. Cardiovascular
      a. Employ basic life support protocols to support ventilation and circulation.
      b. Perform endotracheal intubation and mechanical ventilation as indicated.
      c. Initiate cardiopulmonary resuscitation (CPR) if cardiac arrest is present. Continue until core temperature of 32°C is reached or response achieved.
      d. Ventricular fibrillation may be resistant to defibrillation in severe hypothermia. Attempt single defibrillation; if this is not successful, continue rewarming until temperature >30°C and administer bretylium 5 to 10 mg/kg IV over 5 to 10 minutes, then infusion of 2 mg/min.
   2. Rewarming
      a. For mild and moderate hypothermia (including most cases of secondary hypothermia), passive rewarming is indicated.
         (1) Remove patient from cold environment.
         (2) Apply dry, unheated blankets.
      b. For some cases of moderate hypothermia, use active surface rewarming.
         (1) Heating blankets, hot-water bottles, heat cradles, heat-fluidized beds, warm-water immersion.
         (2) Moderate hypothermia may be associated with afterdrop of core temperature as peripheral vasoconstriction is reversed, producing hypovolemic shock and ventricular fibrillation.
      c. For severe hypothermia, active core rewarming is indicated. Use one or more of the following:
         (1) Infusion of warmed intravenous fluids (temperature not to exceed 40°C).
         (2) Intubation and ventilation with warmed, humidified oxygen. Keep airway temperature <45°C.

(3) Peritoneal dialysis (usually requires 6 to 8 exchanges of potassium-free dialysate heated to 43°C).

(4) Gastric irrigation with warmed fluids with introduction of intragastric balloon. May provoke dysrhythmias.

(5) Mediastinal irrigation (operative technique).

(6) Extracorporeal blood rewarming with a heat exchanger at 40°C.

d. If the patient does not respond to rewarming, consider cerebral edema.

■ VII. SMOKE INHALATION AND CARBON MONOXIDE POISONING

Carbon monoxide (CO) intoxication is the leading cause of death by poisoning in the United States, accounting for 3800 accidental and suicidal deaths annually. It is also the most common cause of death in combustion-related inhalation injury. Many nonlethal exposures may, however, go undetected.

A. Pathophysiology
1. Carbon Monoxide Poisoning
   a. Carbon monoxide combines preferentially with hemoglobin to produce carboxyhemoglobin. This displaces oxygen and reduces systemic arterial content.
   b. Carbon monoxide binds reversibly to hemoglobin with an affinity over 200 times that of oxygen, so a relatively minute concentration of CO in the environment can lead to toxic concentrations in blood.
   c. Mechanisms of toxicity:
      (1) Decreased oxygen-carrying capacity of the blood.
      (2) Alteration of dissociation characteristics of oxyhemoglobin: Shifts oxyhemoglobin dissociation curve to the left.
      (3) Decreased cellular respiration due to binding with cytochrome c oxidase.
      (4) Binding to myoglobin, producing myocardial and skeletal muscle dysfunction.
   d. The half-life of carboxyhemoglobin at room air is 320 minutes; on 100% O_2 at 1 atmosphere, it is 60 minutes; and on 100% O_2 at 3 atmospheres, it is 23 minutes.

Table 5.2. Exogenous Sources of Carbon Monoxide

Smoke from all types of fires
Paint-remover containing methylene chloride
Furnaces
Gasoline-powered engines
Swimming pool heaters
Sterno fuel
Tobacco smoke
Vehicular exhaust fumes
Water heaters

Table 5.3. Acute CO Poisoning

COHb level	Symptoms
10%	Headache
20%	Dizziness, nausea, dyspnea
30%	Visual disturbances
40%	Confusion, syncope
50%	Seizures, coma
>60%	Cardiopulmonary failure and death

2. Smoke Inhalation
   a. Smoke contains carbon particles and various gases (including nitrogen oxide, chlorine, phosgene, ammonia, hydrogen cyanide).
   b. These gases adhere to the respiratory mucosa and produce compounds that are locally and systemically toxic.

B. Predisposition
   1. The most common sources of CO are listed in Table 5.2.
   2. Smoke inhalation from fires accounts for the vast majority of cases.
   3. Vapor of methylene chloride (contained in many paint removers) is readily absorbed through the lungs and is converted to CO by the liver.

C. Clinical Presentation
   1. Carbon Monoxide Poisoning
      a. Symptoms and signs in acute CO poisoning depend on carboxyhemoglobin (COHb) level (see Table 5.3).
         (1) Patients with COHb levels <10% are usually asymptomatic.
         (2) Patients with levels >25% should be considered for hospital admission.

(3) Those with levels >50% commonly have coma and seizures resulting from cerebral edema.

(4) Death is likely if levels >60%.

(5) Determination of treatment only on COHb level is inappropriate, though, because the level alone is a poor predictor of degree of injury. Therefore, clinical assessment is vital to planning treatment.

b. Chronic or subacute poisoning may present with less characteristic symptoms.

2. Smoke Inhalation

Suspect if:

a. Exposure occurred in a closed space.

b. There are facial or pharyngeal burns, or burned nasal vibrissae.

c. There is carbonaceous sputum or hoarseness.

D. Complications

1. Neuropsychiatric problems, such as memory loss, personality changes, mutism, and parkinsonism may occur as long-term sequelae to CO poisoning.

2. Indicators of a poor prognosis include altered level of consciousness, advanced age, metabolic acidosis, and structural abnormalities on computed tomography (CT) or magnetic resonance (MR) scanning.

E. Treatment

1. Carbon Monoxide Poisoning

a. Obtain the COHb level in all patients suspected of having CO exposure (e.g., all victims at a fire scene).

b. Apply supplemental oxygen 100% by mask while awaiting results.

(1) The goal is to improve blood oxygen content by maximizing the fraction dissolved in plasma.

(2) Monitor patients with serial COHb levels. Continue 100% oxygen until the COHb level is <5%. Continue to monitor COHb level thereafter to guard against undetected release of CO from tissue sites.

c. Obtain an ECG, and monitor with serial CK levels if the ECG is suggestive of ischemia.

d. Consider treatment with hyperbaric oxygen (HBO) in the following patients:

(1) Patients with serious CO poisoning (e.g., coma, neurologic deficit, cardiac or hemodynamic instability, history of loss of consciousness)

(2) Pregnant women

          (3) Patients with underlying heart disease or abnormal ECG

   e. Whether HBO alters outcome is still controversial.

   f. If HBO treatment is unavailable, consider intubation and mechanical ventilation with administration of 100% oxygen if clinical findings merit.

   g. Consider transfusion with packed red blood cells in severe poisoning.

2. Smoke Inhalation

   a. If findings of smoke inhalation are present, evaluate the airway with fiberoptic bronchoscopy.

   b. Obtain arterial blood gases and chest radiograph.

   c. Administer humidified oxygen.

   d. Perform early endotracheal intubation in the presence of upper airway edema.

■ VIII. SCORPION ENVENOMATION

Scorpions are arachnids that typically inhabit temperate climates. The only dangerous species of scorpion in the United States is the *Centruroides* genus, which is found primarily in the southwestern states (Arizona, California, New Mexico, Texas).

A. Pathophysiology

   The venom is complex and contains a number of proteins, polypeptides and enzymes (e.g., hyaluronidases, phospholipases), and neurotoxins. The venom affects sodium channels to prolong action potentials and produce spontaneous neural depolarizations of the sympathetic and parasympathetic systems.

B. Predisposition

   Most serious envenomations occur in children.

C. Clinical Presentation

1. The most common finding is severe local pain at the site of the sting. In most cases, this resolves within several hours. There is severe tenderness to palpation or percussion over the site.

2. The sting may be accompanied by wheal and flare reaction, paresthesias at site of sting.

3. Significant envenomation produces tachycardia, hypertension, restlessness, hyperexcitability, diaphoresis, piloerection, nystagmus, diplopia, opisthotonos, muscular fasciculations, or hypersalivation.

4. The most severe cases produce seizures, pulmonary edema, muscular paralysis, respiratory arrest, cardiovascular collapse, and death.

Table 5.4. Severity of *Centruroides* Scorpion Envenomation

Grade	Signs and symptoms
I	Local pain or paresthesias at site; tenderness to touch or percussion
II	Local findings and pain and paresthesias remote from sting site
III	Symptomatic skeletal neuromuscular dysfunction (muscular jerking or shaking) or cranial nerve dysfunction (e.g., blurred vision, difficulty swallowing, hypersalivation, slurred speech, tongue fasciculations)
IV	Somatic skeletal *and* cranial nerve dysfunction

    D. Complications

       These include DI, pancreatitis, jaundice, and renal failure.

    E. Treatment

       1. Maintain airway, and assist ventilations if necessary.

       2. Clean the wound, and administer tetanus prophylaxis if indicated. Do not cool or incise wound.

       3. Classify *Centruroides* sting by severity of involvement according to Table 5.4.

          a. Grade I and II envenomation: Wound care as above, and provide oral analgesics.

          b. Grade III and IV: An antivenin has been produced but is not generally available. Contact your regional poison control center or Central Arizona Regional Poison Management (602) 253-3334. Sedate and provide supportive care. High doses of phenobarbital have been recommended, but care must be taken to prevent respiratory failure.

          c. Treat severe tachycardia with labetolol 10 to 20 mg IV.

    F. Prognosis

       1. Though deaths may occur, none has been reported in the United States since 1968.

       2. If untreated, the sting may be lethal in 1% of adults and as many as 25% of children under age 5 years.

■ IX. SNAKEBITE

Approximately 8000 instances of poisonous snakebite occur annually in the United States, with 9 to 15 deaths resulting. Most bites occur in the southern and southwestern states, with a peak incidence during the summer months.

There are four venomous species in the United States: rattlesnakes (genus *Crotalus* and *Sistruris*), copperheads (*Agkistrodon contortrix*), and cottonmouths (*Agkistrodon piscivorus*)—all of which are pit vipers—and coral snakes (genus *Micrurus*). Rattlesnakes account for 65% of reported venomous snake bites.

A. Pathophysiology

Snake venoms are complex mixtures of toxins that have cytotoxic, hemotoxic, and neurotoxic components. Cytotoxic effects produce tissue necrosis. Hemotoxic venoms interfere with the coagulation system. Rattlesnakes are classically considered to have cytotoxic and hemotoxic venom, but neurotoxic activity may also be present. Coral snake venom has largely neurotoxic activity.

• Snakes are capable of controlling the quantity of venom administered, and approximately 25% to 30% of bites by poisonous snakes do not result in envenomation.

B. Predisposition

1. The majority of victims are males younger than age 20.
2. Severity of a bite depends on
   a. Size and species of snake
   b. Location of bite
   c. Grade of envenomation (see below)
   d. Age and medical condition of the patient

C. Clinical Presentation

1. Pit Vipers
   a. The most important findings of pit viper envenomation are fang punctures at the bite site (usually on the extremities), local pain, and adjacent erythema and edema.
      (1) Edema and erythema are characteristic and usually develop within 30 minutes of envenomation.
      (2) May spread for following 24 hours and develop hemorrhagic bullae.
      (3) If no erythema or edema develops within 4 hours of bite, it is unlikely that envenomation has occurred.
   b. Grade the severity of the bite according to the criteria in Table 5.5.
   c. Swelling resulting from edema and capillary rupture may produce increased fascial compartment pressure.
   d. Severe envenomation produces hypotension due to hemorrhage and third-space fluid loss, shock, pares-

Table 5.5. Severity of Pit Viper Envenomation

Grade	Envenomation	Findings
O	None	Fang marks; minimal pain; <2.5 cm circumferential edema
I	Minimal	2.5–12.5 cm edema and erythema in first 12 hours
II	Moderate	15–36 cm edema and erythema in first 12 hours
III	Severe	Edema >36 cm in 24 hours; systemic symptoms (including coagulation defects) present
IV	Very severe	Systemic symptoms; rapid development of edema, erythema; ecchymoses, bullae; coagulation defects

thesias, and muscular fasciculations. Nausea, vomiting, giddiness, and elevation or depression of temperature may be produced. Coma, convulsions, and death may result.

    e. Hematologic sequelae of severe envenomation include anemia due to hemolysis, hypothrombinemia, thrombocytopenia, hypofibrinogenemia, and hypercoagulability. Gastrointestinal, urinary tract, or intracerebral hemorrhage may result.

    f. CNS effects include seizures, coma, and respiratory paralysis.

  2. Coral Snakes

    a. Coral snake bites do not produce prominent swelling or other local findings.

    b. Neurotoxic venom may cause ptosis, diplopia, dysphagia, dysarthria, salivation, paresthesias, muscular fasciculations, loss of deep tendon reflexes, muscular weakness, and respiratory paralysis.

    c. Onset of symptoms may be delayed by 1 to 5 hours following the bite.

    d. Grade the severity of the bite according to the criteria in Table 5.6. Repeat the evaluation every 15 minutes for the first 4 hours following the bite.

D. Complications

  1. Renal failure may result from DUC or acute tubular necrosis.

  2. Anaphylaxis and serum sickness are potential complications of treatment with antivenin.

E. Treatment

  1. Pit Viper

Table 5.6. Severity of Coral Snake Envenomation

Grade	Envenomation	Findings within 36 hours of bite
O	None	Minimal local swelling; no systemic symptoms
I	Moderate	Systemic symptoms but no respiratory paralysis
II	Severe	Complete respiratory paralysis

   a. Wound care:
     (1) Do not apply ice to bite.
     (2) Use of tourniquets, incision, and suction are traditional but controversial modalities.
     (3) Measure circumference of bitten extremity, and repeat measurement each hour. With massive swelling, measurement of intrafascial pressure may be indicated.
   b. Obtain CBC, platelet count, PT, PTT, thrombin time, fibrinogen level, fibrin split products, electrolytes, BUN, and creatinine. These values should be repeated every 4 hours.
   c. Type and cross match for 4 U packed red blood cells.
   d. Administer intravenous normal saline as indicated by hypotension. Institute Swan-Ganz catheter monitoring in hemodynamically unstable patients.
   e. Antivenin
     (1) Perform skin or eye test for horse serum hypersensitivity. If negative, may proceed with antivenin administration. If positive, consider risk of envenomation against possibility of anaphylactic reaction. In severe envenomation, may precede antivenin infusion with 250 mg methylprednisolone IV. Be prepared to treat anaphylaxis (see Chapter 18, "Allergic and Immunologic Emergencies").
     (2) No universally accepted standard recommendations for antivenin administration exist. Controversy about its use exist.
     (3) No antivenin is required for grades 0 or I pit viper bites.
     (4) Administer to grades II to IV bites. Test dose: 0.2 to 0.5 mL IV over 5 minutes; if no adverse effect, administer remainder over 30 minutes to 2 hours. Individualize dosage to severity and

rate of progression: grade II, up to 5 vials; grade III:, 5 to 15 vials; grade IV, 15 to 20 vials.

    (5) Observe the patient for 3 to 5 hours after initial administration; administer an additional vial every 1 to 2 hours if pain persists or swelling progresses.

  f. Use of fasciotomy in severe envenomation with increased intrafascial pressure is controversial. This may be necessary if intrafascial pressure >30 torr. Obtain surgical consultation as required in instances of massive edema.

  2. Coral Snakes

    a. An antivenin is available for bites of Eastern coral snakes. Administer antivenin to all bite victims of this snake, even before appearance of symptoms. Dosage is 3 to 6 vials in 300 to 500 mL normal saline.

    b. There is no antivenin available for bites of the Arizona coral snake.

    c. Perform endotracheal intubation if there are any signs of bulbar paralysis, such as diplopia or dysphagia.

    d. Institute respiratory support with mechanical ventilation as required. Antivenin may not completely reverse respiratory depression.

■ X. SPIDER BITE

A. Black Widow Spider

The black widow spider is a member of the *Latrodectus* genus and is found throughout the United States. The female, larger and more dangerous than the male, is black or brown, with a characteristic red hourglass marking on the ventral abdomen.

  1. Pathophysiology

Black widow venom is extremely potent. The major activity of the venom lies in provoking the release of catecholamines at adrenergic synaptic terminals and depletion of acetylcholine from motor nerve endings.

  2. Predisposition

There is a high risk for mortality among the following patients:

    a. Patients younger than 16 or older than 65 years.

    b. Those with hypertension or cardiovascular disease (envenomation may cause heart failure, cerebrovascular accident or myocardial ischemia).

3. Clinical Presentation
   a. Pain at the bite site may be minimal, but severe pain may develop in the extremity, along with painful lymphadenopathy, erythema, swelling, and piloerection 20 to 60 minutes following the bite.
   b. Cramping and painful muscular contractions in the back, thigh, abdomen, and chest produce abdominal rigidity, tonic contractions, and tremor.
   c. There may be restlessness, weakness, dizziness, urinary retention, diaphoresis, salivation, nausea, vomiting, priapism, and hypertension.
   d. Distinction must be made from the acute abdomen: despite rigidity, there is minimal tenderness and no rebound tenderness.
4. Complications
   a. Hypertensive crisis
   b. Paralysis and respiratory arrest (especially in children)
   c. Severe envenomation may produce shock and/or coma
5. Treatment
   a. Clean wound, and apply cool compresses (not ice) to the bite site.
   b. Administer diazepam (5 to 10 mg IV q3h as needed) and methocarbamol (1000 mg IV no faster than 100 mg/min, and 1000 mg additionally as IV infusion) for symptomatic treatment of muscular spasm.
   c. Calcium gluconate 10% (1 to 2 mL/kg IV over 20 minutes, maximum 10 mL) may also provide relief of muscular spasm, but this is transient, lasting <30 minutes.
   d. Treat elevated blood pressure if diastolic blood pressure >130 torr (see Chapter 3, "Cardiovascular Disorders").
   e. Antivenin
      (1) Administration of antivenin is recommended for symptomatic patients <16 or >65 years old, those with preexisting hypertension or cardiovascular disease, and those displaying respiratory distress, pronounced hypertension, or persistent severe muscular symptoms despite above treatment.
      (2) Before administration, skin test for horse serum sensitivity (included with antivenin).
      (3) Administer 1 vial antivenin diluted in 50 mL normal saline over 15 to 30 minutes. A

second vial will be required only in severe cases.

6. Prognosis
   a. Prognosis for recovery with treatment is good, and deaths are rare.
   b. There is a 0.5% incidence of anaphylaxis and a 2% incidence of serum sickness associated with antivenin use.

B. BROWN RECLUSE SPIDER

The Brown Recluse spider is of the *Loxosceles* species and is present throughout the southern United States. It is tan or brown, with a violin-shaped mark on the dorsum of the cephalothorax.

1. Pathophysiology

   The venom contains a variety of enzymes, including hyaluronidase, protease, collagenase, and sphingomyelinase D, which are thought to be responsible for dermal necrosis and hemolysis.

2. Predisposition

   Most severe envenomations occur in children.

3. Clinical Presentation
   a. Local pain and burning, bulla formation at site of bite, becoming necrotic over hours to days.
   b. Systemic signs and symptoms: fever, chills, petechiae, nausea, vomiting, and weakness.
   c. Severe cases may produce hemolysis, disseminated intravascular coagulation, thrombocytopenia, jaundice, or shock.

4. Complications
   a. Severe hemolysis may result in death.
   b. Renal failure may result from hemoglobinuria or myoglobinuria.

5. Treatment
   a. There is no commercially available antivenin available in the United States.
   b. Begin intravenous infusion with normal saline.
   c. Obtain CBC, platelet count, electrolytes, BUN, creatinine, PT, PTT, and urinalysis.
   d. Clean the wound, and administer tetanus prophylaxis if indicated. Do not cool or incise wound.
   e. Some recommend the use of dapsone (50 to 200 mg/d), a leukocyte inhibitor, which relieves pain and reduces erythema and induration. Do not administer to children.
   f. Obtain surgical consultation for wound care.

■ XI. USEFUL FACTS AND FORMULAS

A. Temperature

Temperature conversion calculations are often done in the management of critically ill patients. Degrees *Celsius* (°C) and *Fahrenheit* (°F) are most commonly utilized:

°C to °F
°F = (°C × 9/5) + 32

°F to °C
°C = (°F − 32) × 5/9

Occasionally, the *Kelvin* (K) temperature scale is used, primarily in gas law calculations:

K to °C
K = °C + 273

B. Humidity

Relative humidity (RH) is usually measured by hygrometers, thus, eliminating the need of extracting and measuring the humidity content of the air samples:

$$RH = \frac{Content[mg/L \text{ or } mm\,Hg]}{Capacity[mg/L \text{ or } mm\,Hg]} = \%$$

The *humidity deficit* (HD) represents the maximum humidity capacity at body temperature:

HD = Capacity − content = mg/L

where *capacity* = the amount of water the alveolar air can hold at body temperature (also known as absolute humidity); and *content* = the humidity content of inspired air.

The humidity capacity of saturated gases is depicted in Table 5.7

C. Pressure

Pressure is defined as force per unit area, and there are various ways of measuring this force. One way that force can be recorded is in a form of the height of a column, as in the mercury barometer; therefore, it can be recorded in milliliters of mercury (mm Hg) pressure or centimeters of water pressure. To convert *cm H_2O to mm Hg*:

cm H_2O × 0.735 = mm Hg

To convert *mm Hg to cm H_2O*:

mm Hg × 1.36 = cm H_2O

A less commonly used conversion in clinical medicine includes converting *psi to mm Hg*:

Table 5.7. Humidity Capacity of Saturated Gases From 0 to 43°C

Gas temperature (°C)	Water content (mg/L)	Water vapor pressure (mmHg)
0	4.9	4.6
5	6.8	6.6
10	9.4	9.3
17	14.5	14.6
18	15.4	15.6
19	16.3	16.5
20	17.3	17.5
21	18.4	18.7
22	19.4	19.8
23	20.6	21.1
24	21.8	22.4
25	23.1	23.8
26	24.4	25.2
27	25.8	26.7
28	27.2	28.3
29	28.8	30.0
30	30.4	31.8
31	32.0	33.7
32	33.8	35.7
33	35.6	37.7
34	37.6	39.9
35	39.6	42.2
36	41.7	44.6
37	43.9	47.0
38	46.2	49.8
39	48.6	52.5
40	51.1	55.4
41	53.7	58.4
42	56.5	61.6

$Psi \times 51.7 = mmHg$

Other useful pressure-related formulas/facts include the following:

Total Pressure $= P_1 + P_2 + P_3 + \ldots$ *(Dalton's law)*

$$
\begin{aligned}
1 \text{ atmosphere} &= 760\,mmHg \\
&= 29.921\,in\,Hg \\
&= 33.93\,ft\,H_2O \\
&= 1034\,cm\,H_2O \\
&= 1034\,gm/cm^2 \\
&= 14.7\,lb/in^2
\end{aligned}
$$

Useful pressure/volume relationships that can be used in the management of critically ill patients include

Table 5.8. Factors for Converting Gas Volumes From Atps to Btps

Gas temperature (°C)	Factors to convert to 37°C saturated	Water vapor pressure (mmHg)
18	1.112	15.6
19	1.107	16.5
20	1.102	17.5
21	1.096	18.7
22	1.091	19.8
23	1.085	21.1
24	1.080	22.4
25	1.075	23.8
26	1.068	25.2
27	1.063	26.7
28	1.057	28.3
29	1.051	30.0
30	1.045	31.8
31	1.039	33.7
32	1.032	35.7
33	1.026	37.7
34	1.020	39.9
35	1.014	42.2
36	1.007	44.6
37	1.000	47.0
38	0.993	49.8
39	0.986	52.5
40	0.979	55.4
41	0.971	58.4
42	0.964	61.6

Table 5.9. Changes in Density With Altitude Assuming a Constant Temperature

Altitude (Feet)	Standard temperature (°C)	Density ratio Constant temperature	Density ratio Standard temperature
0	15.00	1.0000	1.0000
5000	5.09	0.8320	0.8617
10000	−4.81	0.6877	0.7385
15000	−14.72	0.5643	0.6292

$$\text{Volume}_{BTPS} = \text{Volume}_{ATPS} \times \text{Factor}$$

where $Volume_{BTPS}$ = the gas volume saturated with water at body temperature (37°C) and ambient pressure (BTPS = barometric temperature pressure saturation); $Volume_{ATPS}$ =

the gas volume saturated with water at ambient (room) temperature and pressure (ATPS = ambient temperature pressure saturation); *Factor* = the factors for converting gas volumes from ATPS to BTPS:

$$\text{Conversion factor} = \frac{P_B - PH_2O}{P_B - 47} \times \frac{310}{(273 + °C)}$$

Table 5.8 depicts the conversions factors required to convert Atps to Btps.

D. Altitude

As altitude varies, changes in atmospheric pressure produce alterations in gas density (see Table 5.9).

6

Gastrointestinal Disorders

■ I. GASTROINTESTINAL BLEEDING

A. Classification
   1. Upper gastrointestinal (GI) bleeding is above the ligament of Treitz.
   2. Lower GI bleeding is below the ligament of Treitz.

B. Etiology
   The most common causes of acute GI bleeding requiring admission to the intensive care unit (ICU) are depicted in Table 6.1. The most common sources of GI bleeding in the ICU are gastroduodenal stress ulcerations.

C. Diagnostic Evaluation
   1. History
      Although the history and physical in a critically ill patient with acute GI bleeding may be limited by the patient's clinical condition, the following are points that need to be investigated:
      a. History of hematemesis or melena
      b. Time of onset
      c. Amount of blood
      d. Color and character
      e. Drug or alcohol use (i.e., nonsteroidal anti-inflammatory drug [NSAID], prednisone, coumadin)
      f. Past medical history (i.e., cirrhosis, peptic ulcer disease [PUD], inflammatory bowel disease [IBD], etc.)
   2. Physical Examination
      The precise cause of acute GI bleeding is unlikely to be evident from physical examination alone (except in

Table 6.1. Etiologies of Acute GI Bleeding

Upper	Lower
Esophagus	Small intestine
Mucosal tear	Arteriovenous malformations
Esophageal rupture	Inflammatory bowel disease ischemia
Esophagitis	Meckel's diverticulum
Neoplasms	Neoplasms
Varices	
Stomach	Large intestine
Arteriovenous malformations	Diverticulosis
Gastritis (any etiology)	Hemorrhoids
Neoplasms	Inflammatory bowel disease infections
Peptic ulcer disease	Ischemia
Stress ulcers	Neoplasms
Duodenum	
Arteriovenous malformations	
Neoplasms (*rare*)	
Peptic ulcer disease	

chronic liver disease, Osler-Rendu-Weber syndrome, or hemorrhoids).

  a. General Appearance: This may vary from the patient in no acute distress to the patient in hypovolemic shock.

  b. Vital Signs: Tachycardia, postural hypotension. An increase in heart rate of 10 to 20 beats per minute and drop in blood pressure of >20 mm Hg upon assumption of an upright position are generally indicative of significant, acute volume loss.

  c. Other Signs of Hypovolemia: Altered mental status, low urine output.

  d. Associated Findings: Petechiae, jaundice, hepatomegaly, and splenomegaly.

  e. Rectum: Look for hemorrhoids, fissures, etc. Examine stools for blood even if the patient has an upper GI source.

3. A nasogastric (NG) tube should be placed in *all* patients with acute GI bleeding. The major advantages and disadvantages of NG tubes are shown in Table 6.2.

4. Laboratory Evaluation

All patients admitted to the ICU with GI bleeding should undergo the laboratory tests depicted in Table 6.3.

5. Radiologic Evaluation

All patients should undergo chest radiograph and abdominal x-rays. These may show evidence of perfora-

Table 6.2. Advantages and Disadvantages of NG Tubes in Acute GI Bleeding

Advantages	Disadvantages
1. Document the presence or absence of blood.	1. Patient discomfort.
2. Monitor rate of bleeding.	2. Irritation of esophageal and/or gastric mucosa.
3. To lavage and decompress the stomach.	3. Increased incidence of sinusitis.
	4. Possible esophageal or gastric perforation.

Table 6.3. Initial Laboratory Evaluation in GI Bleeding

Complete blood count (H/H should be repeated every 4 hours until patient is stable or bleeding has been controlled)

BUN, creatinine, and electrolytes

PT, PTT

Type and cross-match for 2–8 U of PRBCs, FFP

Other tests are ordered according to suspected or known underlying disease (i.e., LFTs, CK, etc.)

Abbreviations: BUN, blood urea nitrogen; CK, creatine kinase; FFP, fresh-frozen plasma; H/H, hemoglobin/hematocrit; LFT, liver function tests; PRBCs, packed red blood cells; PT, prothrombin time; PTT, partial thromboplastin time.

tion or obstruction and may indicate ischemic changes. Contrast studies have a low diagnostic yield and may be hazardous for the critically ill patient. They may also interfere with other diagnostic studies (i.e., endoscopy, angiography). Special tests may be required in the evaluation of acute GI bleeding. These include:

   a. Selective angiography may be used as a diagnostic as well as therapeutic tool (e.g., embolization). A bleeding rate at the time of the procedure ≥0.5 mL/min is needed for diagnosis.
   a. Radionuclide scans are sensitive in detecting lesions with lower bleeding rates.

6. Endoscopy is indicated in the vast majority of patients requiring ICU admission for GI bleeding.
   a. Upper endoscopy is indicated when blood is obtained from the NG tube or when frank hematemesis is present.

      b. Flexible sigmoidoscopy should be performed initially if lower GI bleeding is suspected. If this is not diagnostic, colonoscopy should be considered.

D. Initial ICU Management

   1. As in any critically ill patient, the management of acute GI bleeding starts with assessment of the airway, breathing, and circulation (ABCs). A low threshold for endotracheal intubation is recommended in the event of clouding of consciousness or overt shock, to prevent aspiration.

   2. Insert at least 2 large-bore (16-gauge) IV catheters.

   3. Infuse blood, plasma expanders, and/or normal saline to maintain a mean arterial pressure ≥65 mm Hg.

   4. Some authors recommend NG placement in all patients with GI bleeding and lavage of the stomach until the return is clear.

   5. Correction of preexisting coagulopathy (i.e., fresh frozen plasma [FFP], vitamin K, etc.).

   6. H_2-receptor blockers may prevent further hemorrhage. Continuous infusions are preferred (i.e., ranitidine [Zantac] 150 to 300 mg/24 hours IV infusion if the renal function is normal or famotidine [Pepcid] 20 mg IV q12h).

   7. Once the patient's condition is stable, endoscopic and/or angiographic verification of the source of bleeding will allow more definitive therapy.

E. Specific Management of Selected Conditions

   1. Variceal Hemorrhage

      a. Vasopressin Infusion: Start at 0.2 to 0.4 U/min (up to 1 U/min). Some of the major complications of vasopressin (i.e., myocardial ischemia) can be prevented by the co-administration of nitroglycerin.

      b. Sclerotherapy: Indicated at the time of diagnostic endoscopy. Two or three treatments are usually done within a 10-day period.

      c. Balloon Tamponade: Temporizing measure only. It is usually reserved for hemorrhage that fails to stop after therapy with vasopressin and sclerotherapy. Use Sengstaken-Blakemore or Minnesota tubes.

      d. Surgical Therapy: Every patient with a major esophageal bleed should receive surgical consultation in case an emergent intervention is needed. Indications for surgical therapy include the following:

        (1) Child's class A or B patient in whom vital signs can not be stabilized medically.

        (2) Continuous bleeding for ≥48 hours despite sclerotherapy and balloon tamponade.

(3) Third acute episode of esophageal bleeding in spite of previous sclerotherapy.
2. Hemorrhage From Ulcers and Erosive Lesions
   a. Endoscopy therapy with sclerosing agents, or laser coagulation, or heater probe.
   b. Surgical intervention is indicated in cases of
      (1) Visible vascular pedicle on endoscopy
      (2) Transfusion of ≥6 U blood in 24 hours
      (3) Arterial spurting
3. Active Lower GI Bleeding
   a. If a lesion is reachable with sigmoidoscopy or colonoscopy, local therapy may be attempted (e.g., laser coagulation).
   b. Arterial embolization is indicated if the above fails.
   c. All patients with active lower GI bleeding should receive surgical consultation in case an emergent intervention is needed.

■ II. ACUTE MESENTERIC ISCHEMIA

A. Definition
   Acute mesenteric ischemia (AMI) is an acute reduction in blood flow to the intestine leading to inadequate perfusion. AMI may be a reflection of generalized poor perfusion, or it may result from local pathology.

B. Epidemiology
   The incidence of AMI has increased over the past few decades. The rising incidence may be attributable to advances in medical technology and to new therapies extending the life of critically ill patients who are prone to develop AMI (e.g., elderly). The mortality in AMI is between 55% and 100%.

C. Etiology
   1. Occlusive
      a. Atherosclerotic narrowing of the mesenteric bed
      b. Systemic emboli from any source (e.g., endocarditis)
      c. Vasculitis
   2. Nonocclusive
      a. Splanchnic Vasoconstriction
         (1) Hypovolemia
         (2) Hypotension
         (3) Low cardiac output
         (4) Vasopressor agents use

Table 6.4. Risk Factors for the Development of AMI

— Age $\geq$50 years

— Atherosclerotic heart disease

— Congestive heart failure

— Recent myocardial infarction

— Valvular heart disease

D. Risk Factors for AMI

The most common predisposing conditions are depicted in Table 6.4.

E. Diagnostic Evaluation

1. History and Physical Examination

The classic complaint of severe abdominal pain that is out of proportion to the findings of physical examination, in our experience, is rarely seen. If peritoneal signs are present (e.g., rebound tenderness), intestinal infarction is likely to have occurred. Abdominal distention, emesis, and other signs of intestinal obstruction may occur in patients with AMI *in situ.* Lower GI bleeding may occur.

2. Laboratory Studies Reveal

a. Leukocytosis in 75% of patients

b. Metabolic acidosis

c. Elevated amylase, creatine kinase (CK) (6 to 12 hours after infarction has occurred), lactate, and phosphate

3. Radiologic Evaluation

a. Plain Abdominal X-Rays

(1) Useful in excluding other causes of abdominal pain (i.e., mechanical obstruction, perforation)

(2) Seventy percent of patients will show at least one of the following:

(a) Ileus

(b) Ascites

(c) Small bowel dilation

(d) Separation of small bowel loops

(e) Thickening of *valvulae conniventes*

(f) Thumb printing

b. Barium studies are *contraindicated* in these patients, and they interfere with arteriography.

c. Arteriography: For adequate study, the patient needs to be hemodynamically stable. Early use of this test is the key to diagnosis. It provides a "road map" for the surgeon.

F. Therapy
1. As in any critically ill patient, the management of AMI starts with assessment of the ABCs.
2. Adequate hydration. If necessary place a Swan-Ganz catheter to maximize cardiac output, oxygen delivery, and volume status.
3. Patients with suspected embolic or thrombotic occlusion should undergo *urgent* laparotomy for possible resection. Heparin and broad-spectrum antibiotic are indicated before surgery. Most patients will undergo a "second-look" operation within 24 hours of the initial laparotomy.
4. In those cases with nonocclusive AMI, intra-arterial infusions of vasodilators (e.g., papaverine 30 to 60 mg/h) are advocated by some.

■ III. FULMINANT HEPATIC FAILURE AND ENCEPHALOPATHY

A. Definition
1. Acute Fulminant Hepatic Failure
   Acute fulminant hepatic failure (FHF) is defined as acute liver failure associated with the development of hepatic encephalopathy within 8 weeks of the onset of symptoms attributable to hepatocellular dysfunction. This definition assumes that there is no preexisting liver disease.
2. Hepatic Encephalopathy
   Hepatic encephalopathy (HE) is a complex neuropsychiatric syndrome precipitated by abnormal liver function. This syndrome is a feature of acute and/or chronic hepatocellular failure.

B. Etiology
   Common causes of FHF and HE are depicted in Table 6.5.

C. Diagnostic Evaluation
1. History
   A detailed history should be obtained from family members. The following points need to be investigated:
   a. History of preexisting liver disease
   b. Drug or alcohol use
   c. Toxin exposure or ingestion
2. Physical Examination
   This may vary from the patient in no distress to the patient in overt shock.

Table 6.5. Causes of Acute Liver Failure

1. Viral Hepatitis (i.e., A, B, C)

2. Drugs or Toxins
   Acetaminophen
   Acute alcohol intoxication
   Carbon tetrachloride
   Halothane
   Isoniazid
   Monoamine oxidase inhibitors
   Mushroom poisoning

3. Fatty liver of pregnancy

4. Shock of any etiology

5. Massive liver infiltration (i.e., leukemia)

6. Decompensation of chronic liver failure

Table 6.6. Clinical Stages of Hepatic Encephalopathy

Stage	Neurological Findings
I	Confusion, mild changes in personality, psychometric defects
II	Drowsiness to lethargy
III	Somnolent but arousable
IV	Coma

    a. Vital signs: tachycardia, hypotension.

    b. Associated findings: petechiae, jaundice, hepato-megaly, splenomegaly.

    c. The encephalopathy may begin with confusion, disorientation, and irrational behavior. Coma may develop rapidly. (See Table 6.6.)

3. Laboratory and Radiologic Evaluation

    All patients with HE and/or FHF should undergo the following tests:

    a. Chest x-ray, abdominal x-rays.

    b. Blood glucose may reveal hypoglycemia.

    c. Serum bilirubin: A value >23 mg/dL is the best predictor of nonsurvival.

    d. AST and ALT have little prognostic value as levels tend to fall as the patient's condition worsens.

    e. Serum albumin: Its decrease reflects poor outcome.

    f. Serum electrolytes.

    g. Complete blood count.

      h. Head computed tomography (CT) scan to rule out a structural lesion (e.g., hemorrhage).

      i. Lumbar puncture needs to be considered and performed if meningitis is suspected.

      j. If the etiology of FHF is unknown, the following need to be ordered:

          (1) Acetaminophen level

          (2) Hepatitis profile

              (a) Viral hepatitis A is diagnosed by detection of HAV-IgM in the patient's serum.

              (b) Viral hepatitis B is diagnosed by

                 i. Detection of HB_SAg

                ii. Anti-HB_c IgM

              (c) Viral hepatitis C is diagnosed by detection of anti-HCV.

              (d) Delta virus hepatitis is diagnosed by detection of anti-HDV in a patient coinfected with hepatitis B virus.

          (3) Alkaline phosphatase

          (4) Amylase

      k. Serum ammonia level

      l. Electroencephalograms (EEGs) are used to assess clinical response and prognosis in patients with HE.

D. Complications of FHF

When the liver fails acutely, all organ systems are involved to some extent.

  1. Central Nervous System (CNS)

     Hepatic encephalopathy, cerebral edema

  2. Cardiovascular

     Dysrhythmias (particularly in patients with advanced FHF), hypotension

  3. Pulmonary

     Hypoxemia advancing to adult (acute) respiratory distress syndrome (ARDS)

  4. Renal

     The development of renal failure with FHF carries a poor prognosis.

     a. In most instances the renal failure is related to "prerenal" causes.

     b. The *hepatorenal syndrome* is a diagnosis of exclusion. It is associated with a normal urine sediment, a urinary sodium concentration of <20 mmol/L, and resolution if liver function improves.

  5. Hematologic

     Thrombocytopenia, diminished clotting factors with episodes of severe bleeding.

6. Infection
   Susceptibility to infection is increased in patients with FHF.
7. Metabolic
   Hypoglycemia, metabolic acidosis, hypokalemia, hyponatremia.

E. Management
   1. Supportive Therapy
      a. As in any critically ill patient, the management of AMI starts with assessment of the ABCs.
      b. The usual indications for endotracheal intubation and assisted mechanical ventilation apply to these patients.
   2. The use of corticosteroids for patients with FHF has not been proven to improve survival and, indeed, may worsen the clinical picture.
   3. Some authors suggest avoiding parenteral nutrition, as protein and amino acids may worsen the clinical picture. However, new total parenteral nutrition solutions with "branched-chain" amino acids are probably efficacious and help maintain a positive nitrogen balance.
   4. The management of FHF-associated cerebral edema is no different from that for non-hepatic-related causes (see Chapter 9, "Neurologic Disorders").
   5. Some preliminary evidence shows that the benzodiazepine antagonist flumazenil (Romazicon) may have some role in improving the signs and symptoms of HE.
   6. Investigational data have shown some improvement in the hemodynamics of patients with FHF treated with n-acetylcysteine.
   7. Liver transplantation may be an alternative form of therapy (in a few specialized transplant centers) for some patients with no known contraindication to the procedure.
   8. Liver "dialysis": A few specialized centers are currently exploring this form of therapy.

■ IV. PANCREATITIS

A. Definition
   Acute pancreatitis is an inflammatory process of the pancreas with a wide range of clinical severity ranging from self-limited to a lethal disease complicated by multiple organ system failure (10% of cases).

B. Etiology
   The most common causes of pancreatitis are

1. Alcoholism
2. Gallstones
3. Hyperlipidemia
4. Trauma (blunt or penetrating)
5. Infections (i.e., mumps, mycoplasma)
6. Hypoperfusion states (i.e., shock, cardiopulmonary bypass)
7. Hypercalcemia
8. Drugs (i.e., sulfonamides, thiazides)

C. Diagnostic Evaluation
   1. History
      Ninety-five percent of patients with acute pancreatitis present with abdominal pain, of which 50% will present with upper abdominal discomfort radiating to the back. Nausea and vomiting are also present.
   2. Physical Examination
      Depending on the severity of the situation, the patient may have overt signs of shock or may be hemodynamically stable. Other findings include the following:
      a. Abdominal tenderness and distention
      b. Abdominal ileus
      c. Low-grade fever (Note: a fever >39°C should suggest cholangitis, peritonitis, or a pancreatic abscess.)
      d. Mild jaundice
      e. Ascites
      f. Pleural effusion
   3. Laboratory Evaluation
      a. Complete Blood Count (CBC): Shows marked leukocytosis. Thrombocytopenia may be present in those cases complicated by disseminated intravascular coagulation (DIC).
      b. Amylase: Elevated initially, but may decrease after 2 to 3 days if necrosis of the pancreas is widespread. False-positive results may occur in perforation of the esophagus, stomach, intestine, gynecologic disorders, renal failure, severe burns, diabetic ketoacidosis (DKA), salivary gland disorders, and macroamylasemia.
      c. Lipase: Hyperlipasemia persists longer than hyperamylasemia. However, if necrosis of the pancreas is widespread, these values may be normal.
      d. Serum calcium is usually low. When levels are <8 mg/dL, the prognosis is poor.
      e. Other electrolyte imbalances as well as hyperglycemia are usually present.
      f. Metabolic acidosis may be present.

       g. Urinalysis may reveal proteinuria, casts (25% of the cases), and glycosuria.

4. Radiologic Evaluation

Every patient with suspected acute pancreatitis should get a chest x-ray (to rule out free air under the diaphragm, evidence of pleural effusions, etc.) and an abdominal x-ray (signs of intestinal obstruction, ileus, gallstones, the so-called "sentinel loop" of pancreatitis, or the colon "cut-off" sign , etc.). In addition, when the diagnosis remains in doubt, especially in the more severely ill, the following can be obtained:

    a. Ultrasonography (US) is the modality of choice in patients with edematous pancreatitis or suspected biliary pancreatitis and to follow up phlegmon or abscesses. Unfortunately, US cannot be accurately performed in obese patients and in those with moderate-to-severe ileus.

    b. CT is the most useful tool in assessing the retroperitoneum. Its use in acute pancreatitis is mainly to follow up on significant complications (i.e., abscess, phlegmon, pseudoaneurysms).

D. Management

1. As in any critically ill patient, the management of acute pancreatitis starts with assessment of the ABCs.

2. Adequate hydration. When necessary place Swan-Ganz catheter to maximize cardiac output, oxygen delivery and volume status.

3. Correct underlying factors.

4. Control pancreatic enzyme secretion.

    a. Nasogastric suction

    b. H_2-receptor-blocking agents (e.g., ranitidine [Zantac] 300-mg/24 h IV infusion if renal function is normal or famotidine 20 mg IV q12h).

    c. Many clinicians use the following agents in acute pancreatitis; however, clinical studies have not supported the routine use of these agents:

       (1) Calcitonin (300 IU/24 hours)

       (2) Somatostatin (250-µg IV bolus, then 250 µg/h as IV drip).

       (3) Glucagon

    d. Of interest is the use of intramuscular (IM) clonidine (not yet available in the United States) for patients hemodynamically stable with acute pancreatitis. Preliminary data show encouraging results.

5. Sedation and analgesia: Patients may require substantial amounts of analgesia, usually with meperidine (Demerol).

6. Adequate parenteral nutrition (see Chapter 10).
7. Correct hypocalcemia *only* if there is clinical evidence of tetany.

E. Complications

The most common complications of acute pancreatitis are depicted in Table 6.7.

1. Those patients who demonstrate fever >39°C with a white blood cell count >20,000/mm^3 should be evaluated for the presence of a pancreatic abscess (with the use of CT). If there are any fluid collections, CT-guided fine-needle aspiration is then indicated (for Gram's stain and cultures).
2. If the suspected diagnosis is pancreatic abscess, broad-spectrum antibiotics should be started and an emergent surgical consultation obtained.
3. Some authors advocate necrosectomy in patients with necrotizing pancreatitis.

F. Prognosis

1. In assessing the severity of the disease and prognosis, several classifications have been used. The most commonly utilized is the *Ranson's criteria* (initially developed for patients with alcoholic pancreatitis):
   a. Three of more of the following criteria must be met:
      (1) Age >55 years
      (2) White blood cell count >16,000/mm^3
      (3) Glucose >200 mg/dL
      (4) Base deficit >4 mEq/L
      (5) Lactic dehydrogenase (LDH) >350 IU/L
      (6) AST (serum glutamate pyruvate transaminase [SGPT]) >250 IU/L)

Table 6.7. Complications of Acute Pancreatitis

1. Intravascular fluid depletion
   a. Prerenal azotemia
   b. Shock

2. ARDS (3–7 days after the onset)

3. Cardiac dysfunction

4. Pancreatic abscess

5. Pancreatic pseudocysts

6. Chronic pancreatitis

7. Permanent diabetes mellitus

8. Multiorgan system failure

b. Development of the following within 48 hours indicates a worsening prognosis:
  (1) Hematocrit drop >10%
  (2) Serum urea nitrogen (BUN) rise >5 mg/dL
  (3) Partial pressure of O_2 in arterial blood (PaO_2) <60 torr (mm Hg)
  (4) Calcium <8 mg/dL
  (5) Fluid sequestration >6 L
c. Mortality rates correlate with the number of criteria present:
  (1) 0 to 2 criteria, 1% mortality
  (2) 3 to 4 criteria, 16% mortality
  (3) 5 to 6 criteria, 40% mortality
  (4) 7 to 8 criteria, 100% mortality
2. Intensive care management and prompt surgical consultation have lowered the mortality of acute pancreatitis.

■ V. USEFUL FACTS AND FORMULAS

A. Intestinal Transit
The normal 24-hour *intestinal fluid and electrolyte transport* is depicted in Table 6.8.

Table 6.8. Normal 24-Hour Intestinal Fluid and Electrolyte Transport

Site	Fluid received (L)	Amount absorbed (L)	Electrolyte Absorption		
			Na^+	K^+	Cl^-
Duodenum/ jejunum	9.0	4.0	Passive	Passive	Passive
Ileum	5.0	3.5	Active	Passive	Passive
Colon	1.5	1.35	Active	Passive	Active

Table 6.9. Child's Classification of Portal Hypertension

Class	A	B	C
Serum bilirubin (mg/dL)	<2	2–3	>3
Serum albumin (g/dL)	>3.5	3–3.5	<3
Ascites	None	Easily controlled	Poorly controlled
Encephalopathy	None	Minimal	Advanced
Nutrition	Excellent	Good	Poor

B. Stool Formulas

As part of the diagnostic workup of patients with diarrhea, *stool osmolal gap* (SOG) is usually calculated utilizing the following formula:

$$SOG = stool\ osmolality - 2 \times (stool\ Na^+ + stool\ K^+)$$

Normal stool osmolality is <290 mOsm/L. If the SOG >100, it indicates an osmotic diarrhea.

C. Liver Facts

The *Child's classification* for portal hypertension is commonly used in critically ill patients and is depicted in Table 6.9.

7

Hematologic Disorders

■ I. ANEMIA

A. Definition
   Anemia is defined as an absolute decrease in the circulating red blood cell (RBC) mass.

B. Etiology
   1. Decreased RBC Production
      a. Deficiency of hematinic agents (i.e., iron, vitamin B_{12}, folate)
      b. Bone marrow failure
   2. Increased RBC Destruction or Loss
      a. Hemolysis
      b. Hemorrhage

C. Diagnostic Evaluation
   The approach to the anemic patient in the intensive care unit (ICU) will differ depending on whether the patient was admitted with anemia or if the anemia has developed during the ICU stay.
   1. In the Patient Admitted With Anemia
      a. The symptoms of anemia will depend on the degree of anemia, the rapidity of development, cardiopulmonary reserve, and underlying disease.
      b. As a general rule, a hemoglobin <7 g/dL represents severe anemia, and such patients may present with dyspnea on exertion, light headedness, angina, and/or fatigue.
      c. The absence of symptoms in patients with hemoglobin < 7 g/dL suggests a gradual onset.

2. History

Inquire about previous hematologic values, family, and ethnic history (i.e., sickle cell, thalassemia), history of splenectomy, cholelithiasis at an early age, medications, drugs, alcohol use, dietary habits, gastrectomy, and bleeding history.

3. Physical Examination

a. General Appearance: Nutritional status or evidence of specific deficiencies, evidence of chronic illness.

b. Vital Signs: Tachycardia, postural hypotension, other signs of hypoperfusion (i.e., decreased mental status, low urine output), petechiae, purpura.

c. Associated Findings: Jaundice, glossitis (i.e., pernicious anemia, iron deficiency), neurologic abnormalities (i.e., vitamin B_{12}, folate deficiency). Lymphadenopathy, hepatomegaly, splenomegaly (i.e., hemolysis, neoplasms, infiltrative disorders). Heart: Listen for flow murmurs, prosthetic valves (i.e., increased RBC destruction). Rectal: Examine stools for blood.

4. Laboratory Evaluation

Laboratory evaluation usually provides a diagnosis and should always be done in a stepwise manner unless the patient's condition requires emergent transfusion. In this case a blood sample for RBC indices, peripheral blood smear, and iron, folate, and vitamin B_{12} studies should be obtained before transfusion.

a. Hemoglobin and hematocrit (Hct) estimate RBC mass and severity of anemia, and in the patient suspected to have active bleeding, they should be monitored serially. Acute blood loss does not influence the Hct immediately.

b. Mean corpuscular volume (MCV) is a measure of the average size of the RBCs. Classification of the anemia according to the MCV is helpful in generating the differential diagnosis and workup. The smear must be examined to determine whether multiple cell populations are present.

(1) Low MCV (<80): Generally limits the diagnosis to a few disorders: Iron deficiency, thalassemia, sideroblastic anemia, other hemoglobinopathies, and some cases of anemia of chronic disease.

(2) High MCV (<100): Megaloblastic anemias, liver disease, alcoholism, drugs (i.e., methotrexate, AZT), and myelodysplastic syndrome.

(3) Normal MCV: Acute blood loss, hemolytic anemia, pituitary or thyroid failure, aplastic anemia, myelofibrosis, and anemia of chronic disease.

c. Reticulocyte count is also essential in the evaluation of the anemic patient. It reflects the rate of production of RBCs by the bone marrow. According to the reticulocyte count, anemia can be classified into

   (1) Increased RBC destruction (i.e., bleeding, hemolysis) reflected in a high reticulocyte count

   (2) Decreased RBC production (i.e., iron deficiency, anemia of chronic disease) reflected in an abnormally low reticulocyte count

5. Bleeding should be the first concern in patients who develop anemia while in the ICU. Common sites of bleeding are the gastrointestinal (GI) tract, venipunctures, pulmonary tree, genitourinary tract, and the retroperitoneum. Development of anemia in the ICU should prompt additional investigation (i.e., gastric aspiration to look for blood, stools checked for gross or occult blood, prothrombin time [PT], partial thromboplastin time [PTT], and platelet count).

D. Therapy

1. Patient Acutely Bleeding

   a. General Measures

      (1) Airway management: Assess the need for intubation to prevent aspiration, especially in upper GI bleeding.

      (2) Obtain adequate venous access. Large-bore peripheral catheters allow greater volume administration rates than long central lines.

      (3) Obtain blood for type and cross, and diagnostic laboratories as discussed above.

      (4) Fluid resuscitation: Start with colloids or crystalloids, and continue with whole blood or packed red blood cells as required:

         (a) Healthy adult patients can tolerate blood losses up to 20% to 30% of their blood volume if adequate replacement with crystalloid is provided.

         (b) Patients with impaired cardiac reserve, coronary artery disease, or the elderly can develop symptoms with a decrease of about 10% of their blood volume.

      (5) Identify the source of bleeding.

      (6) Monitor endpoints: Patients with acute bleeding should be closely monitored in the ICU for two goals:

         (a) Adequate blood volume replacement: reflected in vital signs, urine output, mental status, central venous pressure (CVP), pulmonary capillary wedge pressure (PCWP), etc.

         (b) Control of bleeding: Follow serial hemoglobin (Hb) and Hct, monitor the bleeding site (GI, genitourinary [GU], etc.).

  b. Specific measures will depend on the cause of the bleeding.

 2. Patient Not Acutely Bleeding

  a. The therapy of anemia will depend on its etiology.

  b. A specific hemoglobin concentration should not be used as the only parameter to decide on the need for transfusion. Transfusion of red cells is usually not necessary in patients with either chronic stable anemia or anemia of acute blood loss unless the patient is symptomatic. Patients with chronic anemia, with hemoglobin levels >7 g/dL rarely require blood transfusion, unless cardiopulmonary or cerebrovascular disease is present.

  c. Randomized, controlled trials in critically ill patients without cardiac ischemia have demonstrated improved outcomes in those patients that are transfused to a target hemoglobin of 7 to 9 g/dL.

■ II. LEUKOPENIA

A. Definitions

Leukopenia is defined by blood leukocyte count below the normal range (in our laboratories < 3800/μL). Neutropenia is defined as absolute neutrophil count < 2000/mL for white patients, and below 1500/mL for patients who are black or are Yemenite Jews. Lymphopenia is defined as an absolute lymphocyte count <1500/μL.

B. Etiology

 1. Neutropenia (see Table 7.1)

 2. Lymphocytopenia (see Table 7.2)

Table 7.1. Neutropenia: Etiology

False decrease in white blood cells	Counts done long after blood has been drawn
	Disintegration of fragile cells (i.e., blasts, immature white blood cells)
	Presence of paraproteins (monoclonal gammopathies), which can produce white blood cell clumping
Decreased production	Bone marrow injury due to ionizing radiation or drugs
	Bone marrow replacement or destruction by tumor or infection
	Nutritional deficiencies: Vitamin B_{12}, folate
	Congenital stem-cell defects
Increased neutrophil destruction, utilization, sequestration	Hypersplenism
	Autoimmune
	Sepsis
Combination (increased destruction and decreased production)	Sepsis
	Antineutrophil antibodies
	Drugs
	Felty's syndrome

Table 7.2. Lymphocytopenia: Etiology

Decreased production	Primary immunodeficiency diseases (HIV)
Increased destruction, utilization, loss	Collagen vascular diseases
	Acute infections or stress
	Ionizing radiation
	Cytotoxic drugs
Unknown mechanisms	Malignancies
	Chronic infection

C. Diagnostic Evaluation
   1. History
      a. Ethnic background: black, Yemenite Jew
      b. Family history: Congenital or hereditary defect
      c. Medications: Chemotherapeutic agents, antibiotics, etc.
      d. Alcohol and dietary history
      e. Diet habits: Nutritional deficiency (B_{12}, folate)
      f. Underlying illness: Malignancies, human immunodeficiency virus (HIV)
   2. Physical Examination
      a. General Appearance: Acute distress, mental status, evidence of chronic illness

    b. Vital Signs: Fever, hypotension, tachycardia, tachypnea, low urine output (e.g., sepsis)

    c. Associated Findings: Hepato- or splenomegaly, lymphadenopathy, abdominal masses, oral thrush, skin rash, purpura, jaundice, etc.

3. Laboratory Evaluation

    a. Complete blood count and differential (CBC) to assess the degree and type of leukopenia.

    b. Bone marrow aspiration and biopsy are pivotal in the evaluation of the leukopenic patient without obvious cause. Analysis of the bone marrow

       (1) Will classify the leukopenia, by revealing the degree of bone marrow cellularity: decreased production, decreased survival, or a combined defect

       (2) May indicate the etiology of the leukopenia as in aplastic anemia, bone marrow infiltration (e.g., leukemia), infection, etc.

    c. Other laboratory tests that may help in identifying the cause of leukopenia are blood and tissue cultures, vitamin levels, and autoantibodies.

4. Therapy

The mainstay of therapy for the leukopenic patient is to treat the underlying disease. For example, in the patient with suspected drug-induced leukopenia, the offending medications should be discontinued. Vitamin deficiency should also be treated when suspected.

    a. Colony-stimulating factors (G-CSF and GM-CSF) represent a line of therapy for the treatment of leukopenia secondary to a decrease in bone marrow production. Currently, they are indicated for chemotherapy-induced severe leukopenia. Other indications for these agents are not well defined.

    b. Transfusions of white blood cell (WBC) concentrates have not been proven to be of benefit in many controlled trials

    c. Supportive therapy for the leukopenic patient requires special consideration, particularly in the ICU environment, where there is a higher risk for nosocomial infections:

       (1) Granulocyte counts <1000/µL result in severe immunocompromise.

       (2) Patients who are immunocompromised should not receive rectal manipulations. Strict hand washing for caregivers should be enforced. Avoid intramuscular (IM) or subcutaneous (SQ) routes.

(3) If the temperature rises >100.5°F (38.5°C), the patient should be fully examined, pan-cultured, and started on broad-spectrum antibiotics.

■ III. THROMBOCYTOPENIA

A. Definition
   Thrombocytopenia is defined as a platelet count <150,000/µL.

B. Etiology (see Table 7.3)

C. Diagnostic Evaluation
   1. History
      Inquire about bleeding, thrombotic events, mental status changes, alcohol use, drugs and medications, and associated illness.
   2. Physical Examination

Table 7.3. Thrombocytopenia: Etiology

Decreased survival or sequestration	Autoimmune—Primary (ITP); Secondary: collagen vascular disease (SLE); viral infections; drug-induced (heparin, quinidine, sulfas); post-transfusion
	Hypersplenism (portal hypertension, infiltrative disorders)
	Thrombotic thrombocytopenic purpura (TTP/HUS)
	Disseminated intravascular coagulation
	Sepsis
Decreased production	Primary bone marrow disorders (aplastic anemia, primary thrombocytopenia)
	Bone marrow infiltration by tumor, infection, etc.
	Drug induced (alcohol, thiazides, alkylating agents)
	Infection
Developed while in ICU	Drug-induced (heparin, H_2-blockers, diuretics, antibodies)
	Disseminated intravascular coagulation
	Sepsis
	Post-transfusion

Abbreviations: HUS, hemolytic uremic syndrome; ITP, idiopathic thrombocytopenic purpura; SLE, systemic lupus erythematosus; TTP, thrombotic thrombocytopenic purpura.

a. Vital Signs: Fever, tachycardia, hypotension, tachypnea, oliguria (i.e., sepsis)
b. Skin: Purpura, hematomas, gingival bleeding, lymphadenopathy, hepato-or splenomegaly, abdominal masses

3. Laboratory Evaluation
   a. Complete Blood Count and Platelet Count
      (1) Platelet counts >50,000/μL in isolation are not associated with significant bleeding problems, and severe spontaneous bleeding is unusual in patients with counts >20,000/μL in the absence of coagulation factor abnormalities.
      (2) Thrombocytopenia associated with anemia suggests thrombotic thrombocytopenic purpura (TTP), hemolytic uremic syndrome (HUS), disseminated intravascular coagulation (DIC), or other microangiopathic process.
      (3) Pancytopenia should suggest leukemia, aplastic anemia, or other bone marrow disorder.
   b. Peripheral Blood Smear: Note platelet size and other abnormalities (i.e., fragmented RBCs may indicate TTP or DIC; increased platelet size suggests accelerated destruction).
   c. Coagulation Evaluation: PT, PTT, D-dimer, fibrin degradation products, may indicate the presence of consumption coagulopathy (e.g., DIC).
   d. Bone Marrow Aspiration and Biopsy (not always necessary): To assess the number of megakaryocytes, and the presence of bone marrow disorders (i.e., leukemia, aplastic anemia, tumor infiltration).

D. Therapy
   Detailed treatment for the various causes of thrombocytopenia is beyond the scope of this chapter. We will concentrate on relevant topics for the acute management of patients in ICU setting.
   1. As hemostasis approaches normal at platelet counts >50,000/μL, patients with active bleeding should be transfused (6 to 10 U) to attempt to achieve levels >50,000/μL.
   2. Lumbar puncture and needle organ biopsies (lung, liver, kidneys, etc.) are more hazardous than thoracentesis, paracentesis, and bone marrow biopsy. Transfusion to 50,000/μL before such procedures is indicated.
   3. Patients with platelet counts <20,000/μL are at higher risk for hemorrhage. However, there is no clear threshold for prophylactic platelet transfusion.

4. Discontinue all nonessential medications including heparin. Consider changing H_2-blockers to coating agents or antacids. Avoid agents known to inhibit platelet function (i.e., nonsteroidal anti-inflammatory drugs [NSAIDs], ticarcillin, etc.).
5. Avoid trauma, IM and SQ injections, rectal manipulations, hard tooth brush, razors, etc., in thrombocytopenic patients.
6. TTP and HUS deserve special consideration because their management differs.
   a. TTP is a syndrome characterized by microangiopathic hemolytic anemia, fever, fluctuating neurologic deficits, and renal insufficiency. HUS is felt to be a variant of this syndrome in which renal failure is the predominant feature. TTP/HUS should be considered a medical emergency.
   b. Patients with TTP/HUS should not receive platelet transfusions, unless life-threatening bleeding occurs.
   c. Therapy for TTP/HUS includes plasma exchange by plasmapheresis if available, otherwise fresh-frozen plasma (FFP) transfusions. Intravenous (IV) steroids can be used, and in unresponsive cases, vincristine has been recommended.

■ IV. ANTICOAGULATION AND FIBRINOLYSIS

Anticoagulants and thrombolytic agents are potentially life-saving drugs when used prophylactically or employed therapeutically in critically ill patients.

A. Anticoagulation
   1. Heparin
      a. Mechanism of Action
         Heparin acts by potentiating the activity of the plasma protease inhibitor antithrombin III, which rapidly inhibits the activity of factors XII_a, XI_a, X_a, IX_a, and thrombin (factor II).
      b. Heparin prolongs the thrombin time (TT), bleeding time, PTT, and to a lesser extent the PT.
      c. Heparin half-life is 1 to 3 hours, but in patients with pulmonary embolism, clearance is accelerated (20% to 40%) compared to normals.
      d. Indications
         (1) Prophylaxis of deep venous thrombosis (DVT) and pulmonary embolism (PE). All patients in

the ICU should be on some form of DVT prophylaxis (commonly, heparin 5000 U SQ q12h or low molecular dose heparin enoxaparin 40 mg SQ qd). Heparin has proved to be an effective agent in DVT prophylaxis, except after major orthopedic procedures (particularly hip and knee replacement) and after prostate surgery.

(2) Full anticoagulation (PTT approximately 2 times normal) in pulmonary embolism or DVT, arterial thrombosis, and other disorders. A 5000 to 8000 U IV bolus is commonly used and infusion rates of 1000 U/h (12 to 25 U/kg/h).

e. Monitoring of Anticoagulation

(1) Not required for prophylactic doses.

(2) For full anticoagulation, the heparin dose should be adjusted to maintain the PTT at 1.5 to 2.0 times control. To avoid the tendency to underanticoagulate patients on heparin therapy, a standardized dosing regimen has been developed (Table 7.4).

(3) Low molecular weight heparin for DVT and acute coronary syndromes (ACS).

Enoxaparin
For DVT   1 mg/kg SQ q12h or
                 1.5 mg/kg SQ qd
For ACS   1 mg/kg SQ q12h

Table 7.4. Standardized Protocol for Dosing of Intravenous Heparin

PTT*	Dose Adjustment†	Repeat PTT
<50	5000-U bolus, increase infusion by 2400 U/24 h	6 hours
50–59	Increase infusion by 2400 U/24 h	6 hours
60–85	Therapeutic range, no change	Next morning
86–95	High therapeutic range, decrease infusion by 1920 U/24 h	Next morning
96–120	Stop infusion for 30 min, decrease infusion by 1920 U/24 h	6 hours
>120	Stop infusion for 60 min, decrease infusion by 3840 U/24 h	6 hours

* Normal PTT range is 27–35 seconds.
† Dosing protocol is based on an initial IV bolus of 5000 to 8000 U, followed by continuous infusion of 24,000 U/24 h. The first PTT should be obtained 6 hours after the bolus of heparin.

f. Complications
   (1) Bleeding: Occurs in 7% to 20% of patients during full-dose heparinization. Hemorrhage typically occurs from the GI, urinary tract, or surgical incisions. Less common sites are intracranial, retroperitoneal, soft tissues, nose, and pleural space. Bleeding is associated with the intensity of the anticoagulation (e.g., when the PTT is more than 3 times normal, the risk of hemorrhage is substantially higher).
   (2) Thrombocytopenia: Heparin use is associated with thrombocytopenia in 5% to 30% of patients, and its incidence is higher with the use of bovine lung heparin.
      (a) If thrombocytopenia is mild (>100,000/μL), not associated with bleeding or thrombotic events, heparin therapy can be continued.
      (b) Severe thrombocytopenia can occur but is rare. It may be associated with bleeding or paradoxic thrombotic events. Diagnosis is made by detection of heparin-dependent immunoglobulin G (IgG). Treatment consists of discontinuation of *all* heparin use, and *avoid* platelet transfusion.
   (3) Osteoporosis can be seen with long-term use of heparin.
   (4) Hypoaldosteronism rarely is seen.
   (5) Antidote: Heparin is generally undetectable in the patient plasma within 3 hours after discontinuation of therapy. In the rare instance in which anticoagulation must be reversed more rapidly, protamine sulfate can be used.

2. Warfarin

Warfarin (Coumadin) is the most frequently used oral anticoagulant in the United States. Sometimes the transition to chronic oral therapy is begun before the patient leaves the ICU or must be initiated because of heparin-induced thrombocytopenia, or as DVT prophylaxis in certain cases. The physician caring for the critically ill can also encounter patients who have accidentally or purposely overdose with warfarin.

a. Mechanism of Action: Warfarin interferes with the hepatic vitamin K- dependent carboxylation of factors II, VII, IX, and X. It also inhibits the synthesis of the anticoagulants factors protein C and S and may thereby be thrombogenic. The antithrombotic effects of warfarin occur only after several days of treatment. In patients on IV anticoagulation therapy who require chronic oral anticoagulation, heparin and warfarin should be overlapped for at least 48 hours.

b. Indications

(1) Prophylaxis of DVT and PE, especially in those patients in whom heparin has not proved to be effective

(2) For chronic anticoagulation therapy

c. Dosing

(1) Loading Dose: 5 to 10 PO qd for 2 to 4 days

(2) Maintenance Dose: 2 to 15 mg PO qd to keep INR (International standardized ratio) therapeutic

d. Complications

(1) Bleeding occurs in 2.4% to 8.1% of patients chronically anticoagulated. The risk is dose related and proportional to the prolongation of the PT. Treatment consists of FFP transfusions. Vitamin K replacement is only recommended for warfarin overdose, because of its delayed onset of action, and because it makes reinstitution of warfarin therapy complicated.

(2) Warfarin skin necrosis secondary to a paradoxic hypercoagulable state due to the warfarin-induced protein C reduction.

B. Fibrinolysis

1. Fibrinolytic therapy has an expanding role in the treatment of many thromboembolic disorders. Six fibrinolytic drugs are currently marketed: streptokinase (SK), anisoylated plasminogen-streptokinase activator complex (APSAC), urokinase (UK), recombinant human tissue-type plasminogen activator (rt-PA), reteplase, and TNK. All six drugs activate the fibrinolytic system by converting plasminogen to the active enzyme plasmin. Plasmin degrades fibrin and dissolves the thrombus.

2. Indications

a. Acute Myocardial Infarction (AMI): Thrombolytic therapy for AMI is discussed in Chapter 3, "Cardiovascular Disorders."

b. Pulmonary Embolism: While the effectiveness and role of thrombolytic agents in AMIs are firmly established, their use in venous thromboembolism remains infrequent and controversial, mainly because of the fear of a negative benefit/risk ratio. SK and UK have both been shown to be more effective than heparin alone in accelerating clot lysis and improving pulmonary tissue perfusion. Current recommendations for the use of fibrinolysis in PE are for patients with massive pulmonary embolism and persistent systemic hypotension in whom rapid resolution of pulmonary obstruction is desired.

   c. Deep Venous Thrombosis: Even more debated is the use of thrombolytic agents in the treatment of DVT. Potential advantages of fibrinolysis over anticoagulation include prevention of PE by lysing the source of thrombus in situ, rapid restoration of normal venous circulation with a prompt resolution of symptoms, and prevention of valve damage, which would otherwise result in chronic venous insufficiency. Risks include a much higher incidence of bleeding.

3. Dosage for Selected Thrombolytic Regimens
   a. Pulmonary Embolism
      UK: 4400-U/kg bolus, followed by 4400 U/kg/h for 24 hours
      UK: 15,000-U/kg bolus over 10 minutes
      SK: 250,000 U over 30 minutes, followed by 100,000 U/h for 24 hours
      rt-PA: 100 mg as continuous peripheral infusion over 2 hours
   b. Deep Venous Thrombosis
      SK: 250,000 U over 30 minutes, followed by 100,000 U/h for 48 to 72 hours
      rt-PA: 0.5 mg/kg over 4 to 8 hours
      rt-PA: 0.05 mg/kg/hour for 24 hours
   c. Myocardial Infarction (See Section III)

4. Monitoring
   a. Clinical monitoring should include serial neurologic examinations to detect central nervous system (CNS) bleeding and frequent vital signs to detect bleeding. All puncture sites should be examined frequently.
   b. Laboratory monitoring should include Hb/Hct, platelet, fibrinogen, PT, PTT.

5. Complications
   a. Bleeding: The greatest limitation of the thrombolytic drugs, and the factor that has limited their acceptance for the treatment of DVT and PE is the incidence of bleeding.
   b. Allergic Reactions: Reactions including skin rashes, fever, and hypotension are rare and usually are asso-

ciated with the use of SK and APSAC. The induction of antibodies against streptococcal antigens can occur after the administration of SK or APSAC or after streptococcal infection, which may neutralize the fibrinolytic activity of SK.

■ V. BLOOD AND BLOOD PRODUCTS TRANSFUSION

Transfusion therapy may be associated with several immediate and delayed adverse effects. Therefore, risks and benefits must be carefully weighed before any blood product is administered. The use of blood components should be guided by a rational diagnostic and therapeutic approach.

A. Whole Blood

Whole blood stored > 24 hours contains few viable platelets or granulocytes; factors V and VIII are decreased, but stable clotting factors are maintained. One unit is 450 mL and transfused to an average-sized adult will increase the hemoglobin by 1.0 g/dL, and Hct by 3%.

1. Indications: Symptomatic anemia with massive hemorrhage
2. Risks
   a. Allergic reactions
   b. Infectious diseases (i.e., HIV, hepatitis B)
   c. Febrile reactions
   d. Volume overload
   e. Noncardiogenic pulmonary edema

B. Packed Red Blood Cells

Removal of 200 to 250 mL of plasma from whole blood results in packed RBCs (PRBCs). Transfusion of 1 U of PRBCs will increase the Hb and Hct by the same amount as will 1 U of whole blood. One unit is 250 to 300 mL.

1. Indications: Symptomatic anemia
2. Risks: Same as for whole blood (see above).

C. Packed Red Blood Cells, Leukocyte Poor

Most of the WBCs are removed from the packed RBCs by saline washing.

1. Indications
   a. Symptomatic anemia and allergic or febrile reaction from leukocyte antibodies
   b. Patients with paroxysmal nocturnal hemoglobinuria

2. Risks

Same as for whole blood (see above).

D. Fresh-Frozen Plasma

FFP is separated from freshly drawn whole blood and then frozen, with a volume of 200 to 250 mL. Rich in all coagulation factors; 1 mL supplies approximately 1 U of coagulation activity. FFP should be ABO compatible; Rh type or cross-matching is not required.

1. Indications
   a. Bleeding due to coagulation factor deficiency
   b. Treatment of TTP and HUS
   c. Rapid reversal of vitamin K deficiency or warfarin overdose

2. Risks

Same as for whole blood (see above).

E. Cryoprecipitate

Cryoprecipitate is made by thawing a unit of FFP at 4°C. A white precipitate forms; most of supernatant plasma is removed and refrozen. The volume is 10 mL. A pack of cryoprecipitate contains von Willebrand's factor, lesser amounts of factor VIII, fibrinogen, factor XIII, and fibronectin. ABO compatibility is preferred.

1. Indications
   a. von Willebrand's disease
   b. Mild-to-moderate hemophilia A
   c. Factor XIII deficiency
   d. Fibrinogen deficiency

2. Risks
   a. Infectious disease
   b. Hyperfibrinogenemia
   c. Allergic reactions

F. Platelets

Platelet packs are obtained from whole blood; 1 U contains at least 5.5×10^{10} platelets/mm^3 in approximately 50-mL volume. In a normal 70-kg adult, 1 U of platelets should increase platelet count by 5000 to 10,000/mm^3.

1. Indications
   a. To correct bleeding secondary to thrombocytopenia or abnormal platelet function
   b. Prophylactically (e.g., in patients with chemotherapy-induced thrombocytopenia, the threshold is somewhat controversial: 10,000 to 20,000/mm^3), and before invasive procedures (target counts of 50,000/mm^3)

2. Risks
   a. Infectious diseases

b. Allergic reactions
c. Alloimmunization

G. Complications of Transfusion Therapy
   1. Disease transmission: HIV, hepatitis, cytomegalovirus (CMV), Epstein-Barr virus (EBV), Chagas' disease, malaria.
   2. Allergic reactions characterized by fever, chills, urticaria, and respiratory distress. These events are secondary to antileukocyte antibodies or antibodies against antigenic proteins in donor plasma. Therapy is symptomatic (acetaminophen; antihistamines; rarely, epinephrine or glucocorticoids are needed).
   3. Red Cell Transfusion Related
      a. Acute Hemolytic Reactions: Fever, chills, back pain, nausea, vomiting, hypotension, dark urine, chest pain. Acute renal failure with hemoglobinuria and DIC may occur. If suspected:
         (1) Inform the blood bank.
         (2) Stop transfusion.
         (3) Replace all IV tubing.
         (4) Send clotted and ETDA-treated blood samples from patient's blood along with the remainder of the unit of blood to the blood bank for cross-match.
         (5) Send blood samples for DIC screen, bilirubin, and free hemoglobin.
         (6) Management
            (a) Intravascular volume expansion plus mannitol to keep urine output >100 mL/h or 1 cc/kg/h.
            (b) Alkalization of urine with IV bicarbonate to keep urine pH >7.0 to avoid hemoglobin tubular precipitation.
            (c) Treatment of DIC
      b. Delayed Hemolytic Transfusion Reactions: 24 hours to 25 days post-transfusion. These are secondary to an amnestic (1 to 3 days) or primary (7 to 25 days) antibody response to RBC antigens. Patients usually develop a drop in the Hb and Hct with an increase in bilirubin. Coombs' test is positive.
      c. Noncardiogenic pulmonary edema (acute respiratory distress syndrome [ARDS]), caused by antileukocyte antibodies.
      d. Coagulopathy associated with a large volume of PRBC transfusions, secondary to dilution of platelet and coagulation factors. Treatment consists of FFP and platelet transfusions.

   e. Citrate intoxication, also seen with large-volume
      transfusion of PRBCs. Patients present with hypocal-
      cemia, hypotension, and drop in cardiac output.
      Treatment: IV calcium.
4. Volume Overload: Especially in patients with congestive
   heart failure (CHF). Diuretics may be needed after transfusion.
5. Platelet alloimmunization develops in patients who have
   received multiple transfusions. Approximately 75% of
   patients receiving platelets on a regular basis will become
   alloimmunized to platelet antigens. Increments <20% of
   expected generally indicate alloimmunization. Patients
   may respond to single-donor platelets, but HLA-matched
   platelets may be needed.

■ VI. DISSEMINATED INTRAVASCULAR COAGULATION

A. Definition
   DIC is a dynamic pathologic process triggered by activation
   of the clotting cascade with resultant generation of excess
   thrombin within the vascular system. Most consider DIC to
   be a systemic hemorrhagic syndrome; however, this is only
   because hemorrhage is obvious and often impressive. What is
   less commonly appreciated is the significant amount of
   microvascular thrombosis and, in some instances, large-vessel
   thrombosis that occurs. This thrombosis is usually the more
   life-threatening insult.

B. Etiology (see Table 7.5)

C. Diagnostic Evaluation
   Since DIC is associated with an underlying disease state, the
   clinical evaluation will be directed toward identifying (1)
   primary illness; (2) the status of the coagulation system; and

Table 7.5. Disseminated Intravascular Coagulation: Etiology

Obstetric accidents (amniotic fluid embolism, abruptio placentae)
Intravascular hemolysis
Sepsis
Malignancy
Trauma
Vascular disorders

(3) the focal and systemic consequences of the DIC-associated hemorrhage, and/or thrombosis.
1. Clinical Findings Associated With the Primary Illness
   These findings will vary according to the precipitating event: obstetrical accident, infection, malignancy, etc.
2. Clinical Findings Associated With the Coagulation Status
   a. Bleeding from venipuncture sites, mucous membranes, hemorrhagic bullae, hematuria, GI bleeding, etc.
   b. Purpura, petechiae, subcutaneous hematomas
3. Clinical Findings Associated With End-Organ Thrombosis and Hemorrhage
   a. Lungs: respiratory distress, hypoxia, ARDS
   b. Kidneys: proteinuria, renal insufficiency
   c. Liver: Budd-Chiari syndrome, hepatitis, hepatic failure
   d. Skin: necrosis, acrocyanosis
   e. CNS: mental status changes, neurologic deficits
4. Laboratory Evaluation
   a. Peripheral blood smear will show fragmented RBCs, thrombocytopenia, with large platelets.
   b. Prolonged PT and PTT.
   c. Thrombocytopenia is usually around 60,000/μL, but values ranging between 3,000 and 100,000/μL can be seen.
   d. Decreased fibrin level.
   e. Decreased anti-thrombin III level.
   f. Elevated levels of fibrin degradation products (FDP).
   g. Elevation of D-dimer neoantigens is a specific test for degradation products of fibrin, whereas nonspecific FDP may be either fibrinogen or fibrin derived.

D. Therapy
   The treatment of DIC is confusing and still controversial. Therapy must be individualized according to the cause of DIC, severity of hemorrhage, severity of thrombosis, hemodynamic status, and age.
   1. The most important and effective treatment for DIC is removal of the triggering disease process (i.e., evacuate the uterus, control of shock, control of infection, removal of tumors, chemo- or radiotherapy, or other indicated therapy).
   2. In cases of obstetric complications, anticoagulation is rarely needed, and evacuation of the uterus usually stops the intravascular clotting process.
   3. If the patient continues to bleed or clot significantly after 6 hours of initiation of therapy directed to stop or blunt

the triggering event, anticoagulation therapy may be indicated. There is general agreement on the need for anticoagulation in acute promyelocytic leukemia and perhaps DIC with solid tumors. We favor the use of low-dose, subcutaneous heparin at doses of 80 to 100 U/kg q6h. Other anticoagulant modalities available are IV heparin and anti-thrombin III concentrates.

4. If the patient continues to bleed after reasonable attempts to treat the triggering event of the DIC, and if anticoagulation therapy has been initiated, clotting factor depletion is the most probable cause of bleeding and replacement therapy should be considered.

■ VII. HEMOLYTIC SYNDROMES

A. Definition

Premature destruction of red blood cells. This process may occur either because of abnormal factors in the intravascular environment or because of defective red blood cells.

B. Etiology (see Table 7.6)

C. Diagnostic Evaluation

1. History and Physical Examination

Clinical manifestations will depend on the underlying disorder, on the severity of the anemia, and on whether the hemolysis is intravascular or extravascular.

Table 7.6. Hemolytic Syndromes: Etiology

Acquired hemolytic disorders	Immune hemolytic anemia
	Warm-antibody (idiopathic, neoplasia, collagen vascular disorder, drugs)
	Cold-antibody (idiopathic, *mycoplasma* infection, lymphoproliferative disorder, paroxysmal cold hemoglobinuria)
	Microangiopathic hemolytic anemia (TTP, DIC, eclampsia)
	Direct toxic effect (malaria, clostridial infection)
	Splenomegaly
	Membrane defects
	Paroxysmal nocturnal hemoglobinuria
	Spur cell anemia
Hereditary hemolytic disorders	Membrane defects (spherocytosis, elliptosis)
	Enzyme defects (G_6PD deficiency)
	Thalassemias
	Hemoglobinopathies

      a. Intravascular hemolysis can present as an acute event with back pain, dyspnea, chills, fever, tachycardia, dark urine, and hypotension, and it may result in renal failure.

      b. Extravascular hemolysis is usually less dramatic and may be accompanied only by jaundice and splenomegaly.

2. Laboratory Evaluation

      a. Elevated reticulocyte count.

      b. Peripheral blood smear can provide a diagnosis in cases of spherocytosis; microangiopathic disorders will show the presence of fragmented RBCs; Heinz bodies suggest enzymatic defects; or the presence of anisocytosis or sickle cells is consistent with hemoglobinopathies.

      c. Other laboratory data suggestive of hemolysis are

          (1) Hemoglobinuria (indicative of intravascular hemolysis)

          (2) Hemoglobinemia (indicative of intravascular hemolysis)

          (3) Low levels of haptoglobin

          (4) Elevated lactic dehydrogenase (LDH)

          (5) Positive Coombs' test

D. Sickle Cell Disease

Sickle cell disease is a heterogeneous group of defects of hemoglobin synthesis, all of which can cause clinically significant illness due to sickling of red cells. Sickle hemoglobin (HbS) is less soluble when deoxygenated and forms polymers that precipitate inside the RBCs, leading to membrane abnormalities, decreased deformability, and increased blood viscosity.

1. Clinical Manifestations

The clinical manifestations of sickle cell disease are secondary to vasoocclusive phenomena, which may lead to microinfarctions with resultant painful crises, and eventually, chronic organ damage.

2. Diagnosis

Demonstration of sickling under reduced oxygen tension. Hemoglobin electrophoresis should be performed to discriminate homozygous SS from AS and to determine the presence of other abnormal hemoglobins.

3. Treatment

The treatment of sickle cell disease is supportive and limited to management of acute and chronic complications. Frequently, these patients need to be admitted to the ICU due to the severity and life-threatening dimensions of their acute attacks.

a. Early antibiotic treatment at the first evidence of infection. Pneumococcal sepsis is a leading cause of mortality. Other prevalent pathogens include: *Escherichia coli, Haemophilus influenzae, Salmonella* sp., *Shigella* sp., *and Mycoplasma pneumoniae.*

b. Painful crises: IV hydration; adequate analgesia (usually, a regular schedule of opioids is necessary); oxygen administration is indicated when hypoxemia is present; correction of acidosis.

c. Look for precipitating events (i.e., infections, surgery, dehydration, trauma, cold temperatures, alcohol ingestion). When abdominal pain is one of the manifestations, other causes of abdominal pain must be ruled out (i.e., acute abdomen, hepatobiliary disease).

d. Acute chest syndrome: Characterized by pleuritic chest pain, fever, cough, hypoxia, and pulmonary infiltrates. Lung scans and pulmonary angiograms are usually of no help. In addition, the latter test is associated with added risk because of possible induction of sickling by the hypertonic contrast media. Differentiation between pneumonia and infarction is often difficult. Features favoring infarction include painful bone crisis, clear chest radiograph at onset, lower lobe disease, and negative blood cultures. Treatment includes oxygen therapy, mechanical ventilation when indicated, empiric antibiotic therapy, and correction of acidosis.

e. Sickle cell crisis associated with cerebrovascular accidents, or repeated venooclusive crisis may benefit from transfusion or exchange transfusion to keep the Hb S levels <39%.

E. Autoimmune Hemolytic Anemia

  1. Warm-Antibody Autoimmune Hemolytic Anemia

     Warm-antibody autoimmune hemolytic anemia (AHA) is usually extravascular and IgG mediated. This type of hemolytic anemia can be seen in the ICU not only in patients admitted with collagen vascular diseases or lymphomas but also in drug-induced hemolytic anemias.

     a. Diagnosis is made by signs of hemolysis and positive direct Coombs' test.

     b. Treatment

        (1) If the suspected mechanisms drug induced, all non-essential medications should be discontinued.

        (2) Sixty percent of cases will respond to steroid therapy (e.g., prednisone 1.0 to 1.5 mg/kg PO daily).

        (3) Splenectomy will increase the success rate to ≈ 80% to 90%.

        (4) Cytotoxic drugs are reserved for patients who fail to respond to steroid plus splenectomy.

        (5) Transfusions are indicated only in severe cases of anemia. In emergency situations, most patients can be managed with careful transfusion (ABO & Rh-compatible blood) administered slowly while watching for reactions.

2. Microangiopathic Hemolytic Anemia

    Microangiopathic hemolytic anemia (MAHA) is a syndrome caused by traumatic intravascular hemolysis. Intraluminal deposition of fibrin strands in small vessels is presumed to be responsible for the red cell destruction.

    a. Etiology includes DIC, TTP, HUS, malignant hypertension, vasculitis, and eclampsia.

    b. Diagnosis

        (1) Evidence of hemolysis (reticulocytosis, elevated LDH, depressed haptoglobin, etc.)

        (2) Fragmented RBCs in the peripheral blood smear

    c. Treatment

    Therapy is directed toward the underlying disorder. Management of TTP, HUS, DIC is discussed elsewhere. Transfusion is rarely indicated.

3. Glucose-6-Phosphate Dehydrogenase Deficiency

    This is a hereditary deficiency of the enzyme glucose-6-phosphate dehydrogenase deficiency (G-6PD) in the red cells. It is a sex-linked disorder that affects men and rarely women of Mediterranean, African, or Chinese ancestry. The disease is associated with episodic hemolysis.

    a. Clinical Manifestations

        (1) Hemolytic episodes are sometimes triggered by infections or the ingestion of some drugs (e.g., sulfonamides, antimalarials, nitrofurantoin, nalidixic acid), etc.

        (2) Patients present with acute intravascular hemolysis associated with hemoglobinemia, hemoglobinuria, decreased haptoglobin, and jaundice.

        (3) Peripheral vascular collapse can occur in severe cases.

(4) Hemolysis is usually self-limited, even if the exposure to the oxidant agent continues, since only the older G-6PD-depleted population of RBCs is affected.

b. Diagnosis

Definitive diagnosis requires measurement of levels of the enzyme. Diagnosis must be made several weeks after the episode, because enzyme levels can be normal during the hemolytic event due to the presence of high numbers of young red cells that are relatively rich in G-6PD.

c. Therapy

(1) Transfusion therapy as indicated.

(2) Protection of renal function during hemolytic episodes: IV hydration to maintain a good urine output, alkalinization of urine (to keep urine pH >7.0).

(3) Prevention of hemolytic episodes can be accomplished by identifying deficient individuals, treating infections promptly, and avoiding exposure to oxidant agents.

■ VIII. USEFUL FACTS AND FORMULAS

Patients in the ICU frequently have hematologic problems. These include anemia, coagulopathies, and thrombocytosis to name just a few. In evaluation of these patients, many laboratory tests and indices are obtained. The following formulas will aid the critical care practitioner in evaluating these hematologic parameters:

A. Red Blood Cells

The *mean corpuscular volume* (*MCV*) indicates the average volume of a single RBC in a given blood sample and is calculated as follows:

$$MCV = \frac{Hct\,(\%) \times 10}{RBC\,(10^{12}/L)}$$

The *mean corpuscular hemoglobin* (*MCH*) indicates the average weight of hemoglobin per erythrocyte:

$$MCH = \frac{Hb\,(g/dL) \times 10}{RBC\,(10^{12}/L)}$$

The *mean corpuscular hemoglobin concentration* (*MCHC*) indicates the average concentration of hemoglobin in the RBCs of any specimen:

$$MCHC = \frac{Hb\,(g/dL)}{Hct\,(\%)} \times 100$$

The *red blood cell volume* can be calculated via a radionuclide study:

$$RBC\ volume = \frac{cpm\ of\ isotope\ injected}{cpm/mL\ RBC\ in\ sample}$$

where cpm = counts per million.

B. Reticulocyte Counts

To calculate the *percentage of reticulocytes* usually based on counting 1000 RBCs, the following formula is commonly utilized:

$$Reticulocytes\,(\%) = \frac{Number\ of\ reticulocytes}{Number\ of\ RBCs\ observed} \times 100$$

The *actual reticulocyte count (ARC)* reflects the actual number of reticulocytes in 1 L of whole blood:

$$ARC = \frac{Reticulocytes\,(\%)}{100} \times RBC\ count\,(\times 10^{12}/L) \times 1000$$

The corrected reticulocyte count (CRC) is calculated as

$$CRC = Reticulocytes\,(\%) \times \frac{Hct\,(L/L)}{0.45\,L/L}$$

The reticulocyte count is usually viewed in relation to the degree of anemia. The *reticulocyte production index (RPI)* is a frequently used correction method:

$$RPI = \frac{(Measured\ Hct/Normal\ Hct) \times Reticulocyte\ count}{Maturation\ time\ in\ peripheral\ blood}$$

The *maturation factor* varies according to the hematocrit in the manner shown in Table 7.7.

A normal RPI is 1.0, an RPI of 3.0 or more represents adequate response of the marrow to anemia. An RPI of < 2.0 represents an inadequate response in the presence of anemia.

Table 7.7. Maturation of Reticulocytes in Peripheral Blood

Hematocrit	Maturation time in days
0.41–0.50	1
0.30–0.40	1.5
0.20–0.39	2
0.10–0.19	2.5

C. **Anemias**

The RBC indices (MCV, MCHC, MCH) are frequently utilized to classify anemias (see Table 7.8).

Table 7.9 depicts the laboratory differentiation of microcytic anemias.

D. **Hemolytic Disorders**

Table 7.10 depicts some of the common RBC morphologic abnormalities encountered in patients with *hemolytic disorders*:

E. **Human Hemoglobins**

Table 7.11 depicts the normal human hemoglobins at different stages of life.

To convert colorimetric readings into grams of Hb/dL (g/dL) using a standard curve set up with the same equipment and reagents used for specimen or calculate specimen concentration (C_u) based on *Beer's law*, the following formula is utilized:

$$C_u(g/dL) = 301 \frac{(A_u \times C_s)}{A_s} \times \frac{1}{1000} = \frac{0.301(A_u \times C_s)}{A_s}$$

where A_u = the absorbance of the unknown; C_s = the concentration of the standard (usually 80 mg/dL); and A_s = the absorbance of the standard run most recently under the same conditions as the patient specimen.

Table 7.8. RBC Indices in Hypochromic and Microcytic Anemias

	MCV (fl)	MCHC (g/dL)	MCH (pg)
Normal	83–96	32–36	28–34
Hypochromic	83–100	28–31	23–31
Microcytic	70–82	32–36	22–27
Hypochromic-microcytic	50–79	24–31	11–29

Table 7.9. Differentiation of Microcytic Anemias

Abnormality	Ferritin	Serum Iron	TIBC	RDW
Chronic disease	N/↑	↓	↓	N
Iron deficiency	↓	↓	↑	↑
Sideroblastic anemia	N/↑	↑	N	N
Thalassemia	N/↑	N/↑	N	N/↑

N = Normal; ↑ = increased; ↓ = decreased
Abbreviations: RDW, red cell distribution width; TIBC, total iron-binding capacity.

Table 7.10. RBC Morphologic Abnormalities in Hemolytic Disorders

Abnormality	Hemolytic Disorder	
	Congenital	Acquired
Fragmented cells (schistocytes)	Unstable hemoglobins (Heinz body anemias)	Microangiopathic processes Prosthetic heart valves
Permanently sickled cells	Sickle cell anemia	
Spur cells (acanthocytes)	Abetalipoproteinemia	Severe liver disease
Spherocytes	Hereditary spherocytosis	Immune, warm-antibody type
Target cells	Thalassemia Hemoglobinopathies (Hb C)	Liver disease
Agglutinated cells		Immune, cold agglutinin disease

Table 7.11. Normal Human Hemoglobins at Different Stages of Life

Hemoglobin	Molecular structure	Stage	Proportion (%)	
			Newborns	Adults
Portland	$\zeta_2\gamma_2$	Embryonic	0	0
Gower I	$\zeta_2\varepsilon_2$	Embryonic	0	0
Gower II	$\alpha_2\varepsilon_2$	Embryonic	0	0
Fetal (F)	$\alpha_2\gamma_2$	Newborn/adult	80	<1
A$_1$	$\alpha_2\beta_2$	Newborn/adult	20	97
A$_2$	$\alpha_2\delta_2$	Newborn/adult	<0.5	2.5

To calculate the fraction of *hemoglobin F as a percentage*, the following formula is used:

$$\text{Hb F (\%)} = \frac{A_{\text{test}}}{A_{\text{diluted total}} \times 5} \times 100$$

where A = absorbance; 5 = the additional dilution factor.
To calculate the *percentage of hemoglobin A$_2$*:

$$\text{Hb A}_2 \text{ (\% of total)} = \text{A fraction I} \times 100\%$$

8

Infections

The number of infectious complications encountered in the intensive care unit (ICU) continues to increase. Patients who otherwise would have not survived in the past are now improving due to new technical advancements. However, the length of stay, as well as the large number of devices employed for this purpose, predispose patients to difficult and often fatal infections. Clinical characteristics of patients who are treated in the ICU have evolved in recent years. Those who are immunocompromised, post-transplant, and the geriatric population are now regularly treated in the ICU with the consequent increase in morbidity, mortality, and cost.

From the infectious diseases point of view, the approach to a critically ill patient who is admitted to the ICU should immediately differentiate if the patient was transferred from the floor versus if the patient was directly admitted to the ICU from the community. This constitutes a paramount parameter to categorize the etiologic agents, to understand the pathophysiology of their processes, and mostly to decide which therapeutic antimicrobial interventions are needed.

■ I. PNEUMONIA (NOSOCOMIAL)

A. If the patient is transferred to the ICU after being in the hospital for several days, then treatment should address the nosocomial aspect of infection and the following important facts:

1. Mortality rates among these patients are 20% to 60%.
2. These patients represent 15% of all hospital deaths.

3. Successful treatment depends upon underlying disease, specific causative organisms, and timely institution of therapy.

B. Predisposing Factors
   1. Intubation.
   2. ICU: Especially the patient who is receiving sedation.
   3. Antibiotics: Broad-spectrum agents will rapidly change normal flora of the mouth and gastrointestinal (GI) tract.
   4. Surgery: Especially thoracic, abdominal or neurosurgery, which increases the risk of aspiration.
   5. Chronic lung disease.
   6. Advanced age.
   7. Immunosuppression.

C. Etiologic Agents
   1. Common
      a. *Klebsiella* sp.
      b. *Escherichia coli*
      c. *Pseudomonas aeruginosa*
      d. *Staphylococcus aureus*
      e. *Enterobacter* sp.
      f. *Acinetobacter* sp.
   2. Less Common
      a. Anaerobic mouth flora (i.e., *streptococci*)
      b. Other gram-negative bacilli (i.e., *Serratia* sp., *Xanthomonas* sp.)
      c. *Haemophilus influenzae*
      d. *Legionella* sp.
      e. *Candida* sp.
      f. *Aspergillus* sp.
      g. Influenza virus
      h. *Streptococcus pneumoniae*
      i. Miscellaneous: according to prevalent organisms in each hospital
      j. Tuberculosis (TB, typical and atypical)

D. Clinical Manifestations
   Patients in the ICU, especially those who are intubated or sedated, will not manifest the usual symptoms of pneumonia such as cough, chest pain, or dyspnea. Patients who are neutropenic cannot mount an inflammatory response, and, therefore, the sputum will not show purulent material. Subtle changes in oxygenation, fever, and clinical deterioration are clues for the diagnosis of pneumonia in intubated patients. Leukocytosis or leukopenia can be the first manifestation of occult pneumonia. In some instances, i.e., pneumocystis pneu-

monia, the presence of spontaneous pneumothorax can be the first indication of pulmonary involvement. Thick, foul-smelling sputum is characteristic of anaerobic and aspiration pneumonia.

E. Diagnosis
1. On chest x-ray, look for new or changing infiltrates.
2. Obtain sputum for Gram's stain *immediately* on every patient.
3. Remember the concept of "colonization" versus true infection; this distinction is sometimes very difficult.
4. Be aggressive in trying to obtain diagnosis (i.e., bronchoalveolar lavage[BAL]). Transtracheal aspirates are not commonly employed.
5. Obtain other stains (i.e., acid-fast bacilli stain [AFB], Giemsa, wet prep).
6. Order serologies if appropriate (i.e., *Legionella,* fungal serologies, cryptococcal antigen, CIE).
7. Remember the microbiological pattern of your hospital.

F. Treatment Options
1. Empiric
These are the most commonly utilized options in the ICU.
2. Common Regimens
a. Beta-lactam plus aminoglycoside (i.e., piperacillin and tobramycin).
b. Cephalosporin plus aminoglycoside (i.e., ceftazidime and gentamicin).
c. Clindamycin plus gentamicin.
d. Clindamycin plus quinolone (i.e., ciprofloxacin).
e. Imipenem/cilastatin plus aminoglycoside.
f. Cephalosporin plus fluorquinolone.
g. Add trimethoprim-sulfametoxasole [TMP-SMX] if *Pneumocystis carinii* pneumonia is suspected.
h. Add erythromycin or azythromycin 500 mg IV qd or erythromycin 0.5 to 1 g IV q6h
b. TMP-SMX 15 to 20 mg/kg/d TMP
c. Doxycycline 100 mg IV q12h
d. Rifampin 300 mg IV q12h
e. Amphotericin B 0.6 to 1 mg/kg/d
Duration of therapy is not well defined, but most authors agree on treating gram-negative and anaerobic pneumonia for 2 to 3 weeks. Gram-positive processes are usually treated between 10 and 14 days, and atypical pneumonias receive 2 weeks of antimicrobial therapy. *Candida* pneumonia requires prolonged treatment with up to 1.5 g of amphotericin B as a total dose.

G. Prevention
   1. Preoperative and postoperative measures for prevention of pneumonia
      a. Identification of high-risk patients
      b. Treatment of respiratory infections, removal of respiratory secretions
      c. Instruction and therapy to expand patients' lungs (i.e., chest physiotherapy, incentive spirometry)
   2. Proper hand washing
   3. Appropriate maintenance of in-use respiratory therapy equipment
      a. Use of sterile fluids in nebulizers
      b. Proper use of single-dose and multidose medications for respiratory therapy
   4. Proper sterilization and disinfection of reusable respiratory equipment
   5. Proper suctioning of the respiratory tract
   6. Protection of patients from other infected patients or staff

■ II. COMMUNITY-ACQUIRED PNEUMONIA

A. Common Organisms
   1. *Streptococcus pneumoniae*
   2. *Staphylococcus aureus*
   3. *Branhamella catarrhalis*
   4. *Haemophilus influenzae*
   5. *Klebsiella* sp.
   6. Influenza
   7. Respiratory syncytial virus
   8. *Chlamydia pneumoniae*
   9. *Legionella* sp.
   10. *Mycoplasma* sp.

B. Other Less Common Organisms
   1. *Pneumocystis carinii*
   2. *Mycobacterium tuberculosis*
   3. *Cryptococcus* sp.
   4. *Chlamydia psittaci*
   5. *Coxiella burnetii*
   6. *Histoplasma* sp.
   7. *Nocardia* sp.
   8. *Strongyloides stercoralis*

C. Common Manifestations
   1. Fever, cough, dyspnea, sputum production usually purulent but not in all cases.

2. Hypoxemia is common.
3. Anxiety.
4. Leukocytosis; also leukopenia in severe infections.

D. Uncommon Presentations in Patients Who Are . . .
   1. Elderly
   2. Immunocompromised (especially neutropenic)
   3. Post-transplantation
   4. Infected with typical organisms

E. Clinical Clues for Diagnosis
   1. Acute onset: bacterial, viral, aspiration, tularemia, pneumocystis
   2. Subacute onset: viral, *Legionella*, *Hemophilus* sp., *Mycoplasma*, Q fever, Psittacosis, *Chlamydia*, *Pneumocystis*
   3. Aerogenous route: any segment
   4. Hematogenous: most commonly in both bases, as blood flow is preferential to these areas

F. Associations
   1. Birds: psittacosis
   2. Turtles: typhoid
   3. Dogs: *Pasteurella multocida*
   4. Cattle: Q fever
   5. Rabbits: tularemia
   6. Air conditioners: *Legionella*
   7. Hides: anthrax
   8. Foreign travel: *Echinococcus*, paragonimiasis
   9. Barracks: *Neisseria meningitidis*, group A *Streptococcus*

G. Treatment
   Empiric treatment is usually dictated by the geographical background, clinical presentation, and host status. Penicillin or a second- or third-generation cephalosporin, in addition to erythromycin are the preferred initial choices.
   1. *Streptococcus pneumoniae*
      a. Penicillin (resistance increasing)
      b. Erythromycin or azithromycin
      c. Fluorquinolone (i.e., levofloxacin)
      d. Vancomycin
   2. *Haemophilus influenzae*
      a. Second-generation cephalosporin (i.e., cefuroxime 1.5 g IV q8h)
      b. Third-generation cephalosporin (i.e., ceftriaxone 2 g IV q24h)
   3. *Staphylococcus aureus*
      a. Oxacillin (3 g IV q4h)
      b. Cefazolin (2 g IV q8h)

       c. Clindamycin (900 mg IV q8h)
       d. Vancomycin (1 g IV q12h)
   4. *Legionella* sp.
       a. Azithromycin (500 mg IV qd) or erythromycin (0.5 to 1 g IV q6h)
       b. Rifampin (300 mg IV PO q12h)
       c. Levofloxacin 500 mg IV qd, or ciprofloxacin 400 mg IV q12h, or gatifloxacin 400 mg IV qd
   5. *Branhamella catarrhalis*
       a. Beta-lactamase-stable antibiotic (i.e., cefuroxime 1.5 g IV q8h)
       b. Penicillin or cephalosporin
   6. *C. pneumoniae*: Tetracycline (500 mg to 1 g IV q6h for 2 weeks), quinolones, azithromycin
   7. *Mycoplasma* spp.: Erythromycin or azithromycin (preferred), quinolones or tetracycline in adults
   8. Influenza
       a. Amantadine (100 mg PO q12h).
       b. Ribavirin requires a special device for medication delivery. (In addition, inhaled medications in the ICU population are of uncertain benefit.)
H. Complications After 72 Hours
   1. Persistent fever
   2. Empyema
   3. Obstruction
   4. Lung abscess
   5. Resistant organism
   6. Focus of infection

■ III. SEPSIS

A. More than 400,000 cases of sepsis, with an associated mortality of 20% to 60%, are estimated to occur annually. Despite improvements in antimicrobial therapy and supportive care, the incidence of and mortality associated with sepsis have not declined. This is, in part, a consequence of an array of medical advances that can place patients at increased risk for development of infection and, potentially, sepsis.

B. Sepsis and Related Disorders
   1. New Definitions
       a. Bacteremia: Positive blood cultures (may be transient)
       b. Sepsis: Clinical evidence suggestive of infection *plus* signs of a systemic response to the infection (all of the following):

      (1) Tachypnea (respiration >20 breaths per minute; if patient is mechanically ventilated, minute volume >10 L/min)

      (2) Tachycardia (heart rate >90 beats per minute)

      (3) Hyperthermia or hypothermia (core or rectal temperature >38.4°C [101°F] or <35.6°C [96.1°F])

c. Sepsis Syndrome (may also be considered *incipient septic shock* in patients who later become hypotensive): Clinical diagnosis of sepsis outlined above, *plus* evidence of altered organ perfusion (one or more of the following):

      (1) PaO_2/FiO_2 no higher than 280 (in the absence of other pulmonary or cardiovascular disease).

      (2) Lactate level above the upper limit of normal.

      (3) Oliguria (documented urine output <0.5 mL/kg body weight for at least 1 hour in patients with urinary catheters in place).

      (4) Acute alteration in mental status.

      (5) Positive blood cultures are not required.

d. Early Septic Shock: Clinical diagnosis of sepsis syndrome as outlined above, *plus* hypotension (systolic blood pressure <90 mm Hg or a 40-mm Hg decrease below baseline systolic blood pressure) that lasts for <1 hour and is responsive to conventional therapy (intravenous fluid administration or pharmacologic intervention)

e. Refractory Septic Shock: Clinical diagnosis of the sepsis syndrome outlined above, *plus* hypotension (systolic blood pressure <90 mm Hg or a 40-mm Hg decrease below baseline systolic blood pressure) that lasts for >1 hour despite adequate volume resuscitation and that requires vasopressors

C. Pathophysiology

Cell walls of gram-negative bacteria contain proteins, lipids, and lipopolysaccharides. Endotoxin (lipopolysaccharide) has three components: an O-specific polysaccharide, the R-core, and lipid A. Lipid A may be the major culprit in initiating the endotoxic symptoms. It is this component of endotoxin that stimulates the release of tissue necrosis factor (TNF) and can also activate the complement pathway. The sepsis syndrome is caused by endothelial damage following endotoxin-stimulated activation of neutrophils, coagulation, complement, and macrophages. Macrophages are stimulated to release TNF, interleukins, leukotrienes, thromboxane, and other cardioactive substances. Endotoxemia markedly increases the risk of myocardial depression and multiple organ failure. In patients who have positive blood cultures, those with severe endotoxemia have 5 times the mortality of those who do not have endotoxemia.

D. Priorities in the Treatment of Sepsis
    a. Early recognition.
    b. Cardiovascular/pulmonary support.
    c. Fluid resuscitation.
    d. Pressor agents.
    e. Empiric antibiotic therapy.
    f. Monoclonal antibodies (not yet proven to be effective).
    g. Other immunotherapeutic agents (investigational).
    h. Corticosteroids are *not effective*.
    i. Drainage of any foci of infection.

E. Prognosis
Mortality in sepsis is a function of the severity of physiologic derangements, the duration of illness, and the number of organ system failures. These organ systems include, but are not limited to, the lungs, kidneys, and liver. When the pulmonary system becomes dysfunctional, the resultant clinical entity is known as the adult respiratory distress syndrome (ARDS). The sequence has been termed the multiple-organ dysfunction syndrome (MODS). MODS is the most common cause of demise in patients who experience uncontrolled inflammation and infection.

■ IV. TOXIC SHOCK SYNDROME

A. Clinical Case Definition (See Table 8.1)
    1. Severe febrile (>38.9°C) illness with rash (erythroderma followed by desquamation), hypotension or syncope, and multiple organ system involvement (at least 4 of the following: mucous membrane, GI, muscular, central nervous system [CNS], renal, hepatic, hematologic, cardiopulmonary, metabolic).
    2. Hypotension: probably due to small-vessel and capillary leakage with extravascular accumulation of fluid (edema).
    3. Blood cultures are usually negative.
    4. Acute episode followed by desquamation
    5. No evidence of other causes: scarlet fever, Kawasaki's disease, Rocky Mountain spotted fever, etc.

B. Epidemiology and Other Clinical Features
    1. Affects mostly young menstruating women. Tampon use, especially continuous use and Rely brand in some studies.

Table 8.1. Toxic Shock Syndrome

Criteria for Diagnosis
    Temperature <38.9°C
    Systolic blood pressure <90 mm Hg
    Rash with subsequent desquamation especially on palms and soles

Involvement of >3 of following organ systems:
    Gastrointestinal: vomiting or severe diarrhea
    Muscular: severe myalgias or fivefold increase in creatine kinase
    Mucous membranes: frank hyperemia
    Renal insufficiency: serum urea nitrogen, creatinine double of normal
    Liver: enzymes twice upper limits of normal
    Blood: thrombocytopenia <100,000/mm^3
    CNS: disorientation without focal findings
    Negative tests for leptospirosis, Rocky Mountain spotted fever, and
        measles

S. *aureus* colonization of vagina. Recurrence rate of 30%. Decrease in the number of reported cases.

2. Also occurs in nonmenstruating women, men, and children (colonization or focal infection with S. *aureus*, including postoperative infections). Common occurrence after surgery. Fatality rate: 5% to 10%.

C. Etiology
    Exotoxin(s) of S. *aureus* appear to cause the disease. Recently, streptococci have been shown to cause the same syndrome.

D. Differential Diagnosis
    Kawasaki's disease, scarlet fever, leptospirosis, Rocky Mountain spotted fever, measles.

E. Treatment
    The most important treatment is volume expansion and correction of hypotension; removal of the tampon, if present, in menstruating women; debridement of wounds, etc.; and administration of antistaphylococcal antibiotics (after cultures have been obtained). Steroids have not been proven to be effective or to alter outcome.

■ V. MENINGITIS

A. Acute meningitis is a medical emergency that requires early recognition, rapid diagnosis, precise antimicrobial therapy, and aggressive ICU support.

1. Etiologic Agents
   a. *Streptococcus pneumoniae*: The most common cause in adults.
   b. *Neisseria meningitis*: Common among groups of young individuals and children.
   c. *Hemophilus influenzae*: Common in children up to 12 years of age.
   d. *Staphylococcus aureus* and *S. epidermidis*: Seen in the elderly or postoperatively.
   e. *Listeria monocytogenes*: Usually mistaken with diphtheroids or contaminants.
   f. Streptococci other than *S. pneumoniae*: Especially group B in neonatal disease.
   g. Gram-negative bacilli: After surgery or trauma.
   h. *Mycobacterium tuberculosis*: Increasing in frequency.
   i. *Cryptococcus*: Usually in immunosuppressed patients (i.e., those with acquired immune deficiency syndrome [AIDS], or impaired cell-mediated immunity).
   j. Syphilis: presentation variable.
   k. *Herpes simplex*.
   l. Toxoplasma: can present as meningoencephalitis or brain abscess.
   m. Naegleria: epidemiological history is paramount.
   n. Other viruses (i.e., echovirus, St. Louis, equine, and Western encephalitis).
2. Associations: Epidemiology and Organisms
   a. Summer and fall: Coxsackie or echovirus; leptospira
   b. Previous meningitis: *S. pneumoniae*
   c. Alcoholism: *S. pneumoniae*
   d. Young adults: *N. meningitis*
   e. Elderly: *S. pneumoniae*, listeria, gram negative bacilli
   f. Lymphoma: *Cryptococcus* sp.
   g. Petechia: *N. meningitidis*, echovirus
   h. Sinusitis: *H. influenzae*, *S. pneumoniae*, anaerobic bacteria
   i. Cellulitis: aerobic, gram-positive cocci
   j. Brain abscess: mixed flora
   k. Swimming in fresh water: amoebas
   l. Other family members with meningitis: *N. meningitidis*
   m. Water contact: leptospira
   n. Hospital acquired: gram-negative bacilli, staphylococcus, candida
   o. Head trauma
      (1) Close fracture: *S. pneumoniae*, gram-negative bacilli

Table 8.2. CSF Findings in Meningitis According to Etiology

Bacterial	Tuberculous	Viral	Chronic
Glucose >40 mg/dL (Blood ratio <0.4)	30–45 mg/dL	20–40 mg/dL	30–40 mg/dL
Protein 100–500 mg/dL	100–500 mg/dL	50–100 mg/dL	100–500 mg/dL
White blood cells 1000–10,000/cc^3	100–400/cc^3	10–1000/cc^3	100–500/cc^3
Gram's stain (+) 60%–80% (untreated) 40%–50% (previously treated)	AFB smear (+) in up to 40%	Smears are usually negative	Special stains needed: India ink (+)75% AFB (+)30%

       (2) Craniotomy: gram-negative bacilli, staphylococci

       (3) Cerebrospinal fluid rhinorrhea: *S. pneumoniae*

3. Cerebrospinal Fluid (CSF) Findings (See Table 8.2)
4. Diagnostic Approach
    a. Order antigen detection for *H. influenzae, S. pneumoniae, N. meningitidis*.
    b. Obtain high-volume CSF for AFB concentrate and fungal cultures (20 to 30 mL).
    c. If CSF is normal or viruses are suspected, repeat lumbar puncture (LP) in 24 to 36 hours.
    d. Upon admission, obtain serologies for viral infections (i.e., St. Louis encephalitis, California encephalitis).
    e. Obtain serologies in serum and CSF for fungal infections.
    f. Polymerase chain reaction (PCR) may be helpful (especially for TB and cytomegalovirus [CMV] infections).
5. Treatment
    In acutely ill patients, the goal of therapy is to institute treatment before the pathologic process of inflammation can produce irreversible progression and/or death. Time is essential in this situation. Empiric therapy is instituted immediately after diagnosis is made, and it is based on the recognition of a community versus hospital and/or postoperative process. For community-acquired meningitis, usual treatment includes a third-generation cephalosporin (i.e., cefotaxime 2 g IV q4h or ceftriaxone 2 to 4 g q12-24h). Ampicillin 2 g IV q4h is added if *Listeria* is suspected. In postoperative cases, especially after neurosurgical procedures, ceftazidime 2 g IV q8h and

vancomycin 15 mg/kg q12h are started. If an anaerobic component or brain abscess is part of the differential diagnosis, metronidazole 500 mg to 1 g IV q6h is also given.

B. Pneumococcal Meningitis

1. Pneumococcal meningitis is still the most common cause of bacterial meningitis in adults. Underlying diseases: sickle cell disease, splenectomy and splenic dysfunction, hypogammaglobulinemia, alcoholism, head trauma (CSF fistula), and chronic pulmonary, hepatic, or renal disease.

2. Associated infections: pneumonia, otitis, bacteremia, endocarditis, mastoiditis.

3. Therapy: penicillin 4 million U IV q4h. All other alternatives include ceftriaxone 2 to 4 g/d or cefuroxime 1.5 g IV q8h. If in doubt, perform in vitro susceptibilities.

C. Hemophilus Meningitis

1. Underlying disease (adults): alcoholism, compromised host defenses, head trauma with CSF fistula).

2. Associated infections: pneumonia, sinusitis, otitis. Secondary cases can occur in close contacts.

3. Therapy: Ampicillin (if sensitive) 12 g/d. Other useful antibiotics include cefuroxime, cefotaxime, ceftriaxone, and chloramphenicol.

D. Meningococcal Meningitis

1. Meningococcal meningitis is seen primarily in children, adolescents, and young adults. Secondary infection in close contacts can occur. Predisposing factors include complement defects.

2. Disseminated neisserial infection (often recurrent in persons with C_5–C_8 deficiency). Waterhouse-Friedericksen syndrome is an acute, often fatal, syndrome of septic shock associated with massive adrenal necrosis, associated with bacteremia due to this organism. It requires early recognition, antibiotic therapy, and especially aggressive ICU/hemodynamic support.

3. Early antimicrobial therapy is needed. Penicillin or cephalosporins are the agents of choice.

E. Listeria Meningitis

Not always seen in compromised hosts as once previously thought. Epidemiological history is important. Therapy is with ampicillin or TMP-SMX.

F. *Staphylococcus Aureus* and *Staphylococcus Epidermidis*

Infection with these organisms is common after neurosurgery and/or ventricular peritoneal shunt placement as well as after Ommaya reservoir insertion.

    1. Therapy
       a. Methicillin sensitive: oxacillin 12 g/d
       b. Methicillin resistant: vancomycin 500 mg to 1 g IV q6-12h (plus) rifampin or TMP-SMX
       c. An infected shunt may need to be removed early in the course of therapy if the patient is not responding. Repeat LP at 2 to 3 days is needed in order to reach this decision (persistent growth of organisms, despite adequate therapy).

G. Gram-Negative Bacilli
    1. Infections with gram-negative bacilli is challenging to treat due to their high morbidity and mortality. Development of resistance can occur while on therapy (especially with *Enterobacter* sp.). Most organisms will respond to ceftriaxone, cefotaxime, or ceftazidime. For *Pseudomonas aeruginosa*, ceftazidime 2 g IV q8h is the drug of choice. Intraventricular aminoglycoside is helpful but does not penetrate CSF, and intrathecal does not reach the ventricles.

H. Complications of Bacterial Meningitis
    1. Brain Abscess: Usually follows trauma, contiguous infection, hematogenous dissemination.
    2. Subdural Empyema: Primarily disease of the young but, in elderly, may complicate neurosurgery or subdural hematoma.
    3. Epidural Abscess: Usually accompanied by focal osteomyelitis and subdural empyema.
    4. All of the above are caused by mixed bacteria and usually required drainage, as well as prolonged IV antibiotic therapy.

I. Herpes Meningitis/Encephalitis
Herpes meningitis/encephalitis is a devastating necrotizing type of encephalitis. Temporal spikes on electroencephalogram (EEG) are characteristic. Recently, magnetic resonance imaging (MRI) has been shown to be of great value for diagnosis. PCR in cerebrospi.nal fluid is diagnostic. However, etiologic diagnosis is usually made by brain biopsy. Treatment is given with acyclovir 15 mg/kg q8h (high dose) for 2 weeks. Careful attention to hydration is mandatory to avoid renal insufficiency.

■ VI. INFECTIONS IN PATIENTS WITH AIDS

A. Opportunistic infections are the most common causes of morbidity and mortality in patients with human immunodeficiency

Table 8.3. Approach to HIV Patients With Opportunistic Infections

Clinical presentation	Common organism*	Diagnostic procedure
Pulmonary infiltrates	*P. carinii* (PCP); tuberculosis (TB); *Mycobacterium avium-intracellulare* (MAI); histoplasma, aerobic bacteria, legionella	BAL and/or lung biopsy; appropriate serologies
Seizures, headache, vertigo, facial palsy	Toxoplasma, cryptococcus MAI, herpes, CMV	MRI, head CT, LP, and appropriate serologies
Esophagitis	Candida, herpes, CMV, cryptosporidium	Endoscopy with biopsy and washings
Diarrhea	CMV, cryptosporidium, giardia, MAI, isospora, *C. difficile*, salmonella	Stool culture (initially)† AFB stain, colonoscopy, and biopsy
Persistent fever	MAI, histoplasma, TB, cryptococcus	CT abdomen‡ Bone marrow Blood cultures with special stains (AFB)

* Remember that each one of these syndromes can be caused by noninfectious processes.
† Also useful to obtain fecal leukocytes for diagnosis of colitis.
‡ Performed when fever persists despite initial evolution.

virus (HIV). Patients with CD4 cells <250 are at risk for developing severe infectious complications. Their approach is depicted in Table 8.3.

  B. Summary of Current Therapeutic Approaches
    1. Pulmonary Disease
      a. Disease due to *Pneumocystis carinii* pneumonia (PCP) (Table 8.4)
      b. Disease due to *M. Tuberculosis*
        (1) Start with at least 4 drugs, preferably 5 INH 300 mg/d, rifampin 600 mg/d, pyrazinamide 15/kg/d, ciprofloxacin 750 mg PO bid, ethambutol 15 to 20 mg/kg/d.
        (2) If TB is sensitive to INH and/or rifampin, continue for 12 to 18 months (not in the ICU).
        (3) If TB is resistant to either or both drugs (INH and Rifampin), multiple drug resistant, con-

Table 8.4. Recommended Management for PCP

Antibiotic	Mild to moderate	Severe (Usually in ICU)
TMP-SMX	2–3 double-strength tabs PO tid for 14–21 days	5 mg/kg IV q6h for 3 weeks
Pentamidine	3–4 mg/kg IV-IM qd	4 mg IV qd
Trimethoprim-dapsone	Trimethoprim 100 mg PO tid Dapsone 100 mg PO qid	?
Clindamycin-primaquine	Clindamycin 600 mg PO tid Primaquine 30 mg PO qid	900 mg IV q8h for 3 weeks
Atovaquone	750 mg PO tid	For 2–3 weeks
Trimetrexate-leucovorin	Trimetrexate 45 mg/m^2/d IV for 21 days Leucovorin 30 mg/m^2 IV q6h for 10 days, and then PO q6h for 14 days	Same as mild to moderate Solumedrol
Corticosteroids adjunctive therapy	?	40 mg IV or (equivalent PO bid) for 5 days Wean gradually over 10 days

tinue with 5 to 6 drugs, and adjust according to sensitivities. Prognosis is very poor.

(4) Follow liver function tests initially weekly and later monthly.

(5) If patient cannot use PO drugs, give IV INH and rifampin (same dose) and IM streptomycin (1 g/d).

c. Pulmonary Disease Due to *Histoplasma capsulatum*

(1) Initiate therapy with amphotericin B at 0.8 to 1 mg/kg/d.

(2) Search for other sites of involvement (i.e., bone marrow biopsy, lumbar puncture, chest x-ray, barium enema, and small bowel series).

(3) Once the patient is stable, switch to fluconazole 200 mg PO bid.

    d. Pulmonary Disease Due to *Legionella* sp.
        (1) Initiate therapy with erythromycin 3 to 4 g
            IV/d.
        (2) If the patient is not responding, add rifampin
            (600 mg/d) and/or ciprofloxacin 400 mg IV
            q12h.
    e. Pulmonary Disease Due to Bacteria Common
        Organisms are
        (1) *Streptococcus pneumoniae*
        (2) *Hemophilus influenzae*
        (3) *Pseudomonas* (especially if sinusitis is present)
    f. Add   Antibacterial   Therapy   Empirically   on
        Admission
        (1) Ticarcillin-clavulanic acid 3.1 g IV q6h (will
            also cover anaerobes in the sinuses).
        (2) Cefuroxime 1.5 g IV q8h.
        (3) Adjust when cultures and sensitivities become
            available.
    g. Pulmonary Disease Due to *M. avium-intracellulare*
        (1) Clofazamine 100 to 200 mg/d PO.
        (2) Rifampin 600 mg/d PO.
        (3) Ethambutol 25 mg/kg/d PO.
        (4) Ciprofloxacin 750 mg PO bid or ofloxacin
            500 mg PO bid.
        (5) Amikacin 7.5 mg IM or IV q12h; or clarithro-
            mycin 1 g PO bid; or azithromycin PO.
        (6) Treatment is given for at least 6 months.
2. Enteric Pathogens in Patients With AIDS (See Table 8.5)
3. CNS Infections in AIDS
    a. Cryptococcal Meningitis
        (1) Acute: amphotericin B 0.5 to 0.8 mg/kg/d
            plus 5- fluorocytosine 100 mg/kg/d until the
            patient is stable or improving. Then switch to
            fluconazole 400 mg/d PO for 3 months.
        (2) Maintenance: fluconazole 200 to 400 mg/d PO.
    b. Toxoplasmosis
        (1) Pyrimethamine 200 mg PO: loading dose
            followed by 75 mg PO daily with folinic
            acid 5 mg PO daily. (No IV presentation
            available.)
        (2) Sulfadiazine 1.5 g PO q6h; or clindamycin 900
            mg IV or PO qid
    c. CMV (Including Retinitis)
        (1) Ganciclovir 5 to 10 mg/kg IV q12h for 14 days
            (initial therapy)
        (2) Foscarnet 60 mg/kg IV q8h for 14 days (initial
            therapy)

Table 8.5. Enteric Pathogens Commonly Seen in Patients With Aids

Organism	Antimicrobial agent	Direction of therapy (days)
G. lamblia	Metronidazole 250 mg PO tid	5
E. histolytica	Metronidazole 750 mg tid and diiodohydroxyquin 650 mg PO tid	10
Shigella sp.	Ampicillin 500 mg IV qd Ceftriaxone 2 g IV qd	14
C. jugum	Ciprofloxacin 500 mg IV q12h	7
I. belli	TMP-SMX 1 double-strength qd	14
CMV	Ganciclovir 5 mg/kg IV q12h	30
Herpes simplex	Acyclovir 1200 mg/d	10
Oral thrush	Ketoconazole 200–400 mg/d PO	10
Candida esophagitis	Fluconazole 200–400 mg/d IV	7–10

      d. Herpes Simplex
         (1) Acyclovir 10 to 15 mg/kg IV q8h
      e. Syphilis
         (1) Crystalline penicillin 24 million U/d for 14 days
         (2) Ceftriaxone 2 to 4 g/d IV for 14 days
C. Important Facts to Remember in Treating HIV-Infected Patients in the ICU
    1. Patients may have more than one infection at the same time.
    2. Blood precautions should be instituted *immediately* to avoid unnecessary exposure.
    3. Noninfectious processes (i.e., tumors) can mimic infections.
    4. Patients require a full physical examination daily, including mouth, perirectal area, and eyes.
    5. Superinfections are common (i.e., fungal and resistant bacteria).
    6. When fever persists, consider lumbar puncture, liver, and bone marrow biopsy.
    7. Obtain CD4-CD8 counts if not recently done.
    8. Code status needs to be established early.
    9. Privacy of and respect toward patient are essential and mandatory.

Table 8.6. Selected   Immunological   Defects   and   Clinical Presentations

Defect	Organism	Manifestations
Phagocytes/ neutrophils (i.e., neutropenia)	Gram-positive cocci Gram-negative bacilli *P. aeruginosa* *Candida* sp. *Aspergillus* sp. *Mucor* sp., *Absidia* sp., *Fusarium* sp.	Bacteremia Sepsis Tissue invasion, Pneumonia, rhinocerebral and cutaneous
Complement (i.e., C_5–C_8 deficiency)	*Neisseria* sp. *Strep. pneumoniae* *H. influenzae* *P. aeruginosa* *Brucella* sp.	Fulminant sepsis Recurrent infection Pneumonia Sepsis Recurrent fever
Antibody (i.e., IgA-IgG deficiency)	Gram-positive cocci *H. influenzae* Herpes simplex *Giardia lamblia*	Pneumonia, otitis Meningitis Encephalitis Liver disease Diarrhea
Cell-mediated immunity (i.e., decrease in CD4 counts)	*Salmonella* *Listeria* sp. *Mycobacterium* sp. *Nocardia* sp. *Cryptococcus neoformans* *Histoplasma capsulatum* *Coccidioides immitis* Herpes simplex Varicella zoster CMV *P. carinii* *Strongyloides stercolaris* *Toxoplasma gondii*	Diarrhea, sepsis Meningitis Pneumonia CNS/lungs Lungs Mucocutaneous Disseminated pneumonia CNS/myocardium

■ VII. INFECTIONS IN THE IMMUNOCOMPROMISED HOST

A. The number of critically ill patients with impaired host defense mechanisms who are admitted to the ICU has dramatically increased in recent years. The knowledge and recognition of the basic deficiency enable the physician to predict the type and site of infection and allow the institution of early empiric therapy (see Tables 8.6 and 8.7).

B. Immunocompromised patients admitted to the ICU should be categorized according to the time of acquisition of infection.

Table 8.7. Common Clinical Presentations in Compromised Patients in the ICU

Reason for admission	Common pathogen	Initial therapeutic approach
Fever and neutropenia	Early: Gram-negative bacilli Gram-positive cocci (usually catheter related) Late: Resistant gram-negative bacilli Fungi (*Candida* sp., *Aspergillus* sp., *Fusarium* sp., *Mucor* sp.)	Early empiric therapy mandatory
Sepsis: postsplenectomy	Encapsulated bacterial organisms	Emergency institution of antibacterial therapy
Neurologic deterioration in patient with cell-mediated immune deficit	Intracellular organisms	Obtain CT, LP, and treat for bacteria and possibly for cryptococcus
Sepsis after solid organ transplantation	Immediately after surgery: Common local bacteria Not related to surgery: Virus, fungus, nocardia	Choose antibacterials according to site Empiric therapy with extensive workup needed
Bilateral pulmonary infiltrates	Organism depends on causative defect	Treat empirically, and obtain BAL and biopsy (if possible)
Diabetic ketoacidosis	Bacterial organisms, mucormycosis, aspergillus	Treat for mixed bacterial infection
AIDS	Depends on sites of infection	See section on AIDS
Postoperative status and malnutrition	Antibiotic-resistant gram-negative bacilli Group D streptococci *Candida* sp.	Utilize broad-spectrum therapy

Hospital-acquired infections have different etiologic agents compared to those from the community, despite having the same basic immunologic defect.

■ VIII. ANTIMICROBIALS (See Table 8.8)

Table 8.8. Selected Antimicrobials Commonly Used in the ICU

Drug	Dose	Renal adjustment: Creatinine clearance >80 50–10 <10	Comments and side effects
Aminoglycosides (i.e., gentamicin)	1–2 mg/kg IV q8h	8–12 h 12 h 24–48 h	Monitor levels, renal function, and hearing
Broad-spectrum penicillin (i.e., piperacillin)	3–4 g IV q8h	4–6 h 8–12 h 12–24 h	Monitor Na^+ and coagulation profile
Imipenem	500 mg to 1 g	6 h 12 h 24 h	Seizures, twitching, facial palsies
Cephalosporins (i.e., ceftazidime)	2 g IV q8h	6–12 h 12 h 14 h	Penetrates CSF well
Aztreonam	2 g IV q8h	6–12 h 12 h 24 h	Tolerated in penicillin-allergic patients
Vancomycin	1 g IV q12h	6–12 h 2–3 d weekly	Monitor levels; interstitial nephritis
Oxacillin	6–12 g IV	4–6 h 6–8 h 8–12 h	Infuse in at least 1 h
Acyclovir	2–3 g/d IV	8 h 12–24 h 24–48 h	Monitor WBC and renal function
Ganciclovir	5 mg/kg IV	12 h 12 h 24–48 h	Monitor bone marrow depression

Table 8.8. *Continued*

Drug	Dose	Renal adjustment: Creatinine clearance >80 50–10 <10	Comments and side effects
Clindamycin	600–900 mg IV	8 h 8 h 8 h	Diarrhea
Chloramphenicol	3–4 g IV or PO	6 h 6 h 6 h	Monitor bone marrow function
Metronidazole	30 mg/kg/d IV or PO	6 h 6 h 6 h	Metallic taste
Amphotericin B	0.5–1 mg/kg IV once a day	24 h 24 h 48 h	Monitor renal function
Fluconazole	200–400 mg q12h IV or PO	12 h 24 h 48 h	Interacts with anticoagulants
Itraconazole	2–4 g PO	12–24 h 24 h 24 h	
TMP-SMX	4–5 mg/kg IV (TMP) or higher	6–12 h 12–24 h 24–48 h	Monitor WBC; skin rash
Doxycycline	100–200 mg IV	12–24 h 12–24 h 12–24 h	Impairs neutrophil function
Levofloxacin	500 mg IV	24 h	Do not use in children
Azithromycin	500 mg IV	24 h	
Erythromycin	1–4 g/d IV	6 h 6 h 6 h	Preferably given through central IV line
Ribavirin	Aerosolized 190 mg/mL at 12.5 L/min over 18 h and the rest over 6 h. Repeat daily for 10 days	? ? ?	Requires special device for medication delivery

■ IX. INFECTIOUS DISEASES "PEARLS" FOR ICU CARE

A. Hand washing is the single most important procedure to prevent infection.

B. Improving the nutritional status is of great importance for the outcome of infections.

C. Remove bladder catheters as soon as possible.

D. Complete daily physical examination is mandatory.

E. Gram's stain is the single best and least expensive test for early diagnosis of several infections (i.e., pulmonary, soft tissue, meningitis).

F. Hypothermia, especially in elderly patients, suggests sepsis.

G. Central catheters should be changed every 5 to 7 days.

H. Peripheral lines should be changed every 2 to 3 days.

I. If prolonged ICU stay is expected, early placement of subcutaneous catheters is recommended.

J. Patients with high fever require special attention to fluid management.

K. Antibiotics interact with many other drugs. (See previous tables.)

L. Drug-induced fever is not uncommon (common agents are antibiotics, H_2-antagonists, and phenytoin).

M. Fever may last for several days, even when appropriate antimicrobial therapy has been instituted.

N. Closely follow the clinical situation, which is more important than laboratory results.

■ X. USEFUL FACTS AND FORMULAS

A. Antibiotic Kinetics

The pharmacokinetics of antibiotics depend on several factors.

The *volume of distribution* (V_D) of an antimicrobial is calculated as:

$$V_D = \frac{A}{C_p}$$

where A = total amount of antibiotic in the body; C_p = antibiotic plasma concentration.

Table 8.9. Selected Antibiotics Levels

Antibiotic	Level (µg/mL)	
Amikacin	Peak 20–30	Through <8
Gentamicin	Peak 10–20	Through 5–10
Chloramphenicol	Peak 5–10	Through <2
Tobramycin	Peak 5–10	Through <2
Vancomycin	Peak 30–40	Through 5–10

Table 8.10. Selected Atypical Mycobacteria

Category	Runyon group	Mycobacterial species
Photochromogens	I	M. kansasii M. marinum
Scotochromogens	II	M. scrofulaceum
Nonchromogens	III	M. avium-intracellulare
Rapid growers	IV	M. fortuitum M. chelonae ssp. chelonae M. chelonae ssp. abscessus M. ulcerans

Repetitive dosing of antibiotics depends on the principle of *minimal plasma concentrations* (C_{min}):

$$C_{min} = \frac{D}{(V_D)(2^n - 1)}$$

where D = dose; n = dosing interval expressed in half-lives.

The *plasma concentration at steady state* (C_{ss}) of an antimicrobial can be estimated utilizing the following formula:

$$C_{ss} = \frac{\text{Dose per half-life}}{(0.693)(V_D)}$$

B. Antibiotic Adjustments

Renal dysfunction in critically ill patients is common. In those patients receiving aminoglycosides, dosage modification is required according to the *aminoglycoside clearance*:

$$\text{Aminoglycoside clearance} = (C_{cr})(0.6) + 10$$

where C_{cr} = creatinine clearance in mL/min.

To estimate the *creatinine clearance*, the *Cockcrof and Gault formula* is utilized:

$$C_{cr}(mL/min) = \frac{(140 - age) \times weight}{Cr \times 72}$$

where Cr = serum creatinine in mg/dL. Another modification to this formula is the *Spyker and Guerrant method*:

$$C_{cr}(mL/min) = \frac{(140 - age) \times (1.03 - 0.053 \times Cr)}{Cr}$$

C. Antibiotic Levels

Some of the clinically employed antibiotic levels are depicted in Table 8.9.

D. Other Facts

Some of the atypical mycobacteria commonly encountered in the critical care setting are depicted in Table 8.10.

9

Neurologic Disorders

■ I. BRAIN DEATH

A. Definition

Traditionally, death has been defined as the absence of spontaneous respirations and spontaneous pulse. A more contemporary definition of death includes the concept of *brain death*, defined as the permanent cessation of all brain function. This concept has evolved coincident with the increasing use of transplantation and, thus, is an important concept for the critical care practitioner to master.

B. Legal Status of Brain Death

In the United States, the concept of brain death and criteria for its diagnosis have been codified in the vast majority of states. Physicians operating outside of areas with specific legislation on brain death often rely on common law for legal certification of death, but the judicial acceptance of the brain death concept is universal in the United States.

C. Determination of Brain Death

Specific requirements for determination of brain death vary from institution to institution. In most institutions, specific sets of criteria are established. The recognition of irreversibility in most instances requires that the cause of the coma be established and be sufficient to account for the loss of brain function observed. For example, when drugs or toxins have been implicated, blood levels of these agents must be absent or below therapeutic levels before the determination of brain death by clinical examination.

Table 9.1. Clinical Determination of Brain Death

A. Coma of established cause.
  • Temperature ≥32°C
  • Absence of significant central nervous system depressants or significant metabolic disturbances
  • Patient not in shock

B. Absence of spontaneous movements, decerebrate or decorticate posturing

C. Absence of brain stem responses
  • Pupils fixed
  • Corneal reflex absent
  • Unresponsiveness to pain in the distribution of the cranial nerves (i.e., supraorbital pressure)
  • Absence of cough or gag reflex
  • Absence of "doll's eyes"
  • No eye movement with cold water (caloric test) bilaterally

D. Absence of respiratory activity for at least 3 minutes (See apnea test)

Table 9.2. Cold Water Caloric Test

A. Elevate patient's head at 30-degree angle.

B. Inject 50 mL of ice water into each external ear canal using an IV catheter (after determination that the ear canal is free of cerumen). The patient should be observed for several minutes for the presence of eye movements.

1. Clinical Determination of Brain Death
   a. A common checklist for the diagnosis of brain death is depicted in Table 9.1.
   b. The specific brain stem functions tested vary from site to site, but every institutional protocol includes a number of simple bedside tests demonstrating the absence of brain stem function. One such example is the cold water caloric test (Table 9.2).
   c. In most institutions, two clinical observers must concur with diagnosis of brain death and so note in the patient's chart.
   d. The final component of the clinical evaluation of brain death is usually the apnea test (Table 9.3).
   e. Ancillary Tests for Brain Death: Other tests used in determining brain death include the following:
      (1) Electroencephalogram (EEG): An isoelectric EEG is not required as a criteria for brain

Table 9.3. The Apnea Test

1. Oxygenate with 100% FiO_2 for 5–10 min before the test.

2. Keep O_2 at 4–8 L/min delivered through a cannula in the endotracheal tube while the patient is disconnected from the ventilator.* (If hypotension and/or dysrhythmias develop, immediately reconnect to the ventilator. Consider other confirmatory tests.)

3. Observe for spontaneous respirations.

4. After 10 min, obtain ABG. Patient is apneic if $PCO_2 \geq 60$ torr (mm Hg) and there are no respiratory movements.

* In patients with COPD, the PaO_2 must be <50 torr at the end of the apnea test.
Abbreviations: ABG, arterial blood gas; COPD, chronic obstructive pulmonary disease; FiO_2, fraction of inspired O_2; PaO_2, partial pressure of O_2 in arterial blood; PCO_2, partial pressure of CO_2 in arterial blood.

death in most institutions. However, it may be used as a confirmatory test.

(2) Cerebral Angiography: In the presence of toxic substances or sedative agents, the irreversibility of coma may not be determined clinically. The four-vessel cerebral angiogram may be used to determine the absence of brain blood flow; and thus, the irreversible nature of coma, confirming the diagnosis of brain death.

(3) Cerebral Radionuclide Studies: Technetium 99 (T^{99}) nuclear imaging studies of the cerebral circulation have been used in some centers as corroborative tests in determination of brain death. This procedure is not as sensitive for cerebral blood flow as four-vessel arteriography in determination of brain death.

f. The patient who is brain dead is ***DEAD***. The physician does not require any permission of the family or other individuals to remove a dead patient from mechanical ventilation or other life support maneuvers.

■ II. COMA

A. Definition

Coma is a term denoting neurologic unresponsiveness. It represents part of a continuum from normal functioning to the absence of neurologic functioning with intermediate states of drowsiness and stupor. Consciousness is separated into two components: level of arousal and the content of consciousness.

1. Level of Arousal

    Level of arousal depends upon the interaction between the reticular activating system of the brain stem and the cerebral hemispheres bilaterally.

2. Content of Consciousness Exists Within the Cerebrum

    These two components—content and consciousness—may be affected individually. For example, *dyskinetic mutism* is a term applied to patients who appear awake (with open eyes, which, on occasion, may even track movements within the room) but have an absence of the content of consciousness. An individual who suffers basilar artery occlusion may develop the "locked-in" syndrome. In this syndrome, the content of consciousness is preserved, but the ability to communicate directly with the environment is absent.

B. Etiology

    Coma is a frequent cause of hospital admission. Common causes of coma are depicted in Table 9.4.

C. Diagnosis

1. Careful History and Physical Examination

    History should include information leading up to the discovery of the comatose patient. Pertinent points in the physical examination include evidence of head trauma (e.g., hemotympanum), cerebrospinal fluid (CSF) rhinorrhea, contusions, or lacerations. A complete neurologic examination looking for focal signs should be recorded.

Table 9.4. Common Causes of Coma

— Cerebrovascular Accidents

— Central Nervous System (CNS) Trauma

— CNS Infections

— Drug Intoxication

— Metabolic

— Metastatic or Primary CNS Neoplasia

— Systemic Infection (sepsis)

— Unknown

2. Toxic-Metabolic Phenomena

Toxic-metabolic phenomena are found eventually to be responsible for the majority of patients with coma without obvious cause; and thus, evaluation for hypo- or hyperglycemia, hypo- or hypernatremia, renal failure, liver dysfunction with subsequent hepatic encephalopathy, and toxin ingestions as the cause of coma should be sought.

3. Computed Tomography (CT) Scan of the Head

Mass lesions, supratentorial or in the posterior fossa, may be found unexpectedly at CT scan and account for unconsciousness. Thus, all patients with coma of unknown etiology should have neuroimaging studies completed.

4. Lumbar Puncture

Patients without evidence of mass lesion should undergo CSF examination primarily to rule out infection. Specific diagnostic studies are noted in Table 9.5.

D. Treatment

Always remember the ABCs (airway, breathing, and circulation).

1. Comatose patients with absent airway-protective reflexes should undergo endotracheal intubation (with assisted mechanical ventilation in those patients with inadequate spontaneous ventilations).

   a. Circulation: Assessment of blood pressure and pulse rate to determine the adequacy of cardiovascular function.

2. Specific management is dictated by the clinical condition of the patient.

Table 9.5. CSF Studies in Patients With Coma of Unknown Etiology

— Tube I
   Cell count with differential

— Tube II
   Glucose, protein

— Tube III
   Gram's stain, acid fast bacilli (AFB) stain, routine cultures, India ink or cryptococcal antigen, pneumococcal antigen, meningococcal antigen, VDRL

— Tube IV
   Special studies as indicated (lactic acid, rheumatoid factor, etc.)

    a. The patient with an infectious source should be treated aggressively with intravenous (IV) antibiotics. Patients with mass lesions should be considered for early surgical intervention.

    b. Patients with toxic-metabolic events should receive appropriate therapy with close monitoring of electrolytes and/or drug levels.

    c. Many clinicians recommend empiric therapy of the comatose patient with naloxone, a narcotic antagonist (2 to 8 mg IV), and dextrose (50-g IV push). However, some data suggest that high levels of glucose may be deleterious to injured neurons, and thus, with the advent of bedside glucose testing, many would advocate the determination of blood glucose before the administration of dextrose.

    d. Flumazenil: A specific benzodiazepine antagonist is also available; however, in the absence of specific knowledge of benzodiazepine overdose, we do not recommend its administration because of its potential for seizures in patients with tricyclic antidepressant overdose.

3. Nonspecific Management

    a. Intravenous access for the administration of medications.

    b. Nasogastric (NG) decompression should be considered through an NG tube.

    c. A urinary catheter should be placed for urine monitoring and ease of nursing care for the comatose patient.

    d. Deep venous thrombosis prophylaxis should be administered to all patients in whom no contraindications exist (i.e., heparin 5000 U SQ q12h or low molecular weight heparin 1 mg/kg).

    e. Stress ulcer prophylaxis should be administered in every comatose patient (H_2-blockers, sucralfate, proton-pump inhibitors, etc.).

    f. Care and comfort measures (including lubrication of conjunctival spaces and eye taping).

    g. Passive range of motion of upper and lower extremities, for the prevention of contractures.

    h. Skin care (including frequent turning and positioning).

■ III. INTRACRANIAL HYPERTENSION

A. Physiology
  1. The contents of the cranial vault include the brain, CSF, and the cerebral blood volume. These contents are constrained by the skull itself.
  2. The brain is a highly metabolic organ and very dependent on continued blood supply.
  3. Because of the closed nature of the cranial vault, cerebral blood flow is dependent upon the difference between mean arterial pressure and intracranial pressure (ICP).

B. Etiology
   A large number of intracranial processes may result in a rise in ICP and impairment of cerebral blood flow (see Table 9.6). These specific entities may require individualized therapy, and they are discussed in other sections of this book.

C. Management
  1. ABCs
  2. Positioning of the Patient
     A 30-degree head-up tilt is recommended for those patients who do not have a contraindication (i.e., hypotension).
  3. Hyperventilation
     The fastest way to control intracranial pressure is hyperventilation. Acute reductions in arterial PCO_2 result in vasoconstriction and decrease in intracranial blood volume. Specific PCO_2 values of approximately 25 to 35 torr (mm Hg) are commonly advocated, although to our knowledge, no controlled studies have demonstrated the utility of these specific target values.
  4. Osmotic Agents
     Mannitol, at doses of 0.25 g to 1 g/kg of ideal body weight (IBW) intravenously over 10 to 20 minutes, pulls water

Table 9.6. Causes of Intracranial Hypertension

— Brain Tumors

— Fulminant Hepatic Failure

— Head Injury

— Meningitis and/or Encephalitis

— Subarachnoid Hemorrhage

— Vasculitis

— Other

from the brain and results in a decrease in ICP. Plasma osmolality should be maintained below 340 mOsm/L. *Note:* The initial administration of mannitol may result in paradoxical increases in ICP; thus, many authors recommend prior therapy with a loop-acting diuretic (i.e., furosemide).

5. Short-Acting Anesthetics

These agents may result in reduction of cerebral blood flow and, thus, reductions in ICP. Pentobarbital is the most commonly used agent. The usual dose of this agent is 10 mg/kg IBW as the loading dose and 100 mg/h for maintenance.

6. Corticosteroids

The only clear role of corticosteroids in the management of intracranial hypertension is in cerebral edema secondary to certain neoplasms. Their use in trauma, cerebrovascular accidents (CVAs), and metabolic causes has not been demonstrated to improve outcome and therefore cannot be routinely recommended.

7. CSF Drainage

An intraventricular catheter may be placed percutaneously at the bedside and permit simultaneous monitoring and therapy of ICP. Sustained elevations of ICP >20 cm H_2O can be managed by withdrawal of CSF through the intraventricular catheter.

8. Positive End-Expiratory Pressure (PEEP)

Some authors have advocated *not* using PEEP; however, in conditions in which this therapy is required (i.e., low lung compliance), routinely used levels of PEEP (3 to 7 cm H_2O) are not expected to impair cerebral blood drainage.

9. Other Management

Other methods less commonly used to decrease ICP include controlled hypothermia, indomethacin, and flumazenil.

■ IV. CEREBROVASCULAR DISEASE

A. Epidemiology

Approximately 250,000 people die each year of cerebrovascular disease in the United States. Many more develop catastrophic and lesser degrees of neurologic deficits.

B. Classification

A number of different syndromes comprise the disorders labeled *cerebral vascular accidents (CVAs)*. These disorders can be broadly grouped into two large categories: (1) those that produce vascular insufficiency (secondary to thrombosis, embolism, or stenosis leading to focal areas of ischemia) and (2) those that produce ruptures of the vascular tree, causing intracranial hypertension and secondary cerebral ischemia.

1. Vascular Insufficiency

 a. Transient Ischemic Attacks (TIAs): TIAs are defined as the sudden or rapid onset of neurologic deficits secondary to cerebral ischemia that lasts from a few minutes to up to 24 hours without residual signs or symptoms. Atherosclerosis is the most frequent cause.

 b. Stroke

  (1) Definition: Stroke is the rapid onset of neurologic deficits involving a set vascular territory with neurologic signs and symptoms lasting >24 hours.

  (2) Risk Factors: Similar to those for TIA. An increasing frequency of stroke related to vasospasm secondary to cocaine abuse has been noted in the last decade in the United States.

  (3) Classification of Stroke: Both thrombosis and embolism may result in vascular insufficiency and the phenomena of stroke. Clinically, the differentiation of thrombosis and embolism is quite difficult. However, some clinical characteristics of each are noted in Table 9.7.

  (4) Embolic Stroke: The most common causes of embolic stroke include emboli secondary to atrial fibrillation, valvular heart disease, bacterial and nonbacterial endocarditis, trauma, secondary to myocardial infarction or ventricular aneurysm, atrial myxoma, and paradoxical embolism secondary to endocardial disease.

Table 9.7. Clinical Characteristics of Embolic and Thrombotic Strokes

	Embolism	*Thrombosis*
Predisposing Factors	Valvular heart disease Endocarditis Myocardial infarction Atrial fibrillation	Atherosclerosis Diabetes Hypertension Arteritis
History of prior TIA	Uncommon	Common
Onset of symptoms	Rapid onset	Progression over hours

(a) Thrombotic Stroke: Occurs when a clot develops in a cerebral vessel. Intrinsic or extrinsic diseases of the cerebral vessels may contribute to thrombotic strokes. These include

    i. Arteriosclerosis.

    ii. Fibromuscular dysplasia.

    iii. Extension of embolism or dissection into cerebral arteries because of arteritis (Takayasu's disease, giant cell arteritis, and other vascular diseases).

    iv. Increased viscosity secondary to proteins or increased cellular elements (i.e., Waldenstrom's macroglobulinemia, leukemias with elevated blast counts, and erythrocytosis of any cause).

    v. TIAs are a risk factor for completed stroke with the highest risk being in the first 3 months immediately following the onset of TIAs.

(5) Initial evaluation and the management of cerebral ischemic syndromes.

    (a) ABCs: Secure the airway and assist with breathing and circulation as with any other patient presenting with a potentially critical illness.

    (b) Careful Examination of the Patient: Emphasis should be on the neurologic examination to localize the area deficits and on other areas of the physical examination to rule in or rule out secondary causes for the ischemic syndrome.

    (c) Laboratory Evaluation: Complete blood count, prothrombin time (PT), partial thromboplastin time (PTT), glucose, electrolytes, serum urea nitrogen (BUN), and creatinine are routinely ordered. Chest radiograph, ECG, and CT scan of the head (to rule out hemorrhage, infarction, subdural hematoma, or intracranial masses).

    (d) In any patient with new neurologic abnormalities, lumbar puncture should be considered to rule out infectious causes and for the completion of the evaluation for subarachnoid hemorrhage (after head CT scan has ruled out increased intracranial pressure).

(e) Echocardiography: For patients with a history or physical examination suggestive of cardiac abnormality, echocardiography should be ordered.

(f) Other useful studies may include duplex ultrasonography and cerebral angiography.

(6) In patients with embolic CVAs with progressively worsening neurologic deficits (stroke in evolution), anticoagulation, beginning with heparin, is recommended. In addition, heparin is commonly prescribed for patients with recurrent TIAs despite antiplatelet therapy. *Note:* Anticoagulation should be started (with heparin) in patients with worsening neurologic deficits (stroke in evolution or suspected embolic source). Anticoagulation is contraindicated in patients with CT or LP evidence of hemorrhage, and it is relatively contraindicated in patients with gastrointestinal (GI) bleeding or coagulation disorders and in patients with hypertension.

(7) Blood Pressure Control: Therapy to maintain systemic blood pressure at approximately 150/100 mm Hg is advocated. Caution must be exercised, as reductions in blood pressure may worsen the clinical condition by producing ischemia in poorly perfused regions of the central nervous system (CNS).

(a) Thrombolytic therapy for ischemic stroke is now the standard of care. A number of different agents can be utilized in this setting (i.e., tissue-plasminogen activator rt-PA). Most authorities recommend routine administration of thrombolytic therapy for ischemic strokes, provided that the onset of symptoms is within 3 hours. In some institutions, this period is extended up to 6 hours from onset of symptoms.

2. Rupture of the Vascular Tree

a. Subarachnoid hemorrhage (SAH) accounts for about 10% of all strokes and 16% to 20% of cerebral vascular deficits. The etiology of SAH includes ruptured aneurysms of cerebral vessels, bleeding from arteriovenous malformations of the CNS, and trauma.

   (1) Clinical Manifestations

      (a) Neurologic deficits may include focal neurologic signs as well as coma.

      (b) Generalized excruciating headache with neck stiffness is classically described.

   (2) Evaluation and Management

      (a) ABCs as noted previously.

      (b) CT scan of the head demonstrating subarachnoid blood is seen in approximately 90% of the cases.

      (c) Lumbar puncture should be performed in those patients whose CT scan is negative and for whom clinical suspicion of SAH is still high.

      (d) The patient should be kept at bed rest. Cardiac monitoring and frequent (q1-2h) neurologic assessments should be ordered.

      (e) Analgesia for headache should be prescribed (acetaminophen and codeine are commonly used).

      (f) Stool softeners and mild laxatives should be prescribed to prevent constipation (and thus increased ICP).

      (g) Blood pressure control: Keep systolic blood pressure in the range of 140 to 160 mm Hg (ischemia of poorly perfused regions may occur; therefore, clinical status should be carefully followed as blood pressure control is obtained.) Calcium channel blockers (i.e., nimodipine 60 mg q4h × 21 days) have been advocated to prevent cerebral blood vessel spasm following subarachnoid hemorrhage. They should be used in patients without contraindications.

      (h) Surgical management: Considerable controversy exists in the surgical management of patients with SAH and aneurysms. The propensity for bleeding from aneurysms leads to the desire to surgically obliterate any accessible lesions. The timing of operation is debated. Many neurosurgeons prefer to wait 5 to 10 days after the event because of cerebral vasospasm, whereas others advocate early surgery.

- (i) Nonoperative interventions (i.e., embolization of arteriovenous (AV) malformation) are also options.

b. Intracerebral Hemorrhage: Intracerebral hemorrhage commonly occurs following trauma. When it occurs spontaneously, it is frequently accompanied by hypertension. Neurologic abnormalities, as seen in other types of strokes, are usually present, and the specific diagnosis requires neuroimaging studies.

- (1) Management
    - (a) ABCs as required for every critically ill patient.
    - (b) Control severe hypertension: As noted above, cerebral ischemia may occur with reductions in blood pressure. However, control of hypertension may reduce cerebral edema and improve neurologic function. Short-acting IV agents are advocated (labetalol, trimethaphan). Reductions in blood pressure should not exceed 20% of baseline value.
    - (c) Additional management of intracranial hypertension as noted above may be required.
    - (d) Supportive therapy as required for all intensive care unit (ICU) patients should continue.

c. Surgical evacuation of the hematoma should occur in patients with accessible lesions who have progressive signs of deterioration.

■ V. STATUS EPILEPTICUS

A. Definition

Status epilepticus is defined as seizure activity continuing for 30 minutes or intermittently over a 30-minute period without the patient's regaining consciousness. It is a condition that may lead to permanent neurologic damage or even death.

B. General Approach

The management of seizure disorders is based on clinical information.

1. Most seizures stop spontaneously within 30 to 90 seconds.
2. The diagnosis of status epilepticus is straightforward and can be determined through observation of the patient in most cases.
3. Generalized seizure disorders without motor findings may lead to changes in mental status or coma and may not be clinically apparent, and thus further diagnostic testing (i.e., EEG) may be required.
4. Continued seizure disorders may result in enzyme elevation (creatine kinase [CK]), making the diagnosis of other clinical conditions more difficult (i.e., myocardial infarction).

C. Specific Management

1. ABCs: As in all critically ill patients, airway, breathing, and circulation must be maintained. Patients should be positioned so they can not harm themselves from their motor activity. Oxygen should be administered, and continuous observation of the patient should ensue.
2. Blood glucose, calcium, magnesium, and other electrolytes, as well as BUN, liver functions, anticonvulsant levels, complete blood count, and toxicologic screen should be obtained.
3. A normal saline infusion should be established, and 50 cc of 50% glucose and 100 mg of thiamine should be administered intravenously.
4. ECG and blood pressure monitoring should be established.
5. Diazepam (Valium), 5 mg over 1 to 2 minutes IV, repeated every 5 to 10 minutes, or lorazepam (Ativan) 2 to 4 q5min can be administered in those patients continuing to seize.
6. Reoccurrence of seizures within 15 to 20 minutes following administration of benzodiazepines is quite frequent, and other antiepileptic agents should be instituted. Fosphenytair 18 mg/kg given IV, at a rate of ≤ 50 mg/min, should be administered as a loading dose for patients not previously receiving phenytoin. If dysrhythmias and/or hypotension ensue, the infusion should be stopped and resumed at a slower rate.
7. Persistent seizures following phenytoin administration should result in administration of phenobarbital IV at rates of 50 to 100 mg/min until the seizure stops or until a loading dose of 20 mg/kg IBW total has been given.

8. Continued seizures should prompt the administration of other medications: Lidocaine 1 to 3 mg/kg IBW as a loading dose and 2 to 4 mg/min has been advocated; sodium pentobarbital 15 mg/kg IBW as the loading dose followed by 0.5 to 3 mg/kg/h; or inhalation anesthetics (i.e., isoflurane). Intravenous propofol (5 to 30 cc/h) has been used in some cases of refractory seizures with success.

9. EEG monitoring is appropriate for patients receiving general anesthetic control of status epilepticus.

10. Review of laboratory data and additional history and physical examination for underlying disorders that may have resulted in the status epilepticus should be undertaken.

11. Following control of the status epilepticus, careful physical and laboratory evaluation for underlying disease processes should ensue. Patients without a clear etiology should undergo head CT scan and lumbar puncture unless contraindicated.

12. Continuous motor seizures may lead to muscle breakdown and thus release of myoglobin and other intracellular components into the circulation. One must be concerned about maintenance of adequate hydration as well as protection from pigment-induced renal failure. (See Chapter 14, "Renal and Fluid-Electrolyte Disorders.")

■ VI. NEUROMUSCULAR DISORDERS

A. Guillain-Barré Syndrome (GBS)
   1. Definition
      GBS is an acute demyelinating disorder of the peripheral nervous system that results in motor and sensory symptoms with few sensory signs. In the vast majority of cases, it results in complete recovery. However, in up to 25% of patients, respiratory failure due to weakness of the respiratory muscles ensues and mechanical ventilation is required for a period of time. Peaks of occurrence are in the 15- to 35- and 50- to 75-year-old age groups.
   2. Clinical Manifestations
      GBS presents in a typical pattern. The usual history is that of a patient with a normal previous health status interrupted by a mild upper respiratory or GI illness followed by ascending weakness and numbness. Other factors include recent vaccination or surgery. Major clinical manifestations are depicted in Table 9.8.

Table 9.8. Major Clinical Manifestations of Guillain-Barré Syndrome

— Distal paresthesias (initially lower extremities).

— Rapidly progressive motor weakness (ascending neuropathy).

— Symmetry is seldom absolute.

— Facial weakness is common (1/3 of cases).

— Recovery usually begins 2–4 weeks after progression stops.

— Sinus tachycardia and labile blood pressure are common.

— CSF protein elevation (after the first week).

— Nerve conduction abnormalities are detectable.

Atypical presentations may include a descending paralysis.

3. Diagnostic Evaluation
   a. Careful physical examination should be performed, attempting to rule out other causes of neuropathology (spinal cord lesions, infection, metabolic or toxic, etc.).
   b. Lumbar puncture usually reveals elevated protein. There are usually few mononuclear leukocytes in the CSF with lymphocyte counts <10/cc.
   c. Eighty percent of all patients show slow nerve conduction.
4. Management
   a. ABCs.
   b. Supportive measures; close monitoring of respiratory function with frequent measurements of the vital capacity and/or negative inspiratory force (NIF) are indicated.
   c. A vital capacity of <10 mL/kg is an indication to consider intubation and assisted mechanical ventilatory support.
   d. Active and passive range of motion of lower and upper extremities should be performed to prevent the formation of contractures.
   e. Decubitus ulcer prevention and care should be instituted.
   f. Prevention of thromboembolism with appropriate therapy (i.e., heparin 5000 U SQ q12h in patients without contraindications).
   g. Plasma exchange presumably removes or dilutes circulating factors implicated in the pathogenesis of GBS. It has been shown to decrease ventilatory dependence in GBS.

h. Corticosteroids have not been proven to be of value in this syndrome.

B. Other Chronic Neurologic Disorders
1. A number of chronic progressive neurologic disorders may result in patient admission to the ICU for physiologic support. These include amyotrophic lateral sclerosis, multiple sclerosis, severe Parkinson's disease, etc. Many of these patients are admitted because of their need for aggressive tracheobronchial toilet or mechanical ventilation.
2. Major concerns in managing these patients involve the decision to institute aggressive therapy. It is preferable that these decisions be addressed with the patient and their family before the need for these services, so that unwanted supportive measures are not forced upon them.

■ VII. DELIRIUM IN THE ICU

A. Epidemiology
Ten percent of medical and surgical patients become delirious during their hospitalization. These patients are at risk for harm to themselves (by the discontinuation of an IV line, arterial line, NG tubes, etc.) and others. Patients who develop delirium are at greater risk of mortality. Patients at high risk for the development of delirium are
1. Those at the extremes of age (elderly and children)
2. Patients with preexisting brain injury
3. Drug-dependent patients
4. Postcardiotomy patients
5. Patients with human immunodeficiency virus (HIV) disease

B. Clinical Features
1. A prodromal state manifested by restlessness, irritability, anxiety, or sleep difficulty.
2. A rapidly fluctuating course. Patients are intermittently clear thinking and coherent or grossly confused, disoriented, and disorganized.
3. Reversed sleep-wake cycles and increased activity and confusion during the night-time hours.

C. Evaluation and Management
1. ABCs as required for all patients with a critical illness.
2. Careful attention to metabolic problems that may produce CNS disturbances should be sought.

3. Laboratories including blood glucose, electrolytes, calcium, BUN, and liver function tests should be obtained as well as arterial blood gases or pulse oximetry to rule out hypoxemia (a common cause of mental status change in the ICU).

4. ECG should also be obtained to help rule out myocardial ischemia.

5. Patients with unexplained mental status changes should receive CT scanning or magnetic resonance imaging of the brain followed by lumbar puncture to rule out infectious or other causes.

6. Careful review of the medications prescribed for the patient should be undertaken. Drugs commonly associated with delirium are depicted in Table 9.9.

7. Whether or not the etiology is known, some simple interventions that may help control the patient's confusion and behavior are often missed. For example, if the patient normally wears eyeglasses or a hearing aid, return these items. The old practice of placing delirious patients together is not helpful, and indeed, it may increase the aggressive behavior of both patients, thus, making orientation almost impossible.

8. Haloperidol (Haldol) is a highly potent antipsychotic agent that effectively calms agitation, sedates, and reduces hallucinations and paranoid thinking. For the patient with a mild level of delirium or agitation, a starting dose of 0.5 to 2 mg IV or IM is usually enough. However, for patients

Table 9.9. Drugs Commonly Associated With Delirium

Analgesics (e.g., morphine)

Antibiotics (e.g., aminoglycosides)

Antivirals (e.g., amantadine, acyclovir)

Anticholinergics (e.g., atropine)

Anticonvulsants (e.g., phenytoin)

Anti-inflammatory agents (e.g., corticosteroids, nonsteroidal anti-inflammatory drugs)

Antineoplastic drugs

Cardiac drugs (e.g., beta-blockers, angiotensin-converting enzyme inhibitors)

Drug withdrawal (e.g., ethanol, benzodiazepines)

Sympathicomimetics (e.g., amphetamines, cocaine)

Miscellaneous (e.g., disulfiram, lithium)

with severe agitation, a starting dose of 5 to 10 mg may be necessary. An interval between 20 and 30 minutes should be allowed between doses. After giving 3 doses of haloperidol with no improvement in symptomatology, give 1 to 2 mg IV lorazepam (Ativan) concurrently, or alternate with haloperidol every 30 minutes. Assuming the patient is calm, reduce the dose by 15% every 24 hours. *Note:* Haloperidol is not approved for IV use despite its common use for this indication. Large IV doses have been used in critically ill patients without evident harm or side effects. Doses as high as 100 mg IV bolus have been given to medically ill patients without evidence of respiratory depression.

9. Delirium should prompt neuropsychiatric consultation for recommendations in evaluation and therapy.

■ VIII. USEFUL FACTS AND FORMULAS

A. Cerebrospinal Fluid (CSF)

Normal pressures and volumes for human CSF are shown in Table 9.10.

The normal composition of the CSF is depicted in Table 9.11.

Additional normal values for CSF in humans are depicted in Table 9.12.

When there are many red blood cells (RBCs) or white blood cells (WBCs) in the CSF, the total protein of the CSF may be "*corrected*" utilizing the following formula:

Protein actual

$$= \text{Protein CSF} - \frac{\text{Protein}_{\text{serum}} \times (1 - \text{Hct}) \times \text{RBC}_{\text{CSF}}}{\text{RBC}_{\text{blood}}}$$

Table 9.10. Normal CSF Pressures and Volumes

CSF Pressure	
Children	3.0–7.5 mm Hg
Adults	3.5–13.5 mm Hg
Volume	
Infants	40–60 mL
Young children	60–100 mL
Older children	80–120 mL
Adult	100–160 mL

Table 9.11. Normal Composition of the CSF

	CSF Concentration (mean)
Specific gravity	1.007
Osmolality (mOsm/kg H_2O)	289
PH	7.31
PCO_2 (mm Hg)	50.5
Na^+ (mEq/L)	141
K^+ (mEq/L)	2.9
Ca^{++} (mEq/L)	2.5
Mg^{++} (mEq/L)	2.4
Cl^- (mEq/L)	124
Glucose (mg/dL)	61
Protein (mg/dL)	28

Table 9.12. Normal CSF Values

CSF parameter	Newborns	Infants, older children, and adults
Leukocyte count	<32/μL	<6/μL
Differential white cell count	<60% polymorphs	<1 polymorph
Proteins	<170 mg/dL	<45 mg/dL
Glucose	>30 mg/dL	>45 mg/dL
CSF: blood/glucose ratio	>0.44	>0.5

Table 9.13. CSF Abnormalities in Multiple Sclerosis

	Alb	IgG/TP	IgG/Alb	IgG index	Oligoclonal banding of Ig
Multiple sclerosis	25%	67%	60%–73%	70%–90%	85%–95%
Normal subjects	3%	—	3%–6%	3%	0%–7%

Abbreviations: Alb, albumin; IgG/TP, IgG value/total protein; Ig, immunoglobulin.

Common CSF abnormalities in patients with multiple sclerosis are depicted in Table 9.13.

The abnormalities in immunoglobulin G (IgG) production in these patients can be estimated by the *Ig G index*:

$$\text{Ig G index} = \frac{\text{CSF IgG/CSF albumin}}{\text{Serum IgG/serum albumin}} = \text{normal} < 0.66$$

B. Cerebral Blood Flow

The cerebral circulation follows the same physiological principles of other circulatory beds, such as *Ohm's law*:

$$F = \frac{P_i - P_o}{R}$$

where F = flow; P_i = input pressure; P_o = outflow pressure; R = resistance. The term "$P_i - P_o$" is referred to as the *cerebral perfusion pressure (CPP)*.

The CPP can be estimated by the following formula:

CPP = MAP – ICP

where MAP = mean arterial pressure; ICP = intracranial pressure.

The *pressure-volume index (PVI)* can be calculated as follows:

$$PVI = \Delta V / [\log P_p / P_o]$$

where P_p = Peak CSF pressure (increase after volume injection and decrease after volume withdrawal).

The *cerebral blood flow (CQ)* is normally 50 mL/100 g/min and is determined by the *Hagen-Poiseuille equation* of flow through a tube:

$$CQ = \frac{(K \times Pr^4)}{(8L \times \eta)}$$

where P = cerebral perfusion pressure (CPP); r = the arterial radius; η = blood viscosity; L = arterial length; K = constant.

C. Brain Metabolism

Oxygen availability to neural tissue (CDO2) is reflected in the formula:

$CDO_2 = CQ \times PaO_2$

where CQ = cerebral blood flow; PaO_2 = arterial oxygen concentration.

The *cerebral metabolic rate (CMRO2)* can be calculated as follows:

$CMRO_2 = CBF \times AVDO_2$

where CBF = cerebral blood flow; $AVDO_2$ = arteriovenous oxygen content difference.

The *oxygen extraction ratio (OER)* can be utilized to assess the brain metabolism:

$OER = SaO_2 - SjvO_2 / SaO_2$

where SaO_2 = arterial oxygen saturation; $SjvO_2$ = jugular venous oxygen saturation.

$OER \times CaO_2 = CMRO_2 / CBF$

where

$$CaO_2 = (Hb \times 1.39 \times SaO_2) + [0.003 \times PO_2(mm\ Hg)]$$

$$CMRO_2 = CBF \times (CaO_2 - CjvO_2)$$

The *arterial-jugular venous oxygen content difference (AjvDO₂)* is calculated as follows:

$$AjvDO_2 = CMRO_2/CBF$$

10

Nutrition

■ I. AIMS OF NUTRITIONAL SUPPORT

A. Preserve tissue mass, and decrease usage of endogenous nutrient stores.

B. Decrease catabolism.

C. Maintain/improve organ function.
   1. Immune
   2. Renal
   3. Hepatic
   4. Muscle

D. Improve wound healing.

E. Decrease infection.

F. Maintain gut barrier (decrease translocation).

G. Decrease morbidity/mortality.
   1. Decrease ICU/hospital stay.
   2. Decrease hospital costs.

■ II. TIMING OF NUTRITIONAL SUPPORT

A. Optimal timing remains controversial.
   1. Some patients tolerate short periods of starvation by using endogenous stores to support body functions.
   2. Well-nourished patients (nonstressed) have actually survived without food for 6 weeks (ingesting only water).

3. Hypermetabolic and hypercatabolic critically ill patients can probably only tolerate a few weeks of starvation before death.
4. There appears to be no benefit of total starvation.

B. Accumulating data suggest that outcome can be improved with early and optimal nutritional support.
   1. Early nutritional support blunts the hypercatabolic/hypermetabolic response to injury.
   2. In a growing number of studies, patients randomized to receive early vs. delayed feeding had decreased infection rates, fewer complications, and shorter length of stay in the hospital.
   3. Animal studies report improved wound healing and improved hepatic function in several injury models with early feeding.

■ III. ROUTE OF NUTRITIONAL SUPPORT

A. Parenteral Nutrition
   1. Nutrients
      Amino acids, dextrose, soy-based lipids, vitamins, minerals and trace elements (see Table 10.1)
   2. Delivery: via peripheral or central vein
   3. Major complications
      a. Central line placement (pneumothorax, hemothorax, carotid artery perforation)
      b. Metabolic derangements (hyperglycemia, electrolyte disturbances)
      c. Immune suppression
      d. Increased infection rates (catheter-related sepsis, pneumonia, abscesses)
      e. Liver dysfunction (fatty infiltration, cholestasis, liver failure)
      f. Gut atrophy (diarrhea, bacterial translocation)
      g. Venous thrombosis
      h. Overfeeding
   4. Other problems include lack of some conditionally essential amino acids that are not stable in solution (i.e., glutamine, cysteine)
   5. Glucose/fat ratio
      a. Usually 60:40 to 40:60 (ratio of calories from each source)
      b. Large amounts of glucose (>60% of calories) can
         (1) Increase energy expenditure.

Table 10.1. Comparison of Nutrients in Enteral vs. Parenteral Nutrition

Nutrient	Enteral	Parenteral
Nitrogen Source	Intact proteins, peptides, or amino acids	Amino acids*
Carbohydrate	Simple sugars or complex carbohydrates (i.e., starch and fiber)	Simple sugar (dextrose)
Lipids	Long- and medium-chain triglycerides, or long-chain fatty acids (ω-3 or ω-6)	Soy-based lipids
Vitamins	Present	Can be added
Minerals and trace elements	Present	Can be added

* Lacks some conditionally essential amino acids (i.e., glutamine and cysteine).

      (2) Increase CO_2 production and increase pulmonary workload (may delay ventilator weaning).
      (3) Produce liver steatosis.
      (4) Lead to immune compromise.

B. Enteral Nutrition
    1. Nutrients (see Table 10.1)
      a. Nitrogen sources: amino acids, peptides, or intact proteins (e.g., casein, whey, soy, lactalbumin)
      b. Carbohydrates: simple sugars or complex carbohydrates (i.e., starch and fiber)
      c. Lipids: long- or medium-chain triglycerides, w-3 or w-6 long-chain fatty acids
      d. Vitamins
      e. Minerals and trace elements
    2. Delivery
      a. Oral
      b. Gastric tube (i.e., nasogastric, gastric)
      c. Small-bowel feeding tube (i.e., nasoduodenal, gastroduodenal, jejunal)
    3. Major Complications
      a. Aspiration (pneumonia, chemical pneumonitis, adult respiratory distress syndrome [ARDS])
      b. Metabolic derangements (e.g., electrolyte disturbances, hyperglycemia); these are less common than with parenteral nutrition

      c. Diarrhea
      d. Misplaced feeding tubes (e.g., pneumothorax, empyema, bowel perforation)
      e. Overfeeding

C. Enteral vs. Parenteral Nutrition

  1. Enteral nutrition is required for optimal gut function (i.e., maintenance of gut barrier, gut-associated immune system, immunoglobulin A [Ig A] secretion, mucin layer)

  2. Total parenteral nutrition (TPN) is associated with
      a. Immunosuppression (thought to be related to intravenous [IV] lipids, which are high in w-6 long-chain fatty acids)
      b. Increased infection rates (compared to enteral) in patients following trauma, burns, surgery, and cancer chemo/radiotherapy
      c. Higher mortality in patients receiving chemo/radiotherapy and after burn injury

  3. TPN is not superior to enteral nutrition in patients with inflammatory bowel disease or pancreatitis.

  4. TPN may be beneficial in patients with short-gut syndromes and some types of gastrointestinal (GI) fistulas.

  5. Enteral nutrition is the preferred method of feeding in patients receiving chemo/radiotherapy, and following surgery, burns, trauma, sepsis, renal failure, liver failure, and respiratory failure.

  6. Parenteral nutrition is indicated when enteral nutrition is not possible (i.e., inadequate small bowel function).

■ IV. GASTROINTESTINAL FUNCTION DURING CRITICAL ILLNESS

A. Oral nutrition remains the best form of nutritional support; however, in many critically ill patients, this is not possible.

B. Decreased motility of stomach and colon are common and typically last 5 to 7 days in critically ill patients (longer if the patient remains critically ill).

  1. Gastric paresis is best assessed and monitored by measuring gastric residuals.

  2. Gastric residuals of ≥150 mL are usually considered abnormal.

  3. Patients with gastric residuals ≥150 mL should be fed in the small bowel (postpyloric) to decrease risk of aspiration.

C. Motility and nutrient absorptive capability of small bowel is usually preserved (even after severe trauma, burns, or major surgery).

D. Bowel sounds are a poor index of small bowel motility.

■ V. NUTRIENT REQUIREMENTS (QUANTITY)

A. Energy
   1. Caloric Content of Major Nutrients
      a. Lipids provide 9 kcal/g.
      b. Carbohydrates provide 4 kcal/g.
      c. Proteins provide 4 kcal/g.
   2. Studies show that most critically ill patients expend 25 to 35 kcal/kg/d.
   3. One can estimate resting metabolic expenditure (RME) using the Harris-Benedict equation (see Table 10.2).
   4. One can also measure RME by indirect calorimetry (metabolic cart).
   5. Some recommend adjusting RME by multiplying by a correction factor (see Table 10.3); however, correction factors frequently overestimate energy needs.
   6. We prefer to initially administer 25 kcal/kg/d (see Table 10.4).
      a. ≈20% protein (percent refers to percentage of total daily calories)
      b. ≈30% lipids
      c. ≈50% carbohydrates
   7. Patients with organ failure/disease states may have increased or decreased needs and should be considered individually.
   8. Overfeeding (with either enteral or parenteral nutrients) is associated with more adverse side effects than slightly underfeeding during most critical illnesses.

B. Protein
   1. Most critically ill patients need 1.2 to 2.0 g/kg/d.

Table 10.2. Harris-Benedict Equations

Men	RME (kcal/d) = 66 + (13.7 × W) + (5 × H) − (6.8 × A)
Women	RME (kcal/d) = 665 + (9.6 × W) + (1.7 × H) − (4.7 × A)

Abbreviations: A, age in years; H, height in cm; RME, resting metabolic expenditure; W, weight in kg.

Table 10.3. Energy Expenditure Correction Factors

Starvation	0.7
Confined to bed	1.2
Out of bed	1.3
Fever	1 + 0.13 per degree C
Elective surgery	1.0–1.2
Multiple fractures	1.2–1.4
Sepsis	1.4–1.8
Burns	
<20% BSB	1–1.5
20%–40% BSB	1.5–1.9
40%–100% BSB	1.9–2.1

Abbreviation: BSB, body surface area burned.

Table 10.4. Macronutrient Nutritional Requirements

Nutrient	% of total calories	Quantity of nutrients	Example for 70-kg patient
Total calories		25 kcal/kg/d	1750 kcal/d
Protein/amino acids	15–25	1.2–2.0 g/kg/d	95 g/d (380 kcal/d) (based on 1.35 g/kg/d)
Carbohydrates	30–65	50% of calories (avg pt)	220 g/d (880 kcal/d)
Fats	15–30	30% of calories (avg pt)	55 g/d (495 kcal/d)

    2. Protein requirements increase in patients with severe trauma, burns, and with protein-losing enteropathies.

C. Water
    1. Must be individualized, as needs vary greatly between patients (differences in insensible losses, GI losses, and urine losses).
    2. Initially estimate: 1 mL water per kilocalorie of energy in adults.

D. Vitamins
    1. Fat-soluble vitamins: A, D, E, K.
    2. Water-soluble vitamins: ascorbic acid (C), thiamine (B_1), riboflavin (B_2), niacin, folate, pyridoxine (B_6), B_{12}, pantothenic acid, biotin.

Table 10.5. Micronutrient Nutritional Requirements

Micronutrient	Enteral nutrition	Parenteral nutrition	Example for TPN for a 70-kg patient
Minerals			
Sodium	60–140 mmol/d	60–120 mmol/d	80 mmol/d
Potassium	50–140 mmol/d	50–120 mmol/d	50 mmol/d
Magnesium	8–15 mmol/d	8–12 mmol/d	10 mmol/d
Phosphorous	25 mmol/d	14–16 mmol/d	15 mmol/d
Calcium	20 mmol/d	7–10 mmol/d	10 mmol/d
Trace elements			
Iron	10 mg/d	1–2 mg/d	none
Zinc	15 mg/d	2–5 mg/d	5 mg/d
Copper	2–3 mg/d	0.5–1.5 mg/d	1 mg/d
Chromium	50–200 µg/d	10–20 µg/d	10 µg/d
Selenium	50–200 µg/d	80–150 µg/d	100 µg/d
Iodine	150 µg/d	120 µg/d	120 µg/d
Manganese	2.5–5.0 mg/d	0.2–0.8 mg/d	0.5 mg/d
Vitamins*			
Vitamin A	RDA = 4000–5000 IU/d	ND	3300 IU/d
Vitamin D	RDA = 200–400 IU/d	ND	200 IU/d
Vitamin E	RDA = 12–15 IU/d	ND	10 IU/d
Vitamin K	RDA = 60–80 µg/d	ND	10 mg/wk[†]
Thiamine	RDA = 1.1–1.4 mg/d	ND	3 mg/d
Riboflavin	RDA = 1.2–1.7 mg/d	ND	5 mg/d
Niacin	RDA = 13–19 mg/d	ND	40 mg/d
Pantothenic acid	4–7 mg/d[‡]	ND	15 mg/d
Pyridoxine	RDA = 1.6–2.0 mg/d	ND	4 mg/d
Folic acid	RDA = 0.4 mg/d	ND	0.4 mg/d
Vitamin B_{12}	RDA = 3 µg/d	ND	5 µg/d
Vitamin C	RDA = 40 mg/d	ND	100 mg/d
Biotin	RDA = 30–100 µg/d	ND	60 µg/d

Abbreviation: ND, not defined.
* Enteral requirements should always exceed parenteral requirements; most recommend supplying 1–3 times the RDA of each vitamin to patients with critical illness.
[†] None if anticoagulation used.
[‡] RDA not established.

3. Published recommended daily allowances (RDAs) are based on oral intake in healthy individuals.
4. Vitamin needs for critically ill patients have not been determined.
5. See Table 10.5 for estimates of nutritional requirements of the vitamins.

6. Commercial enteral formulas generally supply the RDA of the vitamins (if patients receive their caloric needs).
7. An adult parenteral vitamin formulation was approved by the FDA in 1979 and is available for addition to TPN solutions; this should be added just before administration, since degradation can occur.

E. Minerals (Na, K, Ca, PO₄, Mg)

1. See Table 10.5 for estimates of daily nutritional requirements of the minerals.
2. Minerals are present in sufficient quantities in enteral products (special formulas limit electrolytes for renal failure).
3. Must be supplemented in TPN.

F. Trace Elements (iron, copper, iodine, zinc, selenium, chromium, cobalt, manganese)

1. Needs in critically ill patients have not been determined. (See Table 10.5 for estimates of requirements.)
2. Sufficient quantities are thought to be present in enteral products.
3. Must be supplemented in TPN (all except iron can be added to solution).
   a. Deficiency states have been reported in long-term TPN patients.
   b. Specifics are best managed by specially trained nutritional support teams.

■ VI. ROLE OF SPECIFIC NUTRIENTS (QUALITY)

A. Nitrogen Sources

1. Choices
   a. Amino acids
   b. Hydrolyzed protein (peptides)
   c. Intact proteins
2. Evidence suggests that peptides generated from the diet possess specific physiologic activities.
3. Nitrogen is best delivered as intact protein (if digestion and absorption intact) or hydrolyzed protein (impaired digestion).
4. Protein is absorbed primarily as peptides (60%) and amino acids (33%).
5. Essential amino acid formulas should *not* be used.
6. Some amino acids become essential during critical illness.

       a. These are called *conditionally essential amino acids*.
       b. Examples include glutamine, cysteine, arginine, and taurine.
   7. Some amino acids appear to have specific roles.
       a. Glutamine is a fuel for the GI tract and immune system.
       b. Arginine is required for optimum wound healing and is important in immune function.
       c. Cysteine is needed for synthesis of glutathione.
       d. Branched-chain amino acids (BCAA) may improve mental status in patients with hepatic encephalopathy; it is primarily metabolized by peripheral muscle instead of the liver.
       e. Note that glutamine and cysteine are not stable (or present) in TPN solution.

B. Lipids
   1. Linoleic Acid
       a. Essential fatty acid (need 7% to 12% of total calories supplied as linoleic acid)
       b. ω-6 Polyunsaturated, long-chain fatty acid (immunosuppressive)
       c. Precursor to membrane arachidonic acid
   2. ω-3 Polyunsaturated Fatty Acids (PUFA)
       a. Fish oils and linolenic acid.
       b. Decrease production of dienoic prostaglandins (i.e., PGE_2), tumor necrosis factor, interleukin-1, and other proinflammatory cytokines.
   3. Medium-Chain Triglycerides
       a. Good energy source.
       b. Water-soluble.
       c. Enter circulation via GI tract.
   4. Short-Chain Fatty Acids (SCFA)
       a. Examples: butyric and propionic acid
       b. Major fuel for the gut (especially the colon)
       c. Derived from metabolizable fiber
   5. High-Fat Formulas
       a. If the patient is not overfed, these have little effect on CO_2 production (despite being marketed for decreasing the respiratory quotient [RQ]).
       b. Poor GI tolerance.

C. Carbohydrates
   1. Starches and sugars: good for energy
   2. Fiber
       a. Metabolizable fiber (i.e., pectin, guar) is converted to SCFA in the colon by bacteria.

   b. Bulk increases stool mass, softens stool, adds body to stool, and provides some stimulation of gut mass.

D. Dietary nucleic acids may be important for immune function.

■ VII. MONITORING RESPONSES TO NUTRITIONAL SUPPORT

A. Visceral Proteins
   1. Prealbumin
      a. Half-life ≈ 2 days.
      b. Normal range is 10 to 40 mg/dL.
   2. Transferrin
      a. Half-life ≈ 8 to 9 days.
      b. Normal range is 160 to 355 mg/dL.
   3. Albumin
      a. half-life ≈ 20 days.
      b. Normal range is 3.2 to 5.0 mg/dL.

B. Visceral protein levels are affected by nutritional intake as well as the disease state (especially presence of inflammation).

C. Increasing levels of visceral proteins suggest that nutritional support is adequate.

D. Nitrogen Balance
   1. Determined from 12- to 24-hour urine collections and measurements of total urinary nitrogen (more accurate than total urea nitrogen) compared to total nitrogen intake.
   2. May be inaccurate
      a. In patients with renal failure
      b. If urine is not correctly collected by staff
      c. If the patient has increased nitrogen losses in stool or from wounds (i.e., burns)
   3. N-balance = protein intake (g/d)/6.25 − {total urinary nitrogen (g/d) + 2}.
   4. Negative nitrogen balance is not necessarily detrimental over the short term (i.e., 1 to 2 weeks).
   5. Improvement in nitrogen balance suggests that nutritional support is adequate.
   6. Be aware that nitrogen balance may improve as catabolism decreases despite inadequate nutritional support.

E. Indirect Calorimetry (Metabolic Cart)
   1. Measures oxygen consumption and CO_2 production for 15 to 30 minutes, estimates energy expenditure, then extrapolates to 24 hours.

    2. Keep RQ < 1. Values > 1 suggest lipogenesis from excessive caloric intake; values ≈ 0.7 are found in starvation and reflect fat oxidation.

F. Other Nutritional Parameters Not Generally Useful in the Critically Ill
    1. Weight
    2. Skin-fold thickness
    3. Delayed cutaneous hypersensitivity (DCH)
    4. Lymphocyte counts

■ VIII. NUTRITION FOR SPECIFIC DISEASE PROCESSES

A. Acute Renal Failure
    1. Use intact protein or peptide formula with moderate fat.
    2. Do not restrict protein (it is required for healing and for other organ functions).
    3. May limit fluid intake with double-strength formula (2 cal/mL).
    4. Watch K, Mg, and PO_4 levels.

B. Hepatic Failure
    1. Use intact protein or peptide formula.
    2. Usually 1.0 to 1.2 g/kg/d of protein are needed to support repair and immune function.
    3. BCAA may be of value if encephalopathy persists following use of intact protein or peptide diets.

C. Inflammatory Bowel Disease/Pancreatitis
    1. Postpyloric enteral feeding of a peptide-based diet is usually well tolerated.
    2. Enteral nutrition should be attempted before initiating TPN.

D. Multiple Organ Failure
    1. Nutritional support is usually of marginal value.
    2. Nutritional support needs to be started before organ failure develops.

■ IX. NASODUODENAL FEEDING TUBE PLACEMENT

A. Use in patients who do not tolerate oral or gastric feeding.

B. Patients with abdominal surgery should have the tube placed during surgery under direct visualization.

1. The anesthesiologist inserts the tube into the stomach.
2. The surgeon locates the tube, and directs it into the duo-denum or jejunum.
3. Eliminates need for confirmatory x-rays.
4. Allows immediate feeding upon admission into intensive care unit (ICU).
5. Feeding tubes may also be placed into the small bowel using a gastrostomy or jejunostomy.

C. Tubes placed into the stomach will rarely (5% to 15%) migrate spontaneously into the small bowel in critically ill patients (due to gastroparesis).

D. Bedside Method
   1. Place patient in left lateral decubitus position (if possible).
   2. Lubricate the nostril with generic lubricant or 2% viscous lidocaine.
   3. Insert an 8–10 French small-bore feeding tube (containing wire stylet) into the nostril, and gently advance it through the nasopharynx into the esophagus and then the stomach.
   4. If resistance is met or the patient coughs, becomes agitated, or decreases oxygen saturation, then
      a. Pull the tube back into the nasopharynx.
      b. Repeat step 3, and reinsert the tube into the stomach.
      c. Or, change the position of the patient's neck (slightly flex or extend) before reattempting insertion.
   5. Confirm position of the tube in the stomach.
      a. Auscultate over the abdomen.
      b. Aspirate gastric contents (pH $\approx$ 2 to 5, unless on H_2 blocker).
   6. Remove wire stylet, and place a 45-degree bend approximately 1 inch from the distal end of the wire.
   7. Gently reinsert the wire stylet (should not meet resistance).
   8. Slowly advance the tube while rotating it in a clockwise direction.
   9. Check the position every 10 to 15 cm.
      a. Auscultation will reveal higher pitched sounds when the tube is in the pylorus and proximal small bowel.
      b. Bile may be aspirated from the tube in the small bowel.
      c. Bile/small bowel secretions have pH $\approx$ 6 to 7.
      d. Abdominal x-ray
         (1) Can confirm small bowel location.
         (2) May not be cost-effective.
         (3) Will avoid feeding into lung in rare case of misplaced feeding tube.

E. With this bedside method, we (faculty, residents, and medical students) successfully place >90% of attempted small bowel tubes into the duodenum or jejunum.

F. Aggressive surgical and bedside placement allows us to feed >97% of our critically ill patients enterally within 24 to 48 hours of admission into the ICU.

G. If bedside placement is not possible, place the feeding tube into small intestine using
   1. Endoscopy
   2. Fluoroscopy

■ X. RECOMMENDATIONS FOR TPN USE

1. Use *only* when enteral nutrition is not possible (e.g., short-gut syndrome, chylothorax).
   a. Failure of the stomach to empty is not an indication for TPN but rather for a small bowel feeding tube.
   b. Most patients with diarrhea can be managed with enteral nutrition.

2. Initial TPN orders may be based on recommendations in Tables 10.4 and 10.5.

3. Overall TPN management is best performed by specially trained nutritional support teams.

4. For more specifics, the reader is referred to entire texts written about TPN.

■ XI. APPROACH TO ENTERAL FEEDING

A. Enteral nutritional support should be initiated within 12 to 48 hours of admission to the ICU.

B. The oral route is preferred (but frequently not possible).

C. The gastric route is second choice and should be tried before placing a small bowel tube in most patients.

D. Patients at high risk for aspiration or known gastric paresis should be fed with a small bowel tube.

E. Feeding formulas should *not* be diluted.

F. Keep the head of the patient's bed elevated 30 degrees to decrease the risk of aspiration.

G. Feeding should be started at 25 to 30 mL/h and increased by 25 mL/h every 1 to 4 hours as tolerated by gastric residuals (<150 mL) until the caloric goal (25 to 30 kcal/kg/d) is achieved.

H. If the protein goal is not achieved, use a formula with a higher protein/calorie ratio or add protein to the formula.

I. Gastric residuals should be monitored every 4 hours.

J. If the gastric residual is >150 mL, hold feeds for 2 hours and then resume.

K. May increase feeds at slower rate (i.e., ≈10 mL/h every 6 to 12 hours), but often this is not necessary.

L. The goal rate of infusion should be met by the third day of therapy (frequently earlier).

M. Monitor nutritional response by measuring visceral protein levels.
    1. Prealbumin and transferrin levels should be measured on day 1 and every 3 days thereafter during initial therapy.
    2. Increasing levels suggest that the patient is receiving adequate nutritional support.
    3. Levels usually normalize in 1 to 2 weeks if the disease process is controlled and nutritional support is adequate.
    4. If levels fail to increase,
        a. Consider underlying infection, inflammation, or other disease processes.
        b. Reevaluate the adequacy of nutritional support.
        c. Nitrogen balance and energy balance (i.e., indirect calorimetry) may be informative.
        d. Consult the nutritional support service.

N. Several flow diagrams (for specific patient populations, using enteral products currently on our formulary) are given as examples (see Figures 10.1 to 10.3).
    1. Isolated head injury (see Figure 10.1)
    2. Multitrauma, burn, sepsis, and abdominal surgery (see Figure 10.2)
    3. Severe malnutrition (see Figure 10.3)

O. If peptide-based diets are not available, intact protein diets should be used.

P. Formula Osmolality
    1. 300 to 600 mOsm/kg H_2O.
    2. Rarely causes intolerance/diarrhea.

Q. Diarrhea is unfortunately encountered in patients on enteral and parenteral nutrition.

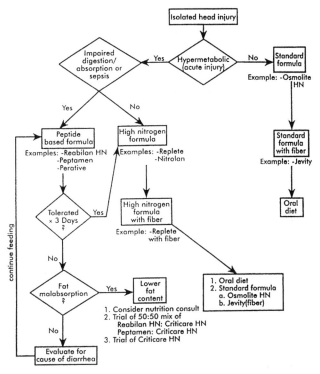

Figure 10.1. Flow diagram for nutritional support in patients with isolated head injury.

1. Generally defined as >300 to 500 mL stool output per day.
2. Most common etiologies are medications and infections. See Table 10.6 for a partial list of etiologies and suggestions for preliminary workup.
3. Note that many elixir forms of medications contain sorbitol.
4. Once the specific etiologies of diarrhea have been evaluated, diarrhea may be treated with antimotility agents (i.e., narcotics). We prefer to add paregoric directly to the feeding formula (30 to 60 cc q4–6h).

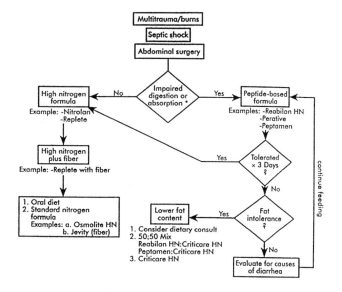

*Shock, resuscitation, major abdominal surgery, gut or
pancreatic injury, sepsis, acute hypoalbuminemia (<2g/dL)

Figure 10.2. Flow diagram for nutritional support in patients with
multiple trauma, burn injury, sepsis/septic shock, or abdominal
surgery.

■ XII. USEFUL FACTS AND FORMULAS

A. Nutritional Assessment

The *total daily energy* (TDE) requirements for a patient can
be calculated using the following formula:

$$\text{TDE for men (kcal/d)} = (66.47 + 13.75W + 5.0H - 6.76A)$$
$$\times (\text{Activity factor}) \times (\text{Injury factor})$$

TDE for women (kcal/day)

$$= (655.10 + 9.56W + 1.85H\ 4.68A)$$
$$\times (\text{Activity factor}) \times (\text{Injury factor})$$

where W = weight (kg), H = height (cm), A = age (years); the
activity factor is derived from Table 10.7.

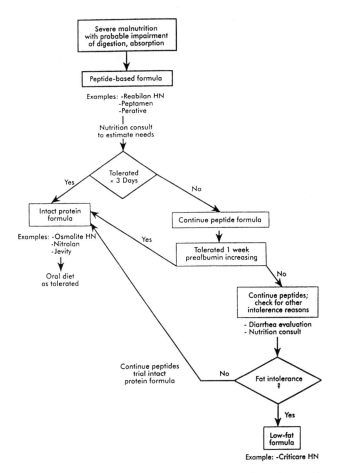

Figure 10.3. Flow diagram for nutritional support in patients with severe malnutrition.

Table 10.6. Etiologies and Evaluation of Diarrhea

Causes	Examples	Workup
Drugs	Sorbitol, antacids, H_2 blockers, antibiotics, lactulose, laxatives, quinidine, theophylline	No specific workup; discontinue any of these medications that are not absolutely necessary
Infections	1. *Clostridium difficile*	1. Specific stool culture, *C. difficile* toxin assay, sigmoidoscopy/colonoscopy for evidence of pseudomembranes
	2. Infectious diarrhea (e.g., typhoid fever, shigellosis)	2. Fecal leukocytes, culture
	3. Other: bacterial overgrowth, parasites, systemic infection, HIV	3. As relevant (e.g., look for ova and parasites; rarely causes new diarrhea in critically ill)
Osmotic		Measure stool osmotic gap (SOG);* SOG >100 suggests osmotic diarrhea
Impaction	May be secondary to narcotics	Rectal exam
Other causes	Inflammatory bowel disease, pancreatic insufficiency, short gut syndrome	

* SOG = stool osmolality − 2(stool Na^+ + K^+).

Table 10.7. Activity Factor

Confined to bed	1.2
Out of bed	1.3

The *injury factors* can be estimated based on the Table 10.8.

The *metabolic rate* (MR) can be calculated in patients with a pulmonary artery catheter as follows:

$$MR\,(kcal/h) = VO_2\,(mL/min) \times 60\,min/h$$
$$\times\,1\,L/1000\,mL \times 4.83\,kcal/L$$

where VO_2 (mL/min) = Cardiac output (L/min) × [arterial oxygen content (CaO_2, mL/L) − mixed venous oxygen content (CmO_2, mL/L)].

Table 10.8. Injury Factors

Surgery	
Minor	1.0–1.1
Major	1.1–1.2
Infection	
Mild	1.0–1.2
Moderate	1.2–1.4
Severe	1.4–1.8
Trauma	
Skeletal	1.2–1.35
Head injury	
with steroid therapy	1.6
Blunt	1.15–1.35
Burns (body surface area)	
Up to 20%	1.0–1.5
20% to 40%	1.5–1.85
Over 40%	1.85–1.95

The *prognostic nutritional index* (PNI) allows for nutritional assessment of the critically ill patient and is calculated as follows:

$$PNI (\% \text{ risk}) = 158\% - 16.6 (\text{alb}) - 0.78 (\text{TSF})$$
$$- 0.2 (\text{tfn}) - 5.8 (\text{DSH})$$

where alb = serum albumin (g/dL); TSF = triceps skin fold (mm); tfn = serum transferrin (mg/dL); DSH = delayed skin hypersensitivity (1 = anergy, 2 = reactive).

The *probability of survival* (POS) based on the nutritional status of a critically ill patient can be calculated as follows:

$$POS = 0.91 (\text{alb}) - 1.0 (\text{DSH}) - 1.44 (\text{SEP})$$
$$+ 0.98 (\text{DIA}) - 1.09$$

where alb = serum albumin (g/dL); DSH = delayed skin hypersensitivity (1 = anergy, 2 = reactive); SEP = sepsis (1 = no sepsis, 2 = sepsis); DIA = diagnosis of cancer (1 = no cancer, 2 = cancer).

Another way to calculate the nutritional deficit is by utilizing the *index of undernutrition* (IOU), as shown in Table 10.9.

The calculation of *daily protein requirements* (PR) can be done utilizing the following formula:

$$PR (g) = (\text{Patient weight}) \text{ in kg} \times (\text{PR for illness in g/kg})$$

Table 10.9. Index of Undernutrition

Assay	Points				
	0	5	10	15	20
Albumin (g/dL)	>3.5	3.1–3.5	2.6–3.0	2.0–2.5	<2.0
Fat area (%)	>70	56–70	46–55	30–45	<30
Muscle area (%)	>80	76–80	61–75	40–60	<40
Transferrin (g/L)	>2.0	1.76–2.0	1.41–1.75	1.0–1.4	<40
Weight lost (%)	0	0–10	11–14	15–20	>20

To determine the nonprotein caloric requirements (NCR):

NCR = (Total required calories)

    −(Required protein calories)

The *nitrogen balance* (NB) reflects the status of the net protein use:

$$NB = (\text{Dietary protein} \times 0.16) - (\text{UUN} + 2\text{ g stool} + 2\text{ g skin})$$

where UUN = urine urea nitrogen.

In patients with renal failure, the increased blood urea pool and extrarenal urea losses must be accounted for:

NB = Nitrogen in

    −(UUN + 2 g stool + 2 g skin + BUN change)

where BUN = serum urea nitrogen.

In addition to the above formulas, the *catabolic index* (CI) can be derived from the same variables:

$$CI = UUN - [(0.5 \times \text{Dietary protein} \times 0.16) + 3\text{ g}]$$

No nutritional stress results in a CI ≥ 0, in moderate nutritional stress CI < 5, and in severe nutritional stress CI > 5.

Another index of the loss of lean tissue in malnourished patients is the *creatinine height index* (CHI) and can be calculated as follows:

CHI = Measured creatinine/expected creatinine

The *body mass index* (BMI) normalizes for height and allows comparisons among diverse populations:

$$BMI = \text{Body weight (kg)}/(\text{height})^2 \text{ (m)}$$

B. Fuel Composition

The body uses different sources of fuel. Table 10.10 depicts some of them.

Table 10.10. Normal Fuel Composition of the Human Body

Fuel	Amount (kg)	Calories (kcal)
Circulating fuels		
Glucose	0.020	80
Free fatty acids (plasma)	0.0003	3
Triglycerides (plasma)	0.003	30
Total		113
Tissue		
Fat (adipose triglycerides)	15	141,000
Protein (muscle)	6	24,000
Glycogen (muscle)	0.150	600
Glycogen (liver)	0.075	300
Total		165,900

Table 10.11. Ideal Body Weight in Males and Females

Height in cm	Males (Weight in kg)	Females (Weight in kg)
145	51.8	47.5
150	54.5	50.4
155	57.2	53.1
160	60.5	56.2
165	63.5	59.5
175	70.1	66.3
180	74.2	
185	78.1	

C. Other Formulas

The *body surface area* (BSA) of a patient can be calculated as follows:

$$BSA\left(m^2\right) = \frac{\left(\text{Weight in Kg}\right)^{0.425} \times \left(\text{height in cm}\right)^{0.725} \times 71.84}{10,000}$$

The *ideal body weight* (IBW) for height in males and females can be estimated based on Table 10.11.

The *percentage of ideal body weight* (%IBW) is calculated as follows:

$$\%IBW = \frac{100 \times \left(\text{height in cm}\right)}{IBW}$$

11

Critical Care Oncology

Cancer is the second leading cause of death in the United States. Enhanced critical care capabilities have contributed substantially to improved survival. Critical care may be needed on a short-term basis for the complications of the underlying malignancy or of aggressive antineoplastic therapy. Postoperative critical care has greatly facilitated major extirpative cancer surgery and is an implicit part of other approaches such as bone marrow transplantation.

The present chapter considers different types of cancer patients likely to need and benefit from treatment in the ICU. Clinical judgment regarding the appropriate use of critical care services is required in all patient populations, not just in patients with cancer. The decision to admit and technologically support critically ill cancer patients should be individualized.

■ I. CENTRAL NERVOUS SYSTEM

A. Altered Mental Status

Alteration in mental status is the most common central nervous system (CNS) presentation for cancer patients in the intensive care unit (ICU). The common differential diagnoses are considered below. If these can be excluded, and the patient has not received excessive sedative or narcotic-analgesic agents, the patient should be treated presumptively for *sepsis*. Altered mental status is a reliable, though nonspecific sign of sepsis, which carries a high mortality rate in cancer patients.

1. Intracranial Mass Lesions

A history of headache, nausea, vomiting, or seizure activity together with papilledema and other signs of raised intracranial pressure suggest an intracranial mass lesion. A moderate increase in intracranial pressure by itself is relatively well tolerated; however, when intracranial pressure becomes critical, brain substance will shift in the direction of least resistance, with resultant herniation through the tentorium or foramen magnum.

2. Primary Tumors of the CNS

These present with focal neurologic signs, depending on location.

3. Secondary (Metastatic) Tumors

Approximately 15% to 30% of secondary tumors will present with new onset seizures. Common malignancies associated with cerebral metastases include breast, lung, kidney, and melanoma.

4. Cerebral Hemorrhage

Cerebral hemorrhage is associated with acute promyelocytic leukemia, as a direct complication of brain metastases, or related thrombocytopenia.

5. Subdural Hematoma

Acute subdural hematomas present with fluctuation in the level of consciousness and hemiparesis.

6. Brain Abscess

Brain abscess accounts for 30% of CNS infections in cancer patients.

a. Clinically apparent raised intracranial pressure and neurologic deficits are late signs.

b. Usually present with fever, headache, drowsiness, confusion, and seizures.

c. Typically seen in patients with leukemias or head and neck tumors.

B. Other Causes of Altered Mental Status in Critically Ill Cancer Patients

1. Leptomeningeal Metastases

a. May present with signs of raised intracranial pressure and hydrocephalus.

b. Acute leukemias, lymphomas, and breast carcinomas are frequent causes.

2. Cerebrovascular accident (CVA)

Commonly occurs in cancer patients. As in all patients, CVA may be thrombotic, hemorrhagic, or embolic in nature.

a. Most patients present with focal neurologic signs and headaches.

b. Seizures are common, especially in hemorrhagic CVA.

    c. Embolic CVA in cancer patients may be related to septic emboli, especially in patients with known fungal infection (i.e., aspergillosis).

3. Metabolic Encephalopathies

Lethargy, weakness, somnolence, coma, agitation or psychosis, focal or generalized seizures can all result from metabolic abnormalities. Lack of focal neurologic signs suggest a metabolic encephalopathy. Examples include

    a. Hypercalcemia (see below)
    b. Hyponatremia
    c. Hypomagnesemia
    d. Hypoglycemia
    e. Uremia

4. Seizures/Postictal State

Patients with primary and secondary tumors (especially hemispheric) commonly present with seizures.

    a. Differential diagnosis includes CVA, CNS infection, or narcotic withdrawal as causes of seizures.
    b. In the immediate postictal period, findings may include evidence of tongue biting, loss of bladder/ bowel control, extensor plantar responses.
    c. The presence of lateralized focal signs suggests that seizures may have a focal origin.
    d. Prolonged coma after a generalized seizure, or transient hemiparesis (Todd's paralysis) following a Jacksonian, focal, or generalized seizure is more common in patients with seizures secondary to mass lesions than in those with seizures secondary to other conditions.

5. Cerebral Leukostasis

Patients with hyperleukocytosis (defined as a peripheral white blood cell [WBC] count >100,000/mm^3), may present with blurred vision, dizziness, ataxia, stupor, or coma, or with an intracranial hemorrhage.

    a. Hemorrhage results from leukostatic plugging of arterioles and capillaries with endothelial cell damage, capillary leak, and small vessel disruption.
    b. Retinal hemorrhages are suggestive of intracranial hemorrhage, and thus fundoscopic examination should be performed frequently.

6. Hyperviscosity Syndrome (HVS)

Excessive elevations of serum paraproteins or marked leukocytosis can result in elevated serum viscosity, sludging, and decreased perfusion of the microcirculation, with stasis. HVS can affect any organ system; however, characteristic clinical findings occur in the lungs and CNS.

a. Patients may present with visual disturbances or visual loss.

b. Characteristic retinopathy is present with venous engorgement (with "sausage-link" or "boxcar" segmentation), microaneurysms, hemorrhages, exudates, and occasionally papilledema.

c. Similar vascular changes may be seen in the bulbar conjunctivae.

d. Other clinical findings may include headache, dizziness, Jacksonian and generalized seizures, somnolence, lethargy, coma, and auditory disturbances, including hearing loss.

7. CNS Infections

Patients with cancer are susceptible to a variety of CNS infections, including meningitis, brain abscess (see above), and encephalitis.

a. Meningitis is most frequently encountered in patient(s) with impaired cell-mediated immunity and is typically caused by *Cryptococcus neoformans* or *Listeria monocytogenes*.

b. Patients with meningitis present with fever, headache, and altered mental status.

c. All cancer patients with fever and altered mental status should have a lumbar puncture preceded by a computed tomography (CT) scan of the head (if a cerebral mass lesion is suspected).

d. Encephalitis is most often caused by Herpes viruses (simplex or zoster) or *Toxoplasma gondii*.

e. Patients with encephalitis commonly present with signs of meningeal irritation (fever, headache, nuchal rigidity) and evidence of altered mental status. Confusion may progress to stupor and coma; focal neurologic signs and seizures are common.

C. Spinal Cord Compression

Significant cord compression results from epidural metastases and is most frequently seen in breast, lung, or prostate cancer with disseminated disease.

Classically, the chief complaint is back pain (90% of patients), which may be associated with weakness, autonomic dysfunction, sensory disturbances, ataxia, and flexor spasms. The neurologic deficit is determined by the level of the involved spinal cord.

1. Compression from metastases typically arises from three locations.

a. Vertebral column (85%)

b. Paravertebral spaces (10% to 15%)

c. Epidural space (rare)

2. The distribution throughout the spine is approximately as follows:
   a. Thoracic (70%)
   b. Lumbar (20%)
   c. Cervical (10%)

D. Central Nervous System: Diagnostic Evaluation in the ICU
   1. History, physical examination, and careful neurologic evaluation, emphasizing lateralizing signs, fundoscopy, and evidence of raised intracranial pressure.
   2. Laboratory tests should include
      a. Arterial blood gases
      b. Serum electrolytes, glucose
      c. Calcium, magnesium, phosphorus
      d. Renal and hepatic function tests
      e. Determination of serum viscosity, especially in cases of multiple myeloma or other paraprotein-producing tumors
   3. Computed Tomography
      Head CT is the diagnostic test of choice for mass lesions, midline shift, intracranial hemorrhage or hydrocephalus.
   4. Magnetic Resonance Imaging (MRI)
      MRI is a sensitive test for detection of intracerebral metastases and to differentiate between vascular and tumor-related masses. It is also the examination of choice for the evaluation of intramedullary, intradural, and extramedullary spine lesion(s).
   5. Myelography
      Myelography provides an indirect image of the spinal cord and nerve roots from the foramen magnum to the sacrum. It is the "gold standard" in the evaluation of spinal cord involvement by tumor.
   6. Lumbar Puncture (LP)
      LP is most useful for the diagnosis of meningeal carcinomatosis, CNS leukemia, and CNS infections.

E. Central Nervous System: Acute Management in the ICU (See also Chapter 9, "Neurologic Disorders")
   1. Raised Intracranial Pressure With Impending Herniation
      a. Glucocorticoid therapy will improve neurologic deficits in 70% of patients with symptomatic brain metastases by reduction of vasogenic brain edema. An initial dose of 10 mg dexamethasone may be given intravenously, followed by 16 mg/d in 3 or 4 divided doses by the most appropriate route. Patients who do not respond to the standard dose may improve when the dose is increased to 100 mg/d.

    b. Osmotherapy with agents such as urea or mannitol is initiated to produce rapid reduction of intracranial pressure in patients with known or suspected intracranial metastases showing signs of herniation.

        Mannitol 1.5 to 2.0 g/kg as a 20% solution can be administered by slow intravenous (IV) infusion. The total dose should not exceed 120 g/d.

    c. Hyperventilation may be instituted in patients who present with signs of brain herniation. They should be intubated expeditiously and ventilated to maintain an arterial PCO_2 of 25 to 30 torr (mm Hg).

    d. Neurosurgical consultation is needed in the vast majority of patients.

  2. Seizures

    a. Position the patient laterally to prevent aspiration and protect the airway.

    b. Correct any metabolic alteration or hypoxemia.

    c. If the seizure is sustained, acute control is achieved with IV diazepam (Valium) 5 to 10 mg, which may be repeated in 5 to 10 minutes up to 30 mg. Alternatively, lorazepam (Ativan) 1 to 10 mg IV or by continuous infusion can be used. Another useful agent that permits rapid cessation of seizures is the administration of IV propofol (Diprivan).

    d. Long-term seizure control can usually be established with IV phenytoin (Dilantin). The loading dose is 15 mg/kg IV (50 mg/min).

    e. Intracerebral metastases should be treated with corticosteroids, chemotherapy, radiation or surgery as indicated by the specific lesion.

  3. Spinal Cord Compression

    Palliation is generally accepted as a reasonable goal in the management of these patients.

    a. Radiotherapy and surgical decompression are the cornerstones of management.

    b. Chemotherapy with nitrogen mustard or cyclophosphamide has been effectively used, generally in combination with radiation, for the management of cord compression caused by lymphoma or Hodgkin's disease.

  4. Other Modalities

    a. Leukophoresis is one of the therapeutic options for severe symptomatic leukocytosis with leukostasis.

    b. If hydrocephalus is present, it should be managed by emergent relief and shunting.

    c. Radiotherapy is currently the most commonly employed therapeutic modality for palliation of cerebral metastases.

5. General Supportive Care
   a. Stress ulcer prophylaxis in the form of antacids, sucralfate, or H_2-receptor antagonists.
   b. Prophylaxis for deep venous thrombosis (DVT) should include, if no contraindication exists, the use of subcutaneous heparin and/or the use of sequential compressive devices (SCDs) on the lower extremities.
   c. Nutritional support should be provided for repletion of malnourished patients, as well as for maintenance of good nutrition in patients at risk for malnutrition due to cancer or its therapy.
   d. Appropriate antimicrobial therapy (see below).

■ II. PULMONARY

The lungs are involved commonly in cancer patients with 75% to 90% of pulmonary complications being secondary to infection. Noninfectious complications include those due to chemotherapy (i.e., bleomycin), thoracic irradiation, and pulmonary resections. Respiratory failure in cancer patients requiring mechanical ventilation is associated with a 75% mortality rate.

A. Pulmonary Infiltrates
   In patients with systemic cancer, the differential diagnosis of pulmonary infiltrates seen on a routine chest film is extensive.
   1. Localized infiltrates that are confined to a lobe or segment in a patient with a compatible history most frequently represent a bacterial process.
   2. Diffuse bilateral infiltrates are more suggestive of opportunistic infection, treatment-induced lung injury, or lymphangitic spread of carcinoma.
   3. Bilateral perihilar infiltrates in patients who have rapidly gained weight support a diagnosis of fluid overload.
   4. Pulmonary infiltrates following bone marrow transplantation.
      a. Life-threatening infections generally occur within the first 100 days post-transplant.
      b. Within the initial 30 days post-transplant, the most common pathogens for pneumonia are bacterial or fungal.
      c. Interstitial pneumonia (diffuse nonbacterial pneumonia) is the predominant problem following transplantation, with the syndrome consisting of dyspnea, nonproductive cough, hypoxemia, diffuse bilateral infiltrates and occurring within 30 to 100 days after transplant.

    d. Cytomegalovirus (CMV) pneumonia comprises the majority of interstitial pneumonitides. The incidence of CMV infection appears to be related to the loss of immunity during pretransplant conditioning and to the development of graft-versus-host disease.

5. Diagnosis
   a. Chest x-ray is never diagnostic of any single entity.
   b. Cultures of sputum and special stains of tracheobronchial secretions (KOH, India ink) should be obtained routinely. Colonization of the upper respiratory tract as well as the inadequacy of sputum production may make identification of the offending organism(s) difficult.
   c. Blood cultures for fungal and bacterial organisms.
   d. Viral titers (especially CMV).
   e. Daily determination of serum lactate levels may be of some value in patients with respiratory failure. An increase in the serum lactate level may precede the deterioration of arterial blood gases and the development of diffuse infiltrates typical of adult respiratory distress syndrome (ARDS).
   f. Bronchoscopy with bronchoalveolar lavage (BAL) has a diagnostic sensitivity of 80% to 90% and is the procedure of choice in cancer patients with diffuse infiltrates.
      (1) BAL is most helpful in diagnosing opportunistic infection (i.e., *Pneumocystis carinii*, viruses such as CMV, fungus and mycobacteria).
      (2) This procedure is also useful for the diagnosis of intraparenchymal pulmonary hemorrhage.
      (3) BAL is safe in thrombocytopenic and mechanically ventilated patients who may not tolerate transbronchial biopsy.
   g. Open lung biopsy is reserved for selected patients due to its attendant morbidity, discomfort, and financial cost.

6. Management
   a. Early empirical use of broad-spectrum antibiotics (see Chapter 8, "Infections").
   b. In patients who remain persistently febrile despite the use of antibiotics, amphotericin B has been shown to reduce the mortality rate due to infection.
   c. Gancyclovir and hyperimmune globulin have recently been shown to improve survival in patients with interstitial pneumonia.

B. Pulmonary Leukostasis

   Leukostasis, with obstructed flow in small pulmonary vessels, is the consequence of the intravascular accumulation of immature, rigid myeloblasts, observed predominantly in acute myelogenous leukemia (AML) and chronic myelogenous leukemia (CML) patients in blast phase. Vascular stasis and distention result in local hypoxia. The release of intracellular enzymes and procoagulants leads to vascular and pulmonary parenchymal damage.

   1. Signs and Symptoms: Progressive dyspnea and/or altered mental status (see discussion on CNS).
   2. Diagnosis
      a. CBC: WBC count is usually >150,000/mm^3.
      b. Arterial Blood Gases (ABGs): True hypoxemia develops as a result of impaired pulmonary gas exchange. Spurious low values for PaO$_2$ may be consistently obtained because the large number of blasts consume oxygen within the ABG specimen itself. The longer the interval between the collection and analysis, the lower the measured PaO$_2$. This may make assessment of gas exchange difficult.
      c. Pulse oximetry may be of benefit to follow the adequacy of arterial oxygenation.
      d. Chest x-ray may be normal or show diffuse nodular infiltrates.
   3. Management
      a. Myeloblast counts >50,000/mm^3 warrant prompt treatment for reduction of the total WBC count to 20% to 60% within hours of recognition of the syndrome.
      b. Leukophoresis.
      c. Chemotherapy (i.e., daunorubicin, cytosine arabinoside, hydroxyurea).
      d. Adequate hydration.
      e. Urate nephropathy prevention should be initiated with allopurinol and urine alkalinization.
      f. Hemodynamic monitoring is suggested.
      g. When ARDS results from leukostasis, the following should be carried out expeditiously:
         (1) Fluid resuscitation to restore blood volume.
         (2) Cardiac output and hemodynamics should be optimized through volume enhancement and inotropic agents as needed.
         (3) Pulmonary vasoconstriction should be treated with a combination of volume expansion, inotropic agents, and supplemental O$_2$.

      (4) DO_2 and VO_2 should be monitored frequently and optimized to $\geq 600\,mL\ O_2/min/m^2$ and $\geq 150\,mL/O_2/min/m^2$, respectively.

      (5) Mechanical ventilation should be instituted when needed to achieve normal pH, pCO_2, and $PO_2 > 60$ on nontoxic FiO_2 (see Chapter 2, "The Basics of Critical Care").

C. Treatment-Induced Lung Injury

  1. Chemotherapy-Induced Lung Injury

    A large number of chemotherapeutic agents can produce pulmonary toxicity, either actively or delayed years after therapy. Commonly used agents with known pulmonary toxicity include alkylating agents (i.e., cyclophosphamide, carmustine, chlorambucil, melphalan, busulfan), antimetabolites (i.e., methotrexate, azathioprine), antitumor antibiotics (i.e., bleomycin, mitomycin), and alkaloids (i.e., vincristine). Pulmonary toxicity may take the following forms:

    a. Noncardiogenic pulmonary edema (ARDS)

    b. Chronic pneumonitis and fibrosis

    c. Hypersensitivity pneumonitis (i.e., procarbazine, methotrexate, bleomycin).

  2. Radiation-Induced Lung Toxicity

    Radiation pneumonitis is a clinical syndrome of dyspnea, cough, and fever developing in association with indistinct, hazy pulmonary infiltrates that may progress to dense alveolar consolidation following treatment with ionizing radiation.

    a. The likelihood of developing radiation-induced lung injury is influenced by a number of variables including the total dose, fractionation of doses, volume of lung irradiated, and a history of prior irradiation and chemotherapy.

    b. Pathophysiology

      (1) Direct effect of ionizing particles on alveolar structure.

      (2) Generation of high-energy oxygen-free radicals in excess of what normal enzymatic systems (peroxidase, superoxide dismutase) can remove.

      (3) The release of vasoactive substances such as histamine and bradykinin affects capillary permeability and pulmonary vascular resistance. The resultant pulmonary damage can exceed the area of radiation.

    c. From 5% to 15% of patients develop radiation pneumonitis.

    d. Symptoms may occur 1 to 6 months following completion of thoracic irradiation.

■ III. CARDIOVASCULAR

A. Cardiac Tamponade (See Also Chapter 3, "Cardiovascular Disorders")

Cardiac tamponade is a life-threatening condition caused by increased intrapericardial pressure, resulting in limitation of ventricular diastolic filling and decreased stroke volume and cardiac output.

1. Common Etiologies in Cancer Patients
    a. Metastatic tumors of the pericardium.
        (1) Much more commonly produce tamponade than primary tumors of the pericardium.
        (2) Cause tamponade by either producing effusions or constriction.
        (3) Cancer of the lungs and breast, lymphoma, leukemia, and melanoma account for 80% of metastatic causes of cardiac tamponade.
    b. Primary tumors of the pericardium.
    c. Postirradiation pericarditis with fibrosis. The pericardium is the most frequent site injured by radiation. The latent period between radiotherapy and onset of clinical pericardial disease may be years.
    d. Encasement of the heart by the tumor.

2. Clinical Findings
    a. Symptoms are often nonspecific but commonly include sensation of fullness in the chest, pericardial pain, or interscapular pain; apprehension; dyspnea, orthopnea.
    b. Clinical signs include altered mental status, hypotension, tachycardia, narrow arterial pulse pressure, distant heart tones with diminished apical impulse, tachypnea, oliguria, and diaphoresis. Other signs include the following:
        (1) Pulsus paradoxus
        (2) Ewart's sign (area of dullness at angle of left scapula)
        (3) Kussmaul's sign (neck veins bulge on inspiration)

3. Diagnosis
    a. Clinical Suspicion: The key to recognizing tamponade is considering the diagnosis.

b. Chest X-Ray
   (1) Large globular heart shadow ("water-bottle" configuration). If the pericardial fluid is <250 mL, the cardiac silhouette may be normal.
   (2) Lung fields are usually clear.
   (3) Pleural effusions are common associated findings.
c. Electrocardiogram (ECG)
   (1) Sinus tachycardia.
   (2) Low voltage QRS (<5 mV).
   (3) Electrical alternans, which result from the heart oscillating in the filled pericardial sac. Alternation of the QRS complexes is most specific for pericardial effusion.
d. Echocardiography makes a quick and definitive diagnosis of tamponade. Two-dimensional echo is more sensitive than M-mode. Findings include the following:
   (1) Prolonged diastolic collapse or inversion of right atrial free wall.
   (2) Early diastolic collapse of the right ventricular free wall.
   (3) Effusions as small as 30 mL are early detected by echocardiography (seen as an echo-free space).
e. Pulmonary Artery (Swan-Ganz) Catheterization
   (1) Elevated pulmonary capillary wedge and right atrial pressures with a prominent x descent with no significant y descent ("square root sign").
   (2) Decreased cardiac output, stroke volume, systemic arterial pressure, and mixed venous oxygen saturation (SvO_2).
   (3) Equalization of all pressures in diastole.
f. MRI is also diagnostic but is expensive and time-consuming compared with echocardiography.
g. Diagnostic Pericardiocentesis
   (1) Cytology to detect presence of malignant cells
   (2) Gram's stain and acid fast bacilli (AFB) smear, culture and sensitivity, cell count and differential
   (3) Protein, lactic dehydrogenase (LDH) content
4. Therapy
   a. Therapeutic pericardiocentesis should be performed immediately in hemodynamically compromised patients.
      (1) Two-dimensional echocardiography-guided pericardiocentesis is successful in 95% of cases with no major complications.

       (2) Reaccumulation of fluid is likely to occur in malignant effusions but can be prevented with chemical sclerosis (i.e., tetracycline), radiation therapy, or surgery (i.e., pleuropericardial window or pericardiectomy).

B. Myocardial Tissue Injury
1. Common Etiologies in Cancer Patients
   a. Anthracycline antibiotics (i.e., doxorubicin and daunorubicin).
   b. Mitoxantrone: A total dose >100 to 140 mg/m^2 can cause congestive heart failure and exacerbate preexisting anthracycline-induced cardiomyopathy.
   c. Cyclophosphamide: Doses >100 to 120 mg/kg over 2 days can result in congestive heart failure and hemorrhagic myocarditis/pericarditis and necrosis.
   d. Busulfan: The conventional oral daily dose may cause endocardial fibrosis.
   e. Interferons: In conventional doses, interferons may exacerbate underlying cardiac disease.
   f. Mitomycin C: Standard doses can cause myocardial damage.
   g. Radiation-induced cardiomyopathy causes a dose-dependent endocardial and myocardial fibrosis, which can result in a restrictive cardiomyopathy.
2. Diagnosis
   a. Endomyocardial Biopsy: Valuable for establishing etiology of cardiac injury in patients who may have received chemotherapy and for detecting subclinical cardiac damage. The anthracyclines cause characteristic degenerative changes in the myocytes.
   b. An ECG-gated blood pool scan for precise measurement of ejection fraction and detecting regional and global myocardial dysfunction.
3. Therapy
   Treatment is the same as for congestive cardiomyopathy of any cause. There is no specific therapy directed at radiation- or chemotherapy-induced myocardial damage.

C. Cardiac Dysrhythmias
1. Etiology
   a. Anthracycline antibiotics cause dysrhythmias unrelated to the cumulative dose; these effects can be seen hours or days after administration. Commonly observed dysrhythmias include supraventricular tachycardia, complete heart block, and ventricular tachycardia. Doxorubicin may also prolong the Q-T interval.

       b. Amacrine produces ventricular dysrhythmias.

       c. Taxol causes bradycardia and in combination with cisplatin may produce ventricular tachycardia.

  2. Diagnosis and treatment are the same as for rhythm disturbances of other etiologies.

D. Superior Vena Cava (SVC) Syndrome

  1. Etiology: Ablation of blood flow from the superior vena cava to the right atrium caused by extravascular compression or intravascular obstruction.

       a. Ninety-five percent of cases are secondary to extrinsic compression of the SVC by mediastinal malignancy (3% from benign disease).

       b. The most common tumors are bronchogenic carcinoma of small cell type (48%) and lymphoma (21%).

  2. Clinical Manifestations

       a. Dyspnea aggravated by lying supine or leaning forward.

       b. Tachypnea and signs of airway obstruction.

       c. Signs and symptoms of increased intracranial pressure (i.e., dizziness, headache, visual disturbance, seizure, altered mental status).

       d. Dysphagia, hoarseness.

       e. Neck vein distention, facial plethora, and edema.

       f. Numerous, dilated, vertically oriented, and tortuous cutaneous venules or veins above the rib cage margin.

       g. Upper body edema with cyanosis and ruddy complexion.

       h. Immediate causes of death are airway obstruction and intracranial hemorrhage. Thrombosis at the SVC may occur in 30% of these patients.

  3. Diagnosis

       a. Clinical suspicion.

       b. CT scan with IV contrast is the diagnostic procedure of choice.

       c. Transesophageal echocardiography is a safe bedside procedure excellent for evaluating the SVC and surrounding structures.

       d. Angiography and radionuclide venography help to localize the obstruction.

  4. Therapy

       a. Symptomatic relief is the rule.

       b. Operative bypass relieves symptoms faster than radiation and is indicated in patients with life-threatening respiratory compromise or advanced cerebral edema.

c. Radiation therapy is the mainstay of treatment for most malignant SVC obstruction, although in small cell carcinoma and lymphomas chemotherapy, it is particularly useful.

d. Temporizing measures may be used in patients without significant airway or neurologic compromise and include corticosteroids to decrease cerebral and laryngeal edema, diuretics, and elevation of the head.

e. Anticoagulation has no definitive role.

■ IV. GASTROENTEROLOGY

A. Neutropenic Enterocolitis (Ileocecal Syndrome)
  1. Incidence
    Neutropenic enterocolitis commonly occurs in patients with hematologic malignancies (leukemia is the most common, with an incidence of 10% to 40%) receiving chemotherapy.
  2. Pathophysiology
    Neutropenic enterocolitis results from mucosal ulceration and necrosis of the ileum, cecum, or ascending colon with overgrowth and mural invasion of bacteria and/or fungi. Thrombocytopenia may predispose patients to hemorrhage into the bowel wall. Enterocolitis typically presents on the seventh day of severe neutropenia.
  3. Clinical Manifestations
    a. Abdominal distention
    b. Right-sided abdominal tenderness
    c. Watery diarrhea
    d. Fever
    e. Thrombocytopenia and neutropenia
  4. Diagnosis
    a. Clinical suspicion.
    b. Plain radiographs of the abdomen may show ileus with distended cecum and pneumatosis coli.
    c. CT of the abdomen: thickened bowel wall containing air.
    d. Sigmoidoscopy.
  5. Differential Diagnosis
    a. Appendicitis
    b. Pseudomembranous colitis
    c. Diverticulitis
    d. Other acute abdominal disorders

6. Medical Therapy
   a. Nutritional support
   b. Nasogastric suction
   c. Broad-spectrum antibiotics with anaerobic, gram-negative, and *Clostridium difficile* coverage
7. Indications for Surgical Exploration
   a. Perforation
   b. Severe bleeding
   c. Abscess
   d. Uncontrolled sepsis
   e. Failure to improve after 2 to 3 days of intensive conservative management

B. Gastrointestinal (GI) Tract Hemorrhage and Perforation
1. GI hemorrhage
   a. The most common cause is hemorrhagic gastritis (32% to 48%), followed by peptic ulcer disease.
   b. Only 12% to 17% of bleeding is from the tumor *per se* (most commonly seen in GI lymphomas).
   c. Less common causes include esophageal varices, Mallory-Weiss tears, candida esophagitis, and enteritis.
2. Perforation
   Lymphomas are the most common malignancies to perforate during chemotherapy.
3. Diagnosis
   A standard diagnostic workup should be performed to identify the source of bleeding with emphasis upon endoscopy.
4. Therapy
   a. Surgical
   b. Temporizing modalities to control bleeding include
      (1) Angiography, with or without vasopressin or embolization.
      (2) Endoscopic intervention.
      (3) These modalities may also be useful in patients with carcinomatosis and previously unresectable disease.

■ V. RENAL/METABOLIC

Many cancer patients develop metabolic abnormalities caused by tumor-produced factors (hormones or locally acting substances) or from tumor destruction by antineoplastic therapy.

A. Hypercalcemia
1. Causes of Hypercalcemia in Cancer Patients
   a. Secondary to malignancy 4%

    b. Etiologies other than the malignancy 77%

    c. With coexistent hyperparathyroidism 2%

    d. Vitamin D intoxication 16%

    e. Idiopathic

2. It is the most common metabolic abnormality of cancer patients (10%).

3. May occur with or without bone metastases.

4. Breast cancer is associated with hypercalcemia in 27% to 35% of patients. Mechanisms include widespread osteolytic metastases, production of parathyroid-like hormone, prostaglandin E_2 (PGE_2) (following hormonal therapy with estrogens or anti-estrogens), humoral osteoclast-activating factor, and coexisting primary hyperparathyroidism.

5. Lung cancer is associated with hypercalcemia in 12.5% to 35% of patients. It is frequently seen in squamous cell carcinoma and is rare in small cell carcinoma. It may occur early or late, with or without bone metastases. Mechanisms include production of osteoclast-activating factor, transforming growth factor alpha, interleukin 1, and tumor necrosis factor.

6. Multiple myeloma produces hypercalcemia in 20% to 40% of patients. Hypercalcemia develops secondary to extensive osteolytic bone destruction osteoclast-activating factor and lymphotoxin. 50% develop renal insufficiency, which can aggravate the hypercalcemia.

7. Lymphoma causes hypercalcemia by humoral mediation and local bone destruction.

8. Head and neck malignancies have an incidence of hypercalcemia of 6%, which is humorally mediated. Hypercalcemia is associated with malignancies of the oropharynx (37%), hypopharynx (24.3%), and tongue (21.5%).

9. Squamous cell, transitional cell, bladder, renal, and ovarian carcinomas may also produce humoral hypercalcemia.

10. Clinical Presentation

    a. Severity of illness depends on the degree of hypercalcemia, concurrent illness or debility, age, and associated metabolic disturbances.

    b. Hypercalcemia of malignancy usually has a rapid onset.

    c. Neuromuscular manifestations often predominate and include lethargy, confusion, stupor, and coma (occurs when serum calcium level is >13 mg/dL). Hallucinations and psychosis, weakness, and decreased deep tendon reflexes (DTRs) are also common.

    d. Cardiovascular manifestations include increased cardiac contractility, increased sensitivity to digitalis, and dysrhythmias.

    e. Renal manifestations include polyuria and polydipsia (earliest symptoms), dehydration, decreased glomerular filtration, loss of urinary concentrating ability, and renal insufficiency.

    f. Gastrointestinal signs and symptoms include nausea and vomiting, anorexia, obstipation/constipation, ileus and abdominal pain.

    g. Skeletal involvement is the hallmark of hypercalcemia from osteolytic metastases or humorally mediated bone resorption resulting in pain, pathologic fractures, deformities, or necrosis.

11. Diagnosis
    a. Laboratory Studies
        (1) Total and ionized serum calcium
        (2) Electrolytes, serum urea nitrogen (BUN), creatinine
        (3) Serum phosphorus and alkaline phosphatase
        (4) Measures of urinary calcium excretion and cyclic adenosine monophosphate (cAMP)
        (5) High alkaline phosphatase level
        (6) Increased urinary calcium excretion
    b. Radiologic Studies
        (1) Radionuclide bone scan
        (2) Skeletal surveys
        (3) Baseline chest x-ray
    c. ECGs should be performed looking for characteristic changes, including prolonged PR and QRS intervals, and shortened QT.

12. Treatment
    Hypercalcemia is often fatal if left untreated, especially when symptomatic or if serum calcium is >13 mg/dL. Treatment goals include promoting urinary calcium excretion, inhibiting bone resorption, and reducing entry of calcium into the extracellular fluid compartment.

    a. Hydration: To restore intravascular volume and increase the urinary output.
        (1) Initially, 5 to 8 L of normal saline IV over the first 24 hours; then, adequate IV fluids to maintain a urine output of 3 to 4 L/day.
        (2) Electrolytes should be monitored during normal saline infusion.
        (3) Monitor urine output and cardiac status to avoid fluid overload.

b. Diuretics: Loop diuretics, such as furosemide, promote calciuresis by blocking calcium reabsorption in the ascending loop of Henle and augment the calciuretic effect of normal saline.

  (1) Furosemide in doses of 40 to 80 mg IV may be given after adequate hydration.

  (2) Monitor electrolytes and urine output to avoid overdiuresis.

c. Inhibitors of bone resorption should be initiated promptly in symptomatic hypercalcemia.

  (1) Mithramycin is an antitumor antibiotic with a direct toxic effect on osteoclasts. The usual dose is 25 μg/kg IV over 6 hours. It generally decreases serum calcium within 6 to 48 hours; it may be repeated if the patient does not respond within 2 days. Use should be restricted to emergency treatment of severe hypercalcemia. Complications include thrombocytopenia, myelosuppression, hypotension, and hepatic and renal toxicity.

  (2) Disodium etidronate (EHDP) is an analog of pyrophosphate that blocks osteoclastic bone resorption and formation of bone crystals. The dose is 7.5 mg/kg/d in 250 mL saline infused over 2 to 6 hours for 3 to 7 days, followed by 20 mg/kg/d orally. The onset of action is slow, with normocalcemia achieved in 4 to 7 days 75% of the time. EHDP is contraindicated in patients with renal failure.

  (3) Glucocorticoids (i.e., prednisone) are most effective in hematologic malignancies (especially multiple myeloma) and breast carcinoma and are of little value in solid tumors. These agents lower serum calcium by inhibition of calcium absorption and the action of vitamin D. Prednisone in a dose of 1 to 2 mg/kg/d has an onset of action in 3 to 5 days. Adverse effects include GI bleeding, hyperglycemia, and osteopenia.

  (4) Calcitonin inhibits osteoclastic bone resorption and enhances calcium excretion. The dose is 4 to 8 IU/kg q6h IM or SQ. It may lower calcium by 2 to 3 mg/dL over 2 to 3 hours. Adverse reactions include nausea and vomiting, flushing, and hypersensitivity reactions (initial skin testing is recommended before administration).

     d. Hemodialysis is useful in patients who present with renal failure or who cannot be treated with normal saline diuresis.

     e. Specific antineoplastic therapy should be initiated in patients for whom treatment exists. It is the most effective means of achieving long-term correction of cancer-related hypercalcemia.

B. Tumor-Lysis Syndrome

Tumor-lysis syndrome is seen when cytotoxic chemotherapy induces rapid tumor cell lysis in patients with a large malignant cell burden of an exquisitely chemosensitive tumor. Intracellular metabolites are released in quantities that exceed the excretory capacity of the kidneys.

1. This syndrome classically occurs in patients with Burkitt's and non-Hodgkin's lymphoma, acute lymphoblastic and nonlymphoblastic leukemia, and chronic myelogenous leukemia.

2. It may occur spontaneously in patients with lymphomas and leukemias, or following treatment with chemotherapy, radiation, glucocorticoids, tamoxifen, and/ or interferon.

3. Manifestations

    a. Related to metabolic abnormalities.

       (1) Hyperkalemia: Generalized weakness, irritability, decreased DTRs, paresthesias, paralysis, cardiac dysrhythmias, and cardiac arrest. The classic ECG changes include peaked T waves, diminished R waves progressing to widened QRS, prolonged PR, loss of P wave, and sine wave pattern as terminal event.

       (2) Hypocalcemia (related to hyperphosphatemia): Muscle spasms, carpopedal spasms, facial grimacing, laryngeal spasm, irritability, depression, psychosis; intestinal cramps, chronic malabsorption; seizures and respiratory arrest. Chvostek's and Trousseau's signs are present in some patients. ECG reveals a prolonged QT interval.

       (3) Hyperuricemia: Gouty arthritis, nephrolithiasis, and urate nephropathy.

    b. Precipitation of calcium salts in tissues.

    c. Acute renal failure.

4. Prevention and Treatment (See Table 11.1)

    a. To prevent acute renal failure, patients who are to undergo treatment for malignancies should receive the following:

Table 11.1. Management of Patients at Risk for Tumor-Lysis Syndrome

---

I. WHEN NO METABOLIC ABERRATION EXISTS:
1. Allopurinol 500 mg/m^2 BSA/d; reduce to 200 mg/m^2 BSA/d 3 days into chemotherapy.
2. Hydration, 3000 mL/m^2 BSA/d.
3. Chemotherapy initiated within 24–48 hours of admission.
4. Monitor electrolytes, BUN, creatinine, uric acid, calcium, phosphorous every 12–14 hours.

II. WHEN METABOLIC ABERRATION EXISTS:
1. Allopurinol initiated as above, reduce dose if hyperuricemia controlled, reduce dose for renal insufficiency.
2. Hydration as above, add nonthiazide diuretics as needed.
3. Urinary alkalinization (urine pH > 7).
 — Sodium bicarbonate 100 mEq/L IV solution initially; adjust as needed.
 — Discontinue when uric acid is normal.
4. Chemotherapy postponed until uric acid controlled or dialysis begun.
5. Monitor same studies, every 6–12 hours until stable (at least 3–5 days).
6. Replace calcium as Ca^{++} gluconate by slow IV infusion for symptomatic hypocalcemia or severe ECG changes.
7. Treat hyperkalemia with exchange resins, bicarbonate.

III. CRITERIA FOR HEMODIALYSIS IN PATIENTS UNRESPONSIVE TO THE ABOVE MEASURES:
1. Serum potassium ≥ 6 mEq/L.
2. Serum uric acid ≥ 10 mg/dL.
3. Serum phosphorus rapidly rising or ≥10 mg/dL.
4. Fluid overload.
5. Symptomatic hypocalcemia.

Abbreviation: BSA, body surface area.

(1) Vigorous IV hydration, often with diuretics or renal dose dopamine to ensure adequate urine output
(2) Alkalinization of the urine during the first 1 to 2 days of cytotoxic therapy to increase the solubility of uric acid
(3) Allopurinol to decrease the formation of uric acid

C. Other Common Metabolic Abnormalities in Cancer Patients
1. Syndrome of Inappropriate Secretion of Antidiuretic Hormone (SIADH)
a. Occurs in 1% to 2% of cancer patients.
b. Common in small cell carcinoma of the lungs as well as prostatic, pancreatic, ureteral, and bladder carcinomas.
c. Occasionally seen in lymphomas and leukemias.

2. Hypoglycemia
   a. Insulinomas: Insulin-secreting, benign, islet-cell tumors
   b. Non-islet-cell tumors (i.e., mesothelioma, fibrosarcoma, hemangiopericytoma, hepatoma, adrenocortical carcinoma, leukemia and lymphoma, pseudomyxoma, pheochromocytoma, anaplastic carcinoma)

■ VI. HEMATOLOGY

Cancer itself, antineoplastic therapy, and the acute conditions that occur in cancer patients all result in hematologic abnormalities. Red blood cells, white blood cells, platelets, and coagulation factors may all be adversely affected quantitatively, qualitatively, or both. Bleeding and infection are the primary life-threatening events in critically ill cancer patients, and they are both the cause and result of hematologic abnormalities. An extensive discussion of these entities can be found in Chapter 7, "Hematological Disorders."

■ VII. CHEMOTHERAPY-INDUCED HYPERSENSITIVITY REACTIONS

A. Etiology and Presentation
   1. Asparaginase has the highest incidence of hypersensitivity reactions (6% to 43%). The incidence is higher when the drug is given intravenously and as a single agent. Common manifestations include
      a. Hypotension or hypertension.
      b. Laryngospasm, respiratory distress.
      c. Agitation.
      d. Facial edema.
      e. Reactions can be life-threatening and are more likely to occur after 2 or more weeks of treatment.
   2. Cisplatin is the second most common antineoplastic agent causing hypersensitivity reactions (1% to 20%). Potentially fatal reactions occur in 5% of patients.
   3. Alkylating agents are much less commonly a cause of hypersensitivity reactions.
      a. Melphalan causes anaphylactic reactions in approximately 2% to 3% of patients.

      b. Bleomycin causes febrile illness in 20% to 25% of patients, which in some cases progresses to a life-threatening syndrome (confusion, chills, respiratory distress, hypotension), seen especially when administered IV to lymphoma patients.

      c. Doxorubicin may cause also anaphylaxis.

B. Therapy

  1. Severe Reactions

      a. Stop the antineoplastic drug infusion immediately.

      b. Epinephrine 0.5- to 0.75-mL (1:1,000 in 10 mL normal saline) IV push every 5 to 15 minutes.

      c. Aminophylline for acute bronchospasm.

      d. Diphenhydramine (or other antihistaminic agent) 25 to 50 mg IV.

      e. Hydrocortisone 500 mg IV initially and repeated every 6 hours for prolonged reactions.

■ VIII. IMMUNE COMPROMISE

The patient with cancer (especially while undergoing chemotherapy) must be considered an immunocompromised host.

A. Types of Immune Defects Recognized in Cancer Patients

  1. Defects in cellular and humoral immunity

      a. T-lymphocyte mononuclear phagocyte defect: Hodgkin's disease, lymphoma, cytotoxic chemotherapy

      b. Decreased or absent B cell function in patients with multiple myeloma, chronic lymphocytic leukemia

  2. Neutropenia

      a. Neutropenia is the most common immunologic defect in patients with neoplastic diseases.

      b. The risk for bacteremia and fungal infection increases with absolute neutrophil counts (ANCs) <1000/mm³.

      c. The most common cause of neutropenia is myelotoxic chemotherapy; neutropenia is also seen with leukemia, aplastic anemia, drug reactions, and when the bone marrow is destroyed by tumor or radiation.

  3. Disruption of the Integument or Mucosal Surfaces

      a. Diagnostic procedures entailing skin puncture and biopsies

      b. Invasive procedures such as the placement of indwelling central venous and pulmonary artery catheters, urinary catheters, or endotracheal tubes

c. Loss of the physical, chemical, and immunologic barrier functions of the gut lining
4. Hyposplenic or Postsplenectomy States
   a. Decreased host responses to infections from encapsulated organisms such as *S. pneumoniae*, *Haemophilus influenza*, and *Neisseria meningitides*

B. Clinical Evaluation
1. Careful attention to patient's history of antineoplastic therapies.
2. Investigate recurring infections, exposure to contagious diseases, and recent travel.
3. The presence of fever without an obvious source should be investigated thoroughly by evaluating the following:
   a. Blood, urine, sputum
   b. Indwelling catheters
   c. Surgical or other skin wounds
   d. Cerebrospinal fluid (CSF)
   e. Stool
   f. Possibility of undrained collections, abscesses
4. Skin lesions should be inspected carefully. *Ecthyma gangrenosum* is a characteristic skin lesion associated with bacterial and fungal sepsis.
5. The oral cavity is another potential source in the immunocompromised hosts. Sinusitis and periodontitis may be sources, especially in orotracheally or nasotracheally intubated patients and those with nasogastric tubes.
6. Fundoscopic examination is essential for detection of fungal infection, especially in patients with central venous and urinary catheters.
7. Perianal lesions may cause severe infection.
8. Panculture is indicated in all febrile patients. All indwelling vascular appliances should be removed and replaced.

The diagnosis and treatment of specific infections in the immunocompromised host is covered in Chapter 8, "Infections."

■ IX. USEFUL FACTS AND FORMULAS

A. Basic Oncology Formulas

Although not clinically useful, these formulas allow a better understanding of the oncogenesis process, its complications, and response to therapy.

The rapidly proliferating component of human tumors is known as the *growth factor (GF)* and is calculated as follows:

Table 11.2. Evaluation of Weight Change Based on the Percent Weight Change Formula

	Significant weight loss (%)	Severe weight loss (%)
7 days	1–2	>2
1 month	5	>5
3 months	7.5	>7.5
6 months	10	>10

$$GF = \frac{\text{Observed fraction of cells in S}}{\text{Expected fraction of cells in S}}$$

where S = part of cell cycle where DNA synthesis occurs predominantly.

The fraction of cells in the "S" phase can be assessed by titrated thymidine labeling and autoradiography. The fraction of labeled cells is known as the *thymidine-labeling index (TLI):*

$$TLI = \frac{\text{Number of labeled cells}}{\text{Total number of cells}}$$

B. Nutrition in Cancer

Also refer to Chapter 10, "Nutrition."

Cancer patients are frequently malnourished and require close nutritional monitoring. To assess the amount of weight loss (*percent weight change*) in these patients, the following formula is utilized

Percent weight change

$$= \frac{(\text{Usual weight} - \text{Actual weight})}{(\text{Usual weight})} \times 100$$

The evaluation of weight change based on the percent weight change formula is depicted in Table 11.2.

A useful formula in the nutritional assessment of these patients relates to the *nitrogen balance:*

Nitrogen balance

$$= \frac{\text{Protein intake (g)}}{6.25} - (24\text{-h urine urea nitrogen} + 4\text{g})$$

The *catabolic index (ID)* aids in the identification of the amount of "nutritional stress" that these patients have:

CI = 24h urine nitrogen excretion
    – [_ dietary nitrogen (g) intake + 3]

Table 11.3. Interpretation of the Catabolic Index

Catabolic index	Interpretation
0	No significant stress
1–5	Mild stress
>5	Moderate to severe stress

Table 11.4. CSF Findings in Patients With Carcinomatous Meningitis

	Percent of abnormal patients	Range
Opening pressure	50	60–450
WBC count	52	0–1800
Glucose	30–38	0–244
Protein	30–81	24–2485
Cytology	41–70	24–2485

The interpretation of the catabolic index is depicted in Table 11.3.

The *arm muscle circumference (AMC)* is another sensitive measure of protein nutritional status in cancer patients:

$$AMC = \text{Arm circumference} - (TSF)$$

where TSF = triceps skinfold measurement.

C. Other Facts

The CSF findings in patients with *carcinomatous meningitis* are depicted in Table 11.4.

The *body surface area* (BSA) of a patient can be calculated as:

$$BSA\,(m^2) = \frac{(\text{Weight in kg})^{0.425} \times (\text{height in cm})^{0.725} \times 71.84}{10,000}$$

12

Critical Care of the Pregnant Patient

Many patients presenting to an intensive care facility will be pregnant. Many patients will have diseases peculiar to pregnancy and will need critical care support. Others, however, will have underlying medical diseases (Table 12.1). Some of those diseases will require consideration of the passenger (fetus) who has created many changes in maternal physiology. The hormonal milieu created by the placenta—progesterone and to a lesser extent estrogen—is responsible for the multifaceted changes in system function.

One change seen early in pregnancy is in pulmonary function. Table 12.2 depicts these modifications. Another organ system with significant change is the kidney. Table 12.3 reflects the serial changes in function. Table 12.4 demonstrates the differential risk of both acquired and congenital heart disease during pregnancy.

Since many books on obstetrical critical care have been published, and a full review of the many changes and diseases is beyond the scope of this chapter, a disease process that reflects the complexity of the severely ill gravida within the intensive care unit (ICU) has been chosen.

Hemodynamic changes during pregnancy and maternal physiologic changes occurring during labor should be kept in mind (see Tables 12.5 and 12.6).

■ I. PREGNANCY-INDUCED HYPERTENSION

A. Definition

Pregnancy-induced hypertension (PIH) is the presence of elevated blood pressure with evidence of end organ dysfunction,

Table 12.1. Preexistent Medical Diseases*

Asthma
Cardiac disease, NYHA class 3/4
Prosthetic valve replacements
Critical mitral stenosis
Aortic stenosis
Eisenmenger's syndrome
Cystic fibrosis
Diabetes mellitus (insulin dependent)
Chronic renal failure
Hypertension
Renal, hepatic, cardiac transplants
Systemic lupus erythematous
Thyrotoxicosis/thyroid storm

* Treatment of these conditions during pregnancy remains unchanged.

most commonly seen as edema, proteinuria, and elevated blood pressure. Table 12.7 presents many of the synonyms for this process. The classification of preeclampsia (PIH) is depicted in Table 12.8.

B. Etiology

No causative agent has been isolated for the development of preeclampsia (PIH). It is most commonly believed to be an end product of antigen-antibody interaction with abnormal ratios of vasoactive agents such as prostacyclines and thromboxanes. The relationship of other agents such as lipid peroxides is under active investigation. Regardless of the exact etiology, the process reflects a diffuse systemic endothelial dysfunction intimately associated with platelet dysfunction. This is seen in the classic HELLP (hemolysis elevated liver enzymes low platelet) syndrome, in which many organ systems have reflected the disease, and if assiduous management does not occur, severe maternal morbidity or mortality may occur. Table 12.9 reflects the panorama of disease manifestations. Table 12.10 depicts those subsets of pregnant women at greatest risk for the disease process. Table 12.11 presents the frequency of preeclampsia in the highest risk populations.

Patients with prior PIH who have underlying chronic hypertension have a 50% to 75% probability of developing PIH in pregnancy. No method exists to predict the severity or to time the onset of the PIH process.

C. Approach to the Preeclamptic Patient
  1. Obtain Patient History
      a. Current gestational age (calculated by LMP, last menstrual period)

Table 12.2. Lung Volumes and Capacities in Pregnancy

	Definition	Change in Pregnancy
Respiratory rate (RR)	Number of breaths per minute	Unchanged
Vital capacity (Vc)	Maximum amount of air that can be forcibly expired after maximum inspiration (IC + ERV)	Unchanged
Inspiratory capacity (IC)	Maximum amount of air that can be inspired from resting expiratory level (TV + IRV)	Increased 5%
Tidal volume (VT)	Amount of air inspired and expired with normal breath	Increased 30%–40%
Inspiratory reserve volume (IRV)	Maximum amount of air that can be inspired at end of normal inspiration	Unchanged
Functional residual capacity (FRC)	Amount of air in lungs at resting expiratory level (ERV + RV)	Decreased 20%
Expiratory reserve volume (ERV)	Maximum amount of air that can be level expired from resting expiratory	Decreased 20%
Residual volume (RV)	Amount of air in lungs after maximum expiration	Decreased 20%
Total lung capacity (TLC)	Total amount of air in lungs at maximal inspiration (VC + RV)	Decreased 5%

Table 12.3. Serial Changes in Renal Hemodynamics

	Nonpregnant	16 wk	26 wk	36 wk	29 wk	37 wk
Effective renal plasma flow (mL/min)	480 ± 72	840 ± 145	891 279	771 ± 175	748 ± 85	677 ± 82
Glomerular filtration rate (mL/min)	99 ± 18	149 ± 17	152 ± 18	150 ± 32	145 ± 19	138 ± 22
Filtration fraction	0.21	0.18	0.18	0.20	0.19	0.21

Table 12.4. Pregnancy Risk With Cardiac Disease

CATEGORY 1: Low Risk During Pregnancy
　　　　　　Small left-to-right shunts
　　　　　　Pulmonary stenosis < 50-mm Hg gradient
　　　　　　Mild mitral/aortic insufficiency
　　　　　　Mild aortic stenosis
　　　　　　Mitral valve prolapse
　　　　　　Rheumatic fever or endocarditis history
　　　　　　Postoperative patients, normal hemodynamics

CATEGORY 2: Moderate Risk During Pregnancy
　　　　　　Large left-to-right shunts, low pulmonary pressure
　　　　　　Moderate pulmonary stenosis
　　　　　　Aortic stenosis (30–60-mm Hg gradient)
　　　　　　Mild hypertrophic cardiomyopathy
　　　　　　Cardiac valve prosthesis
　　　　　　Mild mitral stenosis
　　　　　　Palliated cyanotic heart disease
　　　　　　Moderate aortic/mitral regurgitation

CATEGORY 3: High Risk During Pregnancy
　　　　　　Large left-to-right shunts, mild pulmonary hypertension
　　　　　　Severe aortic/pulmonary stenosis
　　　　　　Mild mitral stenosis with atrial fibrillation
　　　　　　Moderate mitral stenosis
　　　　　　Cardiomyopathy in early stages
　　　　　　Moderate-to-severe IHSS
　　　　　　Cyanotic congenital heart disease, unoperated
　　　　　　Mild Epstein's disease
　　　　　　Postcardiac surgery, mild residual problems

CATEGORY 4: Pregnancy Contraindicated
　　　　　　Congestive heart failure
　　　　　　Pulmonary hypertension
　　　　　　Eisenmenger's syndrome
　　　　　　Severe cyanosis
　　　　　　Advanced coronary artery disease
　　　　　　Marfan's syndrome

Table 12.5. Hemodynamic Changes of Pregnancy

Cardiac output	Increases 30%–40%
Heart rate	Increases 10%–15%
Stroke volume	Increases
Blood volume	Increases 30%–40%
Systemic blood pressure	Decreases
Pulse pressure	Increases
Systemic resistance	Decreases
Pulmonary artery pressure	No Change
Pulmonary resistance	Decreases
Myocardial function	Improves

Table 12.6. Hemodynamic Effects of Labor and Delivery

Cardiac output	Increases with contractions
Blood volume	Increases
Heart rate	Variable
Peripheral resistance	No Change
Systemic artery pressure	Increases

Table 12.7. Synonyms for Pregnancy-Induced Hypertension

Toxemia of pregnancy
PIH
Preeclampsia
Eclampsia
Peripartum hypertension
EPH (edema, proteinuria, hypertension) gestosis

    b. Past medical history: renal or chronic hypertensive
       diseases, systemic lupus erythematosus
    c. Family history of preeclampsia/eclampsia
    d. Symptoms of disease
          (1) Headache, blurred vision, scotoma
          (2) Blindness, diplopia
          (3) Weight gain (>2 lb/wk)
          (4) Right upper quadrant pain, epigastric pain,
              diffuse abdominal pain (ruptured liver)
          (5) Tetanic contractions (abruptio placentae)
          (6) Nausea, emesis
          (7) Unconsciousness or seizure activity
          (8) Vaginal bleeding
          (9) Fetal movement

Table 12.8. Classification of Preeclampsia

	Mild	Severe*
Blood pressure		
Absolute	130/80–140/95 mm Hg	>160/110 mm Hg
	Systolic ≥ 140 mm Hg	
	Diastolic ≥ 90 mm Hg	
Relative	Systolic increased > 30 mm Hg	
	Diastolic increased > 15 mm Hg	
Clinical findings	1 + edema	3–4 + edema
	Normal reflexes	3–4 + reflexes
	No visual symptoms	Scotoma/papilledema diplopia
		May have seizures, altered consciousness
		Severe headaches
		Severe right upper quadrant abdominal pain or tenderness (HELLP)*
		Congestive heart failure
		Pulmonary edema
		Oliguria < 400 cc/24 h
Weight		>5 pounds/week
Lab		
Proteinuria	300 mg/24 h	≥5 g/d; 3+/4+ semiquantitative
Platelets	Normal	May be <150,000
Liver function	Normal	Elevated AST/ALT
Clotting studies	Normal	May be prolonged
Bilirubin	Normal	May be elevated
Anticonvulsants	Intrapartum: yes	Antepartum: yes
		Intrapartum: yes
Abdominal pain	Absent	May be present in epigastrium or RUQ

* HELLP syndrome, reflected by hemolysis, elevated liver enzymes, and low platelet count, comprises the greatest risk group for mortality and morbidity.
Abbreviations: ALT, alanine aminotransferase; AST, aspartate aminotransferase.

Table   12.9. Pregnancy   Induced-Hypertension: Associated Complications

Hypertensive crisis
Pulmonary edema: ARDS
Eclampsia
Intracranial hemorrhage
Amaurosis
Cerebral edema
Acute renal failure
Cortical necrosis
Ruptured liver
Microangiopathic hemolytic anemia
Thrombocytopenia
DIC
HELLP syndrome

Abbreviations: ARDS, adult respiratory distress syndrome; DIC, disseminated intravascular coagulation; HELLP, hemolysis, elevated liver enzymes, low platelets.

Table 12.10. Factors Associated With PIH

Nulligravida
Prior preeclampsia/eclampsia
Family history of preeclampsia, eclampsia
Multifetal pregnancies
Molar pregnancies
Hydrops fetalis (any etiology)
Chronic hypertension/renal disease
Diabetes mellitus, insulin dependent

Table 12.11. Frequency of Preeclampsia

7% of all pregnancies	
70% Nulligravidas	
30% Multigravidas	
Twins	30%
Molar pregnancies	up to 70%
Hydrops fetalis	up to 50%
Diabetes mellitus	up to 50%
Chronic hypertension	20%
Prior severe PIH	up to 50%

2. Physical Examination
   a. Maternal blood pressure, pulse, respiratory rate
   b. Fetal heart rate (FHR) by continuous electronic monitoring
   c. Extensive cardiopulmonary examination
   d. Eyes: scleral icterus, ecchymoses, petechiae
   e. Fundoscopic examination: retinal artery spasm, papilledema, hemorrhages; acute vasospasm is often seen, arteries may be only 50% diameter of veins.
   f. Abdominal examination
      (1) Upper quadrant tenderness
      (2) Uterus size, tone, soft, noncontracting or rigid contracting
      (3) Distension: Is there suggestion of ascites?
   g. Extremities/face: evidence of pathological edema
   h. Pelvic exam: cervical softness, dilatation, position, effacement, fetal presentation
   i. Patellar reflexes: Persistent clonus reflects central nervous system (CNS) hyperactivity and significant potential for seizure activity.
   j. *Please note:* Blood pressure may be taken in both supine and lateral positions. Arm elevation when the patient is turned to the lateral decubitus results in a fall in blood pressure commensurate with the distance in centimeters above the atrial level, roughly, 13.6 mm Hg/10 cm of hydrostatic pressure. This change in pressure is frequently suggested to be the "real blood pressure." A patient may then be considered to be normal when in fact hypertension exists. Table 12.12 reflects these changes in the best study done in normal pregnant patients. (Mean arterial pressure [MAP] is unchanged.)
   The intensivist should remember that because of the vasodilation of pregnancy and decreased systemic vascular resistance (SVR), patients, especially teenagers, with blood pressures (BPs) of 140/90 mm Hg or lesser blood pressures may be significantly hypertensive.
3. Laboratory Evaluation
   a. Type/Rh, indirect Coombs', rapid plasma reagin (RPR), hepatitis B surface antigen (HbsAg), rubella (if not previously obtained)
   b. Complete blood count (CBC), platelets, microscopic examination
   c. Serum urea nitrogen (BUN), creatinine, aspartate aminotransferase (AST), alanine aminotransferase (ALT), glucose, electrolytes, uric acid

Table 12.12. Hemodynamic Alterations in Response to Position Change Late in Third-Trimester of Pregnancy

Hemodynamic parameter	Position			
	LL	SUP	SIT	ST
MAP (mm Hg)	90 ± 6	90 ± 8	90 ± 8	91 ± 14
CO (L/min)	6.6 ± 1.4	6.0 ± 1.4*	6.2 ± 2.0	54 ± 2.0*
P (beats/min)	82 ± 10	84 ± 10	91 ± 11	107 ± 17*
SVR (dyne cm sec^{-5})	1210 ± 266	1437 ± 338	1217 ± 254	1319 ± 394
PVR (dyne cm sec^{-5})	76 ± 16	101 ± 45	102 ± 35	117 ± 35*
PCWP (mm Hg)	8 ± 2	6 ± 3	4 ± 4	4 ± 2
CVP (mm Hg)	4 ± 3	3 ± 2	1 ± 1	1 ± 2
LVSWI (g/m/m^2/beat)	43 ± 9	40 ± 9	44 ± 5	34 ± 7*

Abbreviations: CO, cardiac output; P, pulse; SVR, systemic vascular resistance; PVR, pulmonary vascular resistance; PCWP, pulmonary capillary wedge pressure; CVP, central venous pressure; LVSWI, left ventricular stroke word index; LL, left lateral; SUP, supine; SIT, sitting; ST, standing.
* $P < 0.05$, compared with left lateral position.
Adapted from Clark et al, *Am J Obstet Gynecol* 1991;164:883–887.

Table 12.13. Colloid Osmotic Pressure

Nonpregnant	28 mm Hg
Pregnant, term	23 mm Hg
Postpartum	17 mm Hg
Preeclampsia (PIH)	13.7 mm Hg

    d. Coagulation studies: prothrombin time (PT), partial thromboplastin time (PTT), fibrinogen, fibrin split products (FSPs)

    e. Plasma oncotic pressure (colloid osmotic pressure [COP]) decreases in pregnancy secondary to hemodilution (see Table 12.13)

    f. Urinalysis with rapid screen for proteinuria in intensive care unit (ICU)

    g. Chest x-ray only if pulmonary symptoms or physical examinations suggest its need

    h. Obstetrical ultrasound (in ICU) for fetal age and number, estimated fetal weight, position of fetuses, and placental position

    i. Continuous FHR monitoring

    j. 24-hour urine collection for creatinine clearance and protein excretion

D. Medical Therapy

1. The presentation of a patient with PIH may range from a mild to a life-threatening disease process. The process can only be ended by delivery. The decision to continue or to deliver the pregnancy will be made by consultation between medical and obstetrical personnel.

2. A true rule is that the disease may rapidly progress. Follow up of all maternal and fetal biophysical parameters on a routine basis is required. The frequency will be determined by the disease severity.

3. Most preeclamptic patients are vasoconstricted and hemoconcentrated. After initial therapy, volume expansion and hemodilution occurs.

4. $MgSO_4$ (magnesium sulfate) is considered the standard of therapy as a prophylaxis for seizure activity. The loading dose is 4 to 6 g $MgSO_4 \cdot 7H_2O$ in 100 cc D5 1/4 NS over 15 to 20 minutes. A constant infusion of $MgSO_4$ 1 to 2 g/h will be maintained depending on urine output and reflex activity, which are checked on an hourly basis. Table 12.14 lists the potential effects of the magnesium ion and the average serum level at which they may occur. When $MgSO_4$ is infused, both a Buretrol and an infusion pump normally will be used to enhance patient safety, thus preventing a massive infusion of $MgSO_4$, which could cause maternal death or severe morbidity.

5. Detailed intake and output (I&O) records must be maintained. Since renal function is frequently impaired, an increase in total body water can result in pulmonary edema. In rare cases, if hyponatremia is allowed to occur, cerebral edema may be observed.

6. Postdelivery, I&O must be assiduously maintained to prevent hypovolemia and renal hypoperfusion.

Table 12.14. Magnesium Toxicity

Manifestations	Level (mEq/L)
Loss of patellar reflex	(8–12 mEq/L)
Feeling of warmth, flushing	(9–12 mEq/L)
Somnolence	(10–12 mEq/L)
Slurred speech	(10–12 mEq/L)
Muscular paralysis	(15–17 mEq/L)
Respiratory difficulty	(15–17 mEq/L)
Cardiac arrest	(30–35 mEq/L)

Adapted from Sibai BM: Preeclampsia-eclampsia: Valid treatment approached. *Contemporary OB/GYN* 1990; 35(No.8):84–100.

7. Even in mild disease, diplopia may indicate the development of cerebral edema. Standard therapy with mannitol plus or minus Furosemide (Lasix) (see Chapter 9) may be used. Nimodipine, a specific cerebral Ca^{++} channel blocker, may be given 30 to 60 mg PO q6h with substantial improvement in cerebral autoregulation.

8. Severe pulmonary edema and adult respiratory distress syndrome (ARDS) may occur in preeclamptic patients, as in any other acutely ill patient. Indications for ventilator support are unchanged in this population.

9. Disseminated intravascular coagulation, especially associated with the HELLP syndrome may require extensive blood product transfusion. In preeclampsia, because of vasoconstriction and the increased risk of pulmonary edema, cryoprecipitate is often preferred over fresh frozen plasma (FFP). This reduces the volume of infused blood products. *Note:* There is a higher risk of hepatitis with increasing number of donor exposures.

10. When platelets and FFP are required, it is always advisable to use *jumbo* packs of each to decrease multiple-donor exposure.

11. Swan-Ganz catheter: Invasive pulmonary artery catheter monitoring is sometimes required with preeclampsia, especially when complicated by abruptio placenta, hemorrhage, or ARDS/pulmonary edema. Knowledge of the hemodynamic changes in pregnancy is required in considering selection of therapy (see Tables 12.5 and 12.6). A Swan-Ganz catheter may also be required in other obstetrical disorders (see Table 12.15).

Table 12.15. Acquired Obstetrical Disease That May Require Invasive Hemodynamic Monitoring

Amniotic fluid embolism

Hemorrhagic shock
   Abruptio placenta
   Placenta previa
   Abdominal pregnancy

Pneumonias
   Viral
   Bacterial

Septic shock

Chorioamnionitis

Pyelonephritis

Septic abortion

Table 12.16. Antihypertensive Drugs in Pregnancy

Drug	Onset of action	Duration	Dosage	Mechanism	Side effects
Methyldopa (Aldomet)	3–6 h	7–16 h	IV 250–500 mg q6h PO 250–500 mg q6–8h	Vasodilation	Sedation, dry mouth, nasal congestion, occasional depression, postural Coombs' + hemolytic anemia reflex
Hydralazine (Apresoline)	15–20 min	3–6 h	5–10 mg q30min	Direct smooth muscle relaxation	Reflex tachycardia Headache
Nicardipine* (Cardene)	1–5 min	3–6 h	IV drip 2 mg/h, increase by 2 mg/h each hour; max dosage 10 mg/h	Vasodilation Ca+ channel blocker	Headache, nausea, vomiting, hypotension
Nifedipine† (Procardia)	1–5 min	3–5 h	10-mg capsule 10–20 mg PO, q6h	Vasodilation Ca++ channel blocker	Headache, palpitations, fluid retention Potential for respiratory failure when used with MgSO4 Potential for neuromuscular blockage or potential other drug effects

Labetalol (Trandate)	5–10 min	3–6 h	20 mg by slow IV injection over 2 min. May repeat dose q10–15 min to achieve desired pressure. Maximum dosage 300 mg	Beta-blocker 7-1 vasodilator Ratio of beta-blocker to alpha-blocker (7:1) with IV administration	Hypotension, dizziness, fatigue, nausea, bronchoconstriction in some patients with asthma **Fetal** side effects may include bradycardia, poor temperature control, hypoglycemia, and decreased short-term variability
Sodium Nitroprusside (Nipride)	Immediate	<3 min	50 mg/500 mL D5W Rate of 0.2–0.8 µg/kg/min Titrate to desired blood pressure (Light sensitive). Average of 3 µg/kg/min will usually decrease pressure to desired value.	Vasodilation	Nausea, severe hypotension is not closely watched, thiocyanate toxicity (even when required antepartum, cyanide poisoning does not usually occur)
Trimethaphan (Arfonad)	Immediate	10–15 min	500 mg/500 m: D5W Titrate to desired blood pressure	Ganglionic blocker	Tachycardia, severe hypotension if not carefully titrated Cycloplegia Tachyphylaxis Potential for neuromuscular blockage when >6 mg/min infusion rate May prolong effect time of other neuromuscular blocking drugs

* A reduction of 20% in MAP should be maximal initial target. Following maternal and fetal response to therapy, further decrease in MAP may be desired.

12. Development of seizures (eclampsia) may occur pre- or post-treatment with $MgSO_4$. If seizures develop pretherapy, 4 g of $MgSO_4$ (8 cc of $MgSO_4 \cdot 7H_2O$—50% solution) may be rapidly infused. If seizures develop post-treatment, a second dose of $MgSO_4$ may be given, or some physicians choose to give diazepam (Valium), 2.5 to 5 mg as an IV push as the agent of choice. If the patient does not awaken and become responsive within 60 minutes, then the possibility of an intracranial hemorrhage must be considered and worked up (see Chapter 9).

13. Pulse oximeters and recording dynamaps may be used in many patients. If any concern for an atypical or severe manifestation of PIH is present, an arterial pressure catheter should be placed. Repetitive laboratory studies can be drawn, and continuous blood pressure recording can be achieved.

14. Interactive dialogue between all members of the health-care team will achieve optimum outcome for both mother and child.

E. Major Complications of Preeclampsia/Eclampsia
1. Hypertensive Crises
   a. BPs > 200 systolic or 120 diastolic
   b. May be associated with pulmonary edema, intracranial hemorrhage, or cerebral edema
   c. Rapid treatment is critical (see Table 12.16). An acute reduction of elevated BP should initially be limited to a 20% reduction in mean arterial pressure. A more substantial reduction may create severe uteroplacental hypoperfusion and precipitate acute fetal death or asphyxia. This is especially true if the diastolic blood pressure is acutely dropped to 90 mm Hg or less.
   d. These patients frequently warrant placement of invasive monitoring systems such as pulmonary artery catheters and peripheral arterial cannulas.
2. Cerebral Edema
   a. Initiate fluid restriction
   b. Invasive monitoring
   c. IV mannitol 1 to 2 g/kg of a 20% solution (100 g) of mannitol in 500 mL of 5% D/W) given over 10 to 20 minutes followed by a maintenance dose of 50 to 300 mg/kg IV q6h is effective. The serum osmolality should *not* be allowed to exceed 330 to 340 mOsm.
   d. Complications of osmotic agent use include
      (1) Osmotic diuresis with dehydration and hypernatremia

        (2) Rebound increase in intracranial pressure
        (3) Acute volume expansion
    e. Nimodipine, a calcium channel blocker, has been found to be very effective in cases of subarachnoid hemorrhage associated with cerebral edema to decrease death and permanent neurologic damage. Dosage of 60 mg PO q4–6h may be given. It can be given via a nasogastric tube if required.
    f. If a patient is intubated, hyperventilation may be used. (See Chapter 9.)

3. Hepatic Rupture
    a. Massive intraabdominal hemorrhage results with need for
        (1) Massive blood volume support
        (2) Corrections of disseminated intravascular coagulation (DIC)
        (3) Invasive cardiovascular monitoring
    b. Exploration and surgical repair when necessary. Because of liver dysfunction/damage, packing of the rupture site is often accomplished.
    c. Potential for automatic cell saver at operation can reduce total transfusion requirements.

4. Abruptio Placentae
    a. Frequently associated with fetal distress.
    b. Often accompanied by coagulopathy with prolonged PT, PTT, low fibrinogen, and low platelet count.
    c. Vigorous/massive transfusion support may be required.
    d. Four major complications of hypovolemia and shock in these patients follow:
        (1) Acute tubular necrosis
        (2) Cortical renal necrosis
        (3) Sheehan's syndrome with acute pituitary insufficiency
        (4) ARDS: This has been a major cause of death in our obstetrical ICU.

F. Therapy
1. Magnesium Sulfate
    a. Distribution: extracellular space, bones, and intracellular space.
    b. Unbound to protein.
    c. Excretion by kidney; filtered load excretes T max for reabsorption in most patients treated.
    d. Excretion half-life is ~4 hours.
    e. When used in normal patients for treatment of preterm labor, the earliest manifestations of excessive Ca^{++} antagonism are ocular symptoms of visual

disturbance: blurring of vision, diplopia and difficulty in focusing.

f. $MgSO_4$ does not usually change blood pressure.

g. Measurements of magnesium levels can be achieved in most clinical labs. There is a poor correlation between levels observed and clinical effect. Therefore, no precise level can be stated to be therapeutic.

G. Antihypertensive Therapy (See Table 12.16)

1. In most circumstances, drug therapy in PIH is reserved for those patients with
   a. Persistent systolic BPs >180 mm Hg or
   b. Persistent diastolic BPs >110 mm Hg (105 mm Hg in some institutions)

2. Before delivery, it is desired to maintain the diastolic blood pressure >90 mm Hg. This allows for continued perfusion pressure to provide adequate utero placental perfusion.

3. If diastolic blood pressure decreases <90 mm Hg, frequently, the decreased uteroplacental perfusion will precipitate acute fetal distress, which may progess to an *in utero* death or to perinatal asphyxia.

4. Postdelivery, an acute, rapid decrease in blood pressure usually means substantial blood loss and *not* cure of the disease process. Likewise, a nadir of 90 mm Hg diastolic blood pressure is desired.

5. Medical control of hypertension is often required only for a short period (usually days). No study has ever demonstrated a beneficial long-term outcome with prolonged antihypertensive therapy.

6. The use of calcium channel blockers in a setting of $MgSO_4$ therapy should be considered a significant therapeutic step that may create an adverse impact on cardiovascular function; therefore, an intensive care setting with knowledgeable personnel (internal medicine, OB/GYN maternal fetal medicine, or OB anesthesia) capable of responding to these problems should be present.

■ II. AMNIOTIC FLUID EMBOLISM

A. Definition

Amniotic fluid embolism is the vascular transfer of amniotic fluid containing lanugo hairs, vernix, meconium, thromboplastic substances to the pulmonary circulation. This is a rare (1 in 8000 pregnancies) event that is catastrophic and often associated with death.

    1. It is unpreventable and is most frequent in the second stage of labor.
    2. The mortality rate is 80%; 25% of deaths occur in the first 60 minutes post event.
    3. Old animal models of disease are not applicable to human pathology

B. Presentation
    Sudden onset of maternal distress:
    1. Severe dyspnea, bronchospasm, tachypnea
    2. Tachycardia, hypotension, arrhythmias
    3. Cyanosis, severe hypoxia
    4. Acute cardiovascular collapse, often cardiac arrest
    5. DIC
    6. Seizures, coma

C. Predisposing Factors
    1. Multiple pregnancy
    2. Large fetuses
    3. Short, tumultuous labors
    4. Pitocin administration
    5. Late rupture of membranes with unengaged presenting part

D. Symptoms
    1. Restlessness
    2. Sweating
    3. Anxiety
    4. Coughing
    5. Air hunger

E. Pathophysiology
    1. Pulmonary hypertension; decreased cardiac output
    2. Cor pulmonale with pulmonary edema
    3. Severe hypoxemia and tissue hypoxia
    4. If acute respiratory distress allows survival, thromboplastins yield DIC
    5. Swan-Ganz data reveal predominant left heart failure/dysfunction: 2 degrees to hypoxic injury

F. Differential Diagnosis
    1. Acute pulmonary embolism
    2. Air embolism
    3. Myocardial infarction
    4. Acute aspiration of gastric contents
    5. Massive pneumothorax: uni/bilateral
    6. Reaction to local anesthetic

G. Acute Treatment
    1. Endotracheal tube placement
    2. Mechanical ventilation/positive end expiratory pressure (PEEP)

    3. Volume support with or without blood products
    4. Peripheral and pulmonary arterial catheterization
    5. Central venous pressure (CVP) monitoring
    6. No specific drug therapy: vasopressors and/or bronchodilators of choice

H. Hemodynamic Observations in Humans
    1. Mild-to-moderate increase in pulmonary artery pressure
    2. Variable increase in CVP
    3. Elevated pulmonary capillary wedge pressure

■ III. USEFUL FACTS AND FORMULAS

Uterine oxygen consumption can be calculated by the following formula:

$$O_2 \text{ Uptake by Gravid Uterus} = (A - V) \times F$$

where A = material arterial blood oxygen content; V = uterine venous blood oxygen content; F = uterine blood flow.

The *oxygen saturation of the uterine venous blood* flow (Sv) is another important parameter to follow and is calculated as follows:

$$Sv = \frac{SaO_2 - \dot{V}}{F \times (O_2 \text{ Cap})}$$

where SaO_2 = maternal oxygen saturation; $\dot{V}O_2$ = oxygen consumption rate; F = uterine blood flow; O_2 Cap = oxygen capacity of maternal blood.

If the last menstrual period (LMP) is known, the probable delivery date (DD) can be approximated utilizing *Naegele's rule*:

$$DD = \text{First day of LMP} + 7 \text{ days} - 3 \text{ months}$$

The approximate *weight gain* by a pregnant woman can be calculated after the second trimester as follows:

$$WG = 225 \text{ g} \times \text{weeks of gestation}$$

Occasionally, there is a need for *intraperitoneal fetal transfusion* in a gravid patient. The following formula is used to calculate the volume of red blood cells (RBCs) to be injected into the fetal peritoneal cavity (IPT volume):

$$IPT \text{ volume} = (\text{weeks' gestation} - 20) \times 10 \text{ mL.}$$

To determine the concentration of donor hemoglobin present in the fetus at any time following an intrauterine transfusion, *Bowman's formula* is applied:

$$\text{Hb concentration (g/dL)} = \frac{0.55 \times a}{85 \times b} \times \frac{120 - c}{120}$$

where 0.55 = fraction of transfused RBC in the fetal circulation; a = amount of donor RBC transfused (grams); b = fetal weight (kg); c = interval (days) from the time of transfusion to the time of calculation; 85 = estimation of blood volume (mL/kg) in the fetus; 120 = life span of donor RBC.

The *placental transfer of drugs* can be calculated as follows:

$$Q/t = \frac{KA(C_m - C_f)}{D}$$

where Q/t = rate of diffusion; K = diffusion constant; A = surface area available for exchange; C_m = concentration of free drug in maternal blood; C_f = concentration of free drug in fetal blood; D = thickness of diffusion barrier.

13

Pulmonary Disorders

■ I. CHRONIC OBSTRUCTIVE PULMONARY DISEASE (COPD)

A. Definition

COPD is a disorder characterized by expiratory flow limitation that does not change markedly over periods of several months of observation. The term *COPD* includes the following:

1. Chronic Bronchitis

Chronic bronchitis is a clinical diagnosis made when chronic cough with sputum production is present on most days for at least 3 months of the year for at least 2 consecutive years. Major pathologic findings include airways inflammation and enlargement of the submucosal mucus glands.

2. Emphysema

Emphysema is defined pathologically as an abnormal permanent enlargement of the air spaces distal to the terminal bronchiole, accompanied by destruction of their wall without obvious fibrosis. Clinically, it correlates with a reduction in the diffusing capacity (DLCO).

3. Various degrees of both chronic bronchitis and emphysema coexist in most patients with COPD. The term *COPD* should not be used for other forms of obstructive lung disease such as bronchiectasis, cystic fibrosis, or major airway obstruction.

B. Etiology and Risk Factors

The pathogenesis of most cases of COPD remains unclear. The main risk factor associated with COPD is cigarette smoking, but most smokers do not develop COPD. Less than 1% of patients with emphysema have alpha$_1$-antitrypsin deficiency (serum A1AT < 5 μM; normal values 20 to 48 μM).

C. Diagnostic Evaluation
   1. Clinical Presentation
      a. Cough, sputum production, and dyspnea that usually have been present for several years. Symptoms consistent with severe COPD in a young and/or nonsmoking adult should prompt the consideration of other conditions such as alpha$_1$-antitrypsin deficiency, uncontrolled asthma, or other less common causes of obstructive lung disease (i.e., cystic fibrosis, inmotile cilia syndrome, Young's syndrome [obstructive azoospermia with chronic bronchitis/bronchiectasis], congenital or acquired immunoglobulin deficiency).
      b. During an *acute decompensation* of COPD, there is an increase in dyspnea and cough, and there are changes in sputum volume, color, and consistency. Physical examination may reveal
         (1) Pursed-lip breathing
         (2) Rapid shallow breathing
         (3) Use of respiratory accessory muscles (i.e., sternocleidomastoid, pectoralis, abdominal muscles)
         (4) Thoracoabdominal paradoxical breathing pattern
         (5) Wheezes, coarse crackles, and almost undetectable breath sounds in severe cases
         (6) Increased jugular venous distention, hepatomegaly, peripheral edema, and right-sided S3 and increased P2 sounds are characteristic of patients with cor pulmonale due to severe COPD
         (7) Various degrees of changes in mental status may be present and related to hypoxemia, hypercapnia, infection, and/or drugs
      Other conditions that are commonly associated with or precipitate a worsening of COPD patients are depicted in Table 13.1.
   2. Laboratory Findings
      a. Pulmonary Function Testing (PFT)
         (1) *Spirometry* reveals an obstructive pattern: reduction in the ratio of forced expiratory volume in the first second to forced vital capacity (FEV$_1$/FVC ratio); normal for a 50-year-old person is 70%). The severity of the expiratory

Table 13.1. Common Conditions Associated With COPD Decompensation

Respiratory Infections: Viral upper and lower respiratory tract (i.e., pharyngitis, tracheobronchitis, pneumonitis), aspiration, and bacterial pneumonia

Narcotics and sedatives

Inappropriately high fraction of inspired O_2 (FiO_2) (mainly in "CO_2 retainers")

Heart failure

Excessive diuresis with metabolic alkalosis and compensatory CO_2 retention

Pneumothorax (rupture of a bleb)

Hypophosphatemia, hypomagnesemia

Hypermetabolic states (i.e., sepsis, fever)

Table 13.2. Degree of Impairment in COPD Based on FEV_1

Severity	FEV_1 (% predicted)
Mild	<LLN (i.e., <70%)
Moderate	<60%–40%
Severe	<40%

Abbreviation: LLN, lower limit of normal.

airflow limitation can be assessed by the FEV_1 (as percent of normal predicted according to sex, race, and height). Commonly used values to assign severity of functional impairment are shown in Table 13.2.

(2) In *intubated, mechanically ventilated* patients, the *interrupter technique* can be used to diagnose airflow limitation and assess the improvement of expiratory flow in response to bronchodilators.

b. Radiologic Studies

(1) Chest x-ray may demonstrate evidence of emphysema:

(a) Flattening of the diaphragm

(b) Increased retrosternal air space

(c) Irregular areas of vascular attenuation and radiolucency (bullae: lucent areas in the lung parenchyma >1 to 2 cm in diameter).

           (d) Typical smoker's emphysema is mainly of apical distribution. Predominant lower lung zones changes are consistent with emphysema due to alpha$_1$-antitrypsin deficiency.

    (2) Computed tomography (CT) of the chest is the most sensitive way to detect emphysema, although it is not routinely recommended as a diagnostic test.

    (3) The roentgenographic features of chronic bronchitis are *nonspecific* and may include increased lung markings ("dirty lungs") and thickening of bronchial walls.

    (4) Chest x-ray during an acute COPD exacerbation can be helpful in the detection of associated processes such as pneumonia, atelectasis, or pneumothorax.

c. Arterial Blood Gases (ABGs)

    (1) Various degrees of *hypoxemia* with increased $P(A-a)O_2$ gradient are typical of COPD patients.

    (2) Chronic hypercapnia with compensatory metabolic alkalosis are seen in severe cases ("CO_2 retainers").

    (3) Finding chronic CO_2 retention in moderate COPD with $FEV_1 > 1$ to $1.3\,L$ is unusual and should raise the question of concomitant neuromuscular or sleep apnea disorders.

    (4) Common acid-base disturbances seen during an acute exacerbation of COPD include

        (a) Acute respiratory acidosis.

        (b) Partially compensated respiratory acidosis (acute-on-chronic).

        (c) Chronic respiratory acidosis (mild exacerbation in "CO_2 retainers").

        (d) Metabolic alkalosis induced by diuretics or continuous nasogastric aspiration may be a cause of persistent or worsening hypercapnia in COPD.

D. Management of Acute COPD Exacerbation

    1. Ensure Adequate Oxygenation and Ventilation

        a. For most patients, the goal is to maintain a PaO_2 of 55 to 60 mm Hg (arterial oxyhemoglobin saturation of 88% to 90%). In patients with concomitant coronary artery disease, an arterial saturation >90% is desirable.

(1) *Spontaneously breathing patients* with acute COPD exacerbation can usually achieve those levels using a Venturi mask set to deliver 24% to 35% O_2 (preferred in "mouth breathers") or a nasal cannula with an O_2 flow of 1 to 2 L/min. (See Chapter 2, "The Basics of Critical Care.")

(2) Some COPD patients will develop or worsen hypercapnia during O_2 therapy. A reduction of the hypoxic respiratory drive and a worsening of V/Q mismatch are the underlying mechanisms thought to mediate that response.

b. Patients with significant acidemia, inadequate PaO_2, hypercapnia with changes in mental status, or hemodynamic instability should be assisted with mechanical ventilation (MV).

(1) Noninvasive positive-pressure ventilation (NIPPV) as the initial form of ventilatory assistance has been reported effective in selected patients with acute respiratory failure. Candidates for NIPPV should . . .

(a) Tolerate a facial or nasal mask.

(b) Cooperate with this form of therapy.

(c) Have an intact upper airway function without excessive secretions, regurgitation, or vomiting.

(d) Be hemodynamically stable.

(e) It may also be offered to patients requiring endotracheal intubation who decline invasive procedures.

NIPPV can be administered using a volume-cycled or pressure-controlled ventilator (i.e., BiPAP in S/T mode inspiratory positive airway pressure [IPAP] 10 cm H_2O, expiratory positive airway pressure [EPAP] 5 cm H_2O, rate 10 beats per minute). Close observation with frequent ABGs and continuous monitoring of arterial O_2 saturation (SaO_2) are recommended to determine NIPPV efficacy and to avoid delays in endotracheal intubation.

(2) When volume-cycled MV is instituted in intubated COPD patients, a major goal is to minimize dynamic hyperinflation (auto-positive end-expiratory pressure [PEEP]) and its hemodynamic consequences. In general, the ventilator should be set to lower the mean expiratory flow (VT/Te) through increases

in inspiratory flow (i.e., 90 L/min) and expiratory time (reductions in machine rate, I : E
ratio, or even sedation that leads to failure
to trigger) and reductions in tidal volume (i.e.,
8 mL/kg).

2. Bronchodilators

   a. Inhaled Beta$_2$-Agonists: When delivered by metered
      dose inhalers (MDI), these drugs are as effective as
      nebulized in intubated or spontaneously breathing
      patients (used with a spacer device). Albuterol
      (Proventil, Ventolin) 2 to 4 puffs may be adminis-
      tered initially q20min × 3, followed by q1–2h until
      improvement occurs, and then q4–6h. The dose for
      albuterol nebulization is 2.5 mg (0.5 cc of 0.5%
      solution in 2 to 3 cc of normal saline).

   b. Anticholinergics: Ipratropium bromide (Atrovent)
      has shown to be as effective as beta$_2$-agonists with
      potentially fewer side effects. Ipratropium bromide 2
      to 6 puffs q6h should be added to inhaled albuterol
      during COPD exacerbations.

   c. Methylxanthines: The role of theophylline is still
      controversial. There is no conclusive evidence for its
      routine use during COPD exacerbations. Potential
      drug interactions (i.e., erythromycin, ciprofloxacin,
      cimetidine, isoniazide, Ca^{++} channel blockers),
      increased toxicity in the elderly acutely ill COPD
      patient, and the need for frequent blood level mea-
      surements should be considered when prescribing
      the drug during an acute exacerbation. In patients
      already taking theophylline, a loading dose of 1 mg/
      kg (ideal body weight) of aminophylline for each
      2 μg/mL of desired increase in serum theophylline
      to achieve a target concentration of 12 to 15 μg/mL
      followed by a continuous infusion (0.5 to 0.6 mg/kg/h
      assuming normal half-life) is recommended. For the
      elderly and patients with heart or liver disease, the
      maintenance dose should be reduced to 0.1 to
      0.3 mg/kg/h. When switching to the oral route, 80% of
      the total 24-hour aminophylline infusion that gives a
      therapeutic level is given as theophylline in divided
      doses.

3. Corticosteroids

   Unconfirmed trials have shown benefits from administration of steroids in acute COPD exacerbations.
   Methylprednisolone (SoluMedrol) 0.5 mg/kg IV q6h or
   prednisone 40 to 60 mg/d PO for 3 days and then tapered
   over a 2-week period is recommended.

4. Antibiotics

A recognized upper or lower respiratory infection should be treated adequately. Empiric antibiotic therapy (i.e., trimethoprim-sulfamethoxazole, levofloxacin, doxycycline or amoxicillin for 7 to 10 days) in acute COPD exacerbation has been associated with an earlier resolution and fewer relapses.

5. Correct precipitating or associated problems (Table 13.1).

■ II. ASTHMA

A. Definition

1. Asthma

Asthma is a clinical syndrome characterized by increased responsiveness of the tracheobronchial tree to a variety of stimuli with slowing of forced expiration that changes in severity either spontaneously or as a result of therapy.

2. Status Asthmaticus

Status asthmaticus is a severe episode of asthma that does not respond to usually effective treatment requiring more aggressive therapy for reversal.

B. Pathophysiology

The key feature of asthma is *airway inflammation* with hyperresponsiveness leading to airway obstruction and in severe cases to hyperinflation, increased VD/VT and V/Q mismatch, with subsequent hypoxemia and respiratory insufficiency.

C. Diagnostic Evaluation

1. Clinical Presentation

Dyspnea, wheezing, and coughing are the most common symptoms during an asthma attack. Other diagnostic considerations, especially when a prior history of asthma is absent, should include the following:

a. Heart failure and ischemia with diastolic dysfunction

b. Aspiration of foreign bodies

c. Epiglotitis and croup

d. Pulmonary embolism (rare)

Table 13.3 shows several adverse prognostic indicators obtained by history, physical examination, and routine tests in acute life-threatening asthma.

2. Laboratory Evaluation

a. Spirometry: Bedside spirometry shows an obstructive pattern (see "COPD," section C2a). Serial FEV_1 determinations are indicated to objectively evaluate

Table 13.3. Factors Associated With Severe Acute Asthma Attacks

Previous episode(s) of severe asthma (especially if associated with respiratory failure)

Changes in mental status

Use of accessory muscles of respiration

Very diminished or absent breath sounds

Pulsus paradoxus >10 mm Hg

Tachycardia >130 beats per min

Cyanosis

Hypoxemia

Hypercapnia or normocapnia in the setting of tachypnea

FEV_1 <20% predicted

---

the response to treatment. If spirometry is not available, monitoring peak expiratory flow using a peak flowmeter is recommended.

b. Arterial Blood Gases: Hypoxemia may be seen in cases complicated by respiratory failure, pneumonia, or pneumothorax. The most common acid-base abnormality is acute respiratory alkalosis. *Normocapnia* or *acute respiratory acidosis* indicates impending or established respiratory failure.

c. Chest X-Ray: May show evidence of hyperinflation, increased bronchial markings or associated conditions such as pneumonia or pneumothorax.

d. Other Tests: In addition to the usual admission tests, theophylline level and blood and sputum cultures should be done if clinically indicated.

D. Management of Asthma Attacks

1. Ensure Adequate Oxygenation

a. Most asthma patients will maintain $SaO_2 > 90\%$ to 92% during an acute attack with a low concentration of supplemental O_2 (Venturi mask or nasal cannula 2 L/min). Monitor patient with pulse oximeter, and supplement O_2 as necessary.

b. Mechanical Ventilation: Few patients with severe asthma will not respond to aggressive medical management and will require ventilatory support. The ventilatory strategy in patients with severe airway obstruction should provide adequate oxygenation and at the same time minimize the risk of barotrauma through the use of small tidal volumes (i.e., 5 to 8 mL/kg) and minute ventilation (even if $PaCO_2$ is allowed to climb: "controlled hypoventilation"). As in the case of COPD with expiratory flow limitation, reducing the ventilator's mean expiratory flow (VT/Te) will improve air trapping with its deleterious.

2. Beta-Adrenergic Agonists

Beta-adrenergic agonists are first-line therapy for acute asthma episodes. Selective beta$_2$-agonists such as albuterol and terbutaline administered by MDI with a holding chamber or by nebulization titrated to maximum effect are preferred. For dosing see COPD, section D2a. When drug delivery by aerosol is inadequate, SQ epinephrine (0.3 mL 1:1000 q20 min × 3 max.) or terbutaline (0.25 mg q20 min × 2 max.) can be used.

3. Corticosteroids

Methylprednisolone (Solumedrol) 40 mg q6h IV or prednisone 60 mg orally q8h are recommended for the first 36 to 48 h. Significant clinical benefit are usually present 6 hours later. When the patient is stable, a prednisone-tapering program may consist of 60 mg/d for 4 days, reducing the dose to 40 mg/d and then by 10 mg/d every 4 days. At the same time, the patient should be started on inhaled corticosteroids (i.e., triamcinolone acetonide [Azmacort] 6 to 8 puffs bid).

4. Methylxanthines

The controversy regarding methylxanthines still continues. A recent study showed that aminophylline (theophylline) when added to the above therapy, may benefit patients hospitalized with acute asthma.

5. Complicating Factors

Treat any obvious associated precipitant or complicating conditions such as pneumonia and pneumothorax.

6. Other Forms of Therapy

Other interventions that have been used in status asthmaticus but are not considered standard therapy include magnesium sulfate, general anesthetics, and bronchial lavage of thick secretions.

■ III. PULMONARY EMBOLISM

A. Clinical Presentation and Risk Factors

1. The clinical findings of pulmonary embolism (PE) are nonspecific. It most commonly presents as the acute onset

of dyspnea with or without pleuritic chest pain, minor hemoptysis, tachypnea, and abnormal chest x-ray (although a normal chest x-ray is not uncommon either). Other forms of presentation include the following:

   a. Acute cor pulmonale (>40% of circulation compromised)

   b. Insidious onset of dyspnea (recurrent unrecognized PEs)

   c. Syncope, wheezing, fever, cough, dysrhythmias and cardiopulmonary arrest.

   d. Asymptomatic

2. PE originates from thrombi in the deep venous system of the lower extremities (deep venous thrombosis [DVT]) in most cases. Important risk factors for venous thromboembolism include the following:

   a. Prolonged immobility or paralysis.

   b. Surgery (mainly orthopedic—hip, knee—and lengthy procedures).

   c. Trauma.

   d. Malignancy.

   e. Congestive heart failure (CHF), recent myocardial infarction (MI).

   f. Advanced age.

   g. Obesity.

   h. Pregnancy and estrogen therapy.

   i. Prior history of DVT/PE: Less often, DVT/PE is caused by antithrombin III, protein S and protein C deficiencies, or lupus anticoagulant syndrome.

3. Chest x-ray abnormalities may be subtle or even absent.

   a. Pulmonary Infiltrates

     (1) Only a minority represent pulmonary infarction, and they usually resolve over few days

     (2) A pleural-based triangular infiltrate (Hampton's hump) may be seen with infarction. It usually persist for weeks.

   b. Pleural effusion(s)

   c. Elevated hemidiaphragm

   d. Platelike atelectasis

   e. Oligemia (Westermark's sign)

4. Arterial Blood Gases

   a. Hypoxemia in most cases (but 15% of PEs have $PaO_2 > 80\,mm\,Hg$)

   b. $P(A\text{-}a)O_2$ gradient widened

   c. Hypocapnia

5. Electrocardiogram (ECG)

   a. Nonspecific QRS and ST-T changes

   b. Sinus tachycardia

       c. Atrial dysrhythmias (multifocal atrial tachycardia [MAT], atrial flutter)

       d. S1-Q3-T3 pattern (only 10% of cases)

       e. Pulseless electrical activity in massive PE

B. Diagnostic Tests

   1. Ventilation/Perfusion (V/Q) Scan

      A normal V/Q scan practically rules out pulmonary embolism. On the other hand, an abnormal V/Q scan is nonspecific and should be considered in the context of the clinical probability (see Figure 13.1). The V/Q scan and simultaneous chest x-ray findings are categorized as normal/very low, low, intermediate, or high probability, as depicted in Table 13.4.

   2. Lower Extremities Venous Studies (LEs)

      a. Duplex Ultrasound (DU): DU is Doppler ultrasound combined with real-time two-dimensional ultrasound to study the venous system. When available, it is the method of choice for diagnosing proximal DVT

Table 13.4. V/Q Scan Interpretation Categories

Normal and very low probability
- No perfusion defects present (ventilation study and/or chest x-ray may be abnormal)
- 3 small segmental (<25% of a segment) perfusion defects with normal chest x-ray

Low probability
- >3 small segmental perfusion defects with normal chest x-ray
- Large or moderate segmental perfusion defect involving no >4 segments in 1 lung and no >3 segments in 1 lung region with matching ventilation defects and chest x-ray normal o with abnormalities smaller than the perfusion defects
- Nonsegmental perfusion defect (small pleural effusion, cardiomegaly, enlarged aorta, mediastinum, hila)
- One moderate segmental (>25% to <75%) perfusion defect with normal chest x-ray mismatch)

Intermediate probability
- All V/Q scans not included in the above categories (borderline or difficult to categorize)

High probability
- 2 large segmental (>75%) perfusion defects without corresponding ventilation or chest x-ray abnormality or smaller ventilation or chest x-ray abnormalities (mismatch)
- 2 moderate segmental and one large segmental perfusion-ventilation mismatches
- 4 moderate segmental perfusion-ventilation mismatches

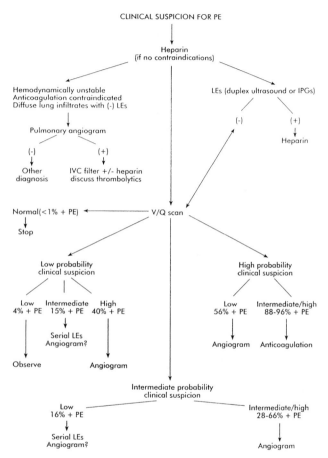

Figure 13.1. Diagnostic/Treatment Approach to Pulmonary Embolism.

(positive predicted value of 94%). Diagnostic criteria of DVT include the inability to collapse the vein and to visualize the clot. DU can also assess flow augmentation, valvular incompetence, and other causes of pain and swelling (i.e., popliteal cysts and hematomas).

    b. Impedance Plethysmography (IPG): IPG determines
       the changes in electrical impedance of the calf in
       response to blood volume changes produced by in-
       flating a pneumatic thigh cuff. It is very sensitive for
       occlusive proximal DVT but insensitive for calf vein
       thrombosis. False-positive results may be found in
       mechanically ventilated patients, CHF, and severe
       arterial insufficiency.
    c. Venography: It is considered the gold standard for
       the diagnosis of leg DVT. Disadvantages include its
       invasiveness, cost, and potential allergic reactions to
       contrast media. Definitive diagnostic findings include
       filling defects in a well-opacified vein and/or partially
       occluding defects surrounded by contrast media.
    d. Other Methods
       (1) I^{125}-Labeled Fibrinogen Scan: very sensitive
           for below-the-knee DVT, but definitive results
           take 6 to 72 hours.
       (2) Isotope Venography: good for above-the-knee
           DVT (including the inferior vena cava [IVC]). It
           can give a perfusion lung scan at the same time.
3. Pulmonary Arteriography
   In general, pulmonary arteriography is a safe procedure
   (mortality <0.2%, morbidity 4%), even in patients with
   significant pulmonary hypertension. Definitive angiographic signs include the presence of intraluminal filling
   defects or cutoffs of pulmonary arteries. It is indicated
   in patients with suspected PE and:
    a. Contraindications for anticoagulation (considering
       IVC filter)
    b. Hemodynamic instability (considering thrombolytic
       therapy or embolectomy)
    c. High clinical suspicion for PE with other than
       high-probability V/Q scan and negative leg venous
       studies
    d. Extensive pulmonary parenchymal disease or CHF

C. Treatment of Acute Thromboembolism
   1. Anticoagulation
      Anticoagulation should be started as soon as the clini-
      cal suspicion for PE is high enough to initiate a diag-
      nostic evaluation.
       a. Heparin: Give an initial bolus of 10,000 U intra-
          venously followed by a continuous infusion of 1300
          U/h (20,000 U in 500 mL D_5W at 33 mL/h). Check the
          first activated partial thromboplastin time (aPTT) in
          6 hours, and maintain it between 1.5 and 2.5 times

control. Modify heparin infusion according to the following:

    (1) If aPTT > 2.5 control, stop infusion for 1 hour, reduce the dose by 100 to 200 U/h, and recheck it in 4 to 6 hours.

    (2) If aPTT is between 1.25 and 1.5 control, increase the dose by 100 U/h, and recheck it in 4 to 6 hours.

    (3) If aPTT is <1.25 control, rebolus with 5000 U IV, increase the dose by 200 U/h, and recheck it in 4 to 6 hours.

In most patients, continue heparin for at least 5 days (provided that coumadin was started on day 1 or 2). Seven to ten days of heparin infusion are recommended for patients with massive PE or extensive iliofemoral thrombosis.

    Low molecular weight heparin has been used instead of unfractionated heparin in PE with excellent results (see Chapter 7, "Hematological Disorders").

  b. Coumadin: Oral anticoagulation started on day 1 or 2 at a dose of 5 to 10 mg/d is recommended. The goal is to prolong the prothrombin time (PT) to an International Normalized Ratio (INR) of 2.0 to 3.0. Coumadin should be continued for at least 3 to 6 months in most patients. For those with a continuing risk factor or recurrent thromboembolism, anticoagulation should be given indefinitely. In cases where coumadin may be contraindicated (i.e., pregnancy during the first and third trimester), adjusted-dose SQ heparin can be effectively used.

2. Thrombolytic Therapy

    Thrombolytic drugs dissolve thrombi by activating plasminogen to plasmin, which in turn degrades fibrin (see Chapter 7, "Hematologic Disorders"). In contrast to thrombolytic therapy for MI, complete emboli resolution in the pulmonary vessels is not accomplished frequently. Although a reduction in PE mortality has not been shown with this form of therapy, it should be considered in patients with acute massive PE and hemodynamic instability without significant risk factors for bleeding. The role of thrombolytic therapy in DVT and submassive PE is less well established. Agents used for PE/DVT include the following:

  a. Streptokinase (SK): 250,000-IU loading dose followed by 100,000 IU/h for 24 hours in PE and 48 to 72 hours in DVT.

  b. Urokinase (UK): 4400-IU/Kg loading dose followed by 4400 IU/kg/h for 12 hours in PE and 24 to 48 hours in DVT.
  c. Tissue Plasminogen Activator (tPA): 100 mg over 2 hours.

The efficacy and bleeding complications of SK, UK, and tPA are equivalent. When using SK or UK, checking a thrombin time or an aPTT 2 to 4 hours into the infusion is recommended to verify a fibrinolytic state. Heparin should be restarted when the aPTT is <2 times control.

3. IVC Filter

Indications for placement of an IVC filter (Greenfield, Mobin-Uddin, Bird's nest) include the following:

  a. Contraindications to anticoagulation
  b. Acute massive PE
  c. Recurrent PE on adequate anticoagulation therapy
  d. Chronic thromboembolism with pulmonary hypertension
  e. Following pulmonary embolectomy or thromboendarterectomy

4. Embolectomy

Embolectomy may be considered for documented massive PE with hemodynamic instability despite heparin, fluids, and vasopressors, and for those patients with contraindications for thrombolytic therapy. This procedure is advised only if an experienced surgical team is immediately available.

■ IV. ADULT RESPIRATORY DISTRESS SYNDROME (ARDS)

A. Definition

ARDS is a form of acute lung injury characterized by a high-permeability (noncardiogenic) pulmonary edema. In clinical practice, it is defined by the presence of the following:

1. Acute respiratory distress in a patient with predisposing conditions
2. Diffuse bilateral infiltrates on chest x-ray (pulmonary edema pattern)
3. Hypoxemia ($PaO_2 < 55$ mm Hg with $FiO_2 > 0.5$)
4. Reduced respiratory system static compliance (<40 to 50 mL/cm H_2O)
5. Low or normal pulmonary artery occlusion pressure (pulmonary capillary wedge pressure [PCWP] <16 cm H_2O)

B. Etiology

ARDS is most commonly associated with

1. Sepsis
2. Bronchial aspiration of gastric content
3. Trauma
4. Nosocomial pneumonia

Major risk factors for the development of ARDS are listed in Table 13.5.

C. Pathophysiology

The basic abnormality in ARDS is the disruption of the alveolar-capillary barrier. The endothelial injury in ARDS is frequently part of a more generalized permeability defect. An initial exudative phase is followed by proliferation of type II pneumocytes and fibrosis seen as early as the end of the first week.

D. Clinical Presentation

1. ARDS may develop insidiously over hours or even days after the initiating insult (i.e., pneumonia evolving into ARDS). Occasionally, it coincides with the precipitating event (i.e., gastric contents aspiration).
2. The signs and symptoms of ARDS are specific and usually include
   a. Dyspnea
   b. Tachypnea (rapid shallow breathing)
   c. Coarse lung crackles
   d. Cyanosis
   e. Agitation
3. Systemic manifestations of other organ dysfunctions may be related to the precipitating cause (i.e., burn, trauma) or

Table 13.5. Conditions Associated With ARDS

Air embolism
Aspiration of gastric contents
Burns
Cardiopulmonary bypass
Disseminated intravascular coagulation
Drugs (cocaine, heroin, methadone, acetylsalicylic acid)
Multiple fractures (fat embolism)
Multiple transfusions
Near drowning
Pancreatitis
Pneumonia (bacterial, viral, fungal)
Prolonged hypotension
Sepsis
Toxin inhalation
Trauma

may represent the generalization of the inflammatory response:

    a. Disseminated intravascular coagulation
    b. Encephalopathy
    c. Acute renal failure
    d. Acute liver failure
    e. Sepsis (gut bacterial translocation)

4. ABGs show marked hypoxemia and hypocapnia with either acute respiratory alkalosis or acute metabolic acidosis.

5. Despite the chest x-ray appearance of diffuse bilateral infiltrates, chest CT reveals a patchy, nonhomogeneous distribution of affected lung mixed with normal parenchyma. Small pleural effusions can be seen in ARDS. Usually, the cardiovascular silhouette on chest x-ray is within normal limits.

6. The pulmonary artery occlusion pressure or wedge pressure measured by a balloon-tipped, flow-directed catheter (Swan-Ganz catheter) in the past was used to detect the hydrostatic component of the pulmonary edema (cardiogenic). In pure ARDS, the wedge pressure should be <16 to 20cm H_2O.

E. Management

1. Treatment of the Precipitating Condition(s)

Specific treatment for the underlying disorder should be instituted as soon as possible (i.e., antimicrobials for infections, sepsis; drainage of abscesses, transfusion for hypovolemic shock, etc.).

2. Supportive Care

    a. Ventilatory Support (see "Acute Respiratory Failure," below)

    b. Hemodynamic Monitoring and Support

       (1) The use of pulmonary artery catheter (PA catheter or Swan-Ganz catheter) is controversial, as no study has ever proved that this technique improves survival in suspected or established ARDS. However, the information derived from hemodynamic monitoring using this catheter can be used in the following:

          (a) Differentiation of cardiogenic vs. non-cardiogenic pulmonary edema.

          (b) Management of intravascular volume (avoiding volume overload).

          (c) Assessment of the cardiovascular effects of PEEP titration (cardiac index, stroke volume).

    (d) Unfortunately, overtreating or confusing parameters is common while using a PA catheter.

   (2) In severe cases of ARDS, where high levels of extrinsic PEEP or dynamic hyperinflation (auto-PEEP) are necessary to maintain adequate oxygenation, a reduced cardiac index should be corrected with the use of inotropes (i.e., dobutamine or dopamine) to maintain an adequate O_2 delivery.

  c. Nutritional Support (see Chapter 10, "Nutrition")

  d. Diagnosis and Treatment of Complications

   (1) Barotrauma (i.e., tube thoracostomy for pneumothorax)

   (2) Acute renal failure (i.e., hemodialysis)

   (3) DIC (i.e., transfusions)

   (4) Infections: line sepsis, urinary tract infection (UTI), cellulitis (i.e., antibiotics, change central lines)

 3. Other Therapeutic Modalities

  a. *Pharmacologic and immunologic agents* targeted to arrest a specific step in the inflammatory cascade or pathophysiologic process characteristic of ARDS and sepsis have been extensively evaluated without success: i.e., monoclonal antibodies against bacterial lipopolysaccharide and tumor necrosis factor (TNF), soluble interleukin-1 (IL-1) and TNF receptors, prostaglandin E1, pentoxifylline, nonsteroidal anti-inflammatory drugs (NSAIDs) (i.e., ibuprofen), synthetic surfactant mixtures (Exosurf), inhaled nitric oxide, etc.

  b. *Extracorporeal oxygenation and CO_2 removal* (IVOX, $ECCO_2R$, ECMO), as currently implemented, have not demonstrated to be superior to conventional supportive care.

F. Prognosis

 1. The mortality of ARDS has remained unchanged over the past two decades in spite of advances in supportive therapy.

 2. Early mortality is usually related to the underlying condition(s); later, mortality is mainly related to multiple organ failure rather than pulmonary dysfunction. (In a study by Montgomery et al., <20% of deaths were attributed to irreversible respiratory failure.)

 3. Most *ARDS survivors* surprisingly have minimal long-term impairment of lung function (mild restrictive and diffusion

capacity [DLCO] defects). Occasionally, reversible airway obstruction may develop).

■ V. ACUTE RESPIRATORY FAILURE

A. Definition

Acute respiratory failure is the inability to maintain adequate blood oxygenation and/or alveolar ventilation in the absence of an intracardiac shunt. Provided the baseline ABGs are close to predicted normal values, this usually means an acute increase in $PaCO_2 > 50\,mm\,Hg$ with arterial acidemia and/or a $PaO_2 < 55\,mm\,Hg$ while breathing room air.

B. Classification and Etiology

Two clinical and pathophysiologic distinct types of acute respiratory failure can be described:

1. Hypoxemic Respiratory Failure

The hallmark of this type of respiratory failure is the inability to adequately oxygenate the blood. The main pathophysiologic mechanisms involved are V/Q mismatch (response to 100% O_2) and intrapulmonary shunting (no significant improvement with 100% O_2). The patients exhibit a rapid shallow breathing pattern and a low or normal $PaCO_2$. This form of respiratory failure is commonly the result of a diffuse acute lung injury with high-permeability pulmonary edema (ARDS), severe pneumonic infiltrates, or cardiogenic pulmonary edema.

2. Hypercapnic Respiratory Failure (Pump Failure)

The hallmark of ventilatory pump failure is hypercapnia with acute respiratory acidosis. The $P(A-a)O_2$ gradient is useful in determining if the hypoxemia present in this form of respiratory failure is due to hypoventilation (normal gradient) only or to additional parenchymal lung disease (elevated gradient). The hypercapnia is the result of abnormalities in one or more of the determinants of the $PaCO_2$:

$$PaCO_2 = k\ VCO_2/VE\ (1-VD/VT)$$

a. *Increased CO_2 production (VCO₂)* in patients with fever, sepsis, agitation, or excessive carbohydrate load, associated with a limited ventilatory capacity (high VD/VT, low VE)

b. *Increased dead space (VD/VT)* in severe COPD, cystic fibrosis, and severe asthma

    c. *Decreased total minute ventilation (VE)* due to ventilatory pump dysfunction:

        (1) Decreased Central Respiratory Drive: CVA, drugs (narcotics, sedatives, anesthetics), central hypoventilation, hypothyroidism

        (2) Abnormal Respiratory Efferents

            (a) Spinal Cord: trauma, poliomyelitis, amyotrophic lateral sclerosis, tetanus, rabies

            (b) Neuromuscular: myasthenia gravis, multiple sclerosis, botulism, Guillain-Barré syndrome, hypophosphatemia, hypomagnesemia, drugs (streptomycin, amikacin, neuromuscular blockers), polyneuropathy of critical illness, bilateral phrenic nerve injury

        (3) Abnormal Chest Wall and/or Muscles: severe kyphoscoliosis, ankylosing spondylitis, massive obesity, muscular dystrophy, polymyositis, respiratory muscles fatigue, acid maltase deficiency

        (4) Airways, Upper Airway Obstruction: epiglotitis, fixed and variable upper airway obstruction due to tumors, post-extubation, tracheomalacia, bilateral vocal cord paralysis

C. Management

The management of acute respiratory failure is initially supportive, aimed at the correction of hypoxemia or hypercapnia until specific actions are implemented to correct, if possible, the factors that lead to the respiratory failure (i.e., antibiotics for pneumonia; diuretics, morphine, nitroglycerin and afterload-reducing agents for cardiogenic pulmonary edema; naloxone for narcotics overdose).

1. Hypoxemic Respiratory Failure

    a. Patients with V/Q mismatch abnormalities without significant intrapulmonary shunt will usually respond to noninvasive O_2 supplementation (i.e., nasal cannula, Venturi mask).

    b. In patients with cardiogenic pulmonary edema, the use of continuous positive airway pressure (CPAP) (5 to 10cm H_2O) via a face mask in addition to O_2 supplementation can be beneficial by reducing the transmural pressure of the left ventricle, and therefore afterload, but also by decreasing the preload.

    c. The ventilatory management of patients with diffuse acute lung injury (i.e., ARDS) requires mechanical ventilation and should be viewed as a balance between *adequate oxygenation* on one hand, and the *risk for barotrauma* and *cardiovascular compromise* on the other. The following section pertains to specific aspects of the ventilatory management of ARDS.

(1) Adequate Oxygenation: For most patients with ARDS, this means a PaO_2 of 55 to 60 mm Hg or O_2 saturation of 88% to 90% with a cardiac index >2.5 L/min/m^2 and hemoglobin 10 g/dL. Arterial O_2 saturation can be increased in ARDS by the following:

(a) *Raising the fraction of inspired oxygen (FiO$_2$):* To avoid potential O_2 toxic effects, it is recommended not to use 100% O_2 for more than a few hours and to maintain an FiO$_2$ ≤ 0.6. A particular effort should be made to decrease FiO$_2$ to the minimum acceptable in patients exposed to drugs that may increase O_2 toxicity (i.e., bleomycin, amiodarone).

(b) *Increasing the end-expiratory lung volume* to recruit collapsed or flooded alveoli. This can be achieved by adding *extrinsic PEEP* and/or setting the ventilator to create *dynamic hyperinflation (auto-PEEP)*. It is unclear if one strategy is more effective that the other in ARDS. The goal is to maximize oxygenation while at the same time *avoiding* hypotension, reduced cardiac pump function, and, a *plateau pressure > 35 cm H$_2$O*. With these considerations:

i. *Extrinsic PEEP* is usually started at a level of 5 cm H$_2$O and titrated up by 2-cm H$_2$O increments to a level of 15 to 20 cm H$_2$O along with the use of other strategies to minimize barotrauma (see "Avoiding Barotrauma," below).

ii. *Extended-ratio ventilation* (prolonged I : E ratio, known as inverse ratio ventilation when I/E > 1 : 1) is a technique used to increase mean alveolar pressure and transpulmonary pressure. It can be implemented with either volume-controlled or pressure-controlled ventilators. Increasing the inspiratory time (see Table 13.6), increases the mean airway pressure (MAP) and allows the recruitment of lung units with long time constants, therefore, improving oxygenation. Extended-ratio ventilation is more easily implemented with volume-controlled than pressure-controlled ventilators. Both require heavy sedation with or without paralysis; i.e., morphine sulfate, midazolam (Versed), lorazepam (Ativan) or propofol (Diprivan) by continuous infusion with or without vecuronium (Norcuron) or atracurium (Tracrium). Monitoring of plateau pressure to keep it <35 cm H_2O, auto-PEEP (end-expiration occlusion method), and hemodynamics by a pulmonary balloon-tipped, flow-directed catheter (Swan-Ganz) is required.

(2) *Avoiding barotrauma*: Barotrauma in the form of extra-alveolar air or worsening of acute lung injury is the result of alveolar overdistention (increased transmural pressure or alveolar pressure [Palv] – pleural pressure [Ppl]). Thus, it seems reasonable to avoid lung volumes above total lung capacity (TLC) to prevent lung damage.

Table 13.6. Prolonging Inspiratory Time (Ti) and I/E Ratio in Volume-Controlled Ventilators*

Reduce inspiratory flow (i.e., to 40 L/min)
Use decelerating inspiratory flow waveform
Add an inspiratory pause (i.e., 0.2–0.5 s)
Increase the percent inspiratory time[†]

* Applying these changes in a stepwise manner will allow progressive extension of Ti and I : E ratio to the degree that is tolerated or needed. Adjustment in tidal volume (VT) as recommended (see below) and monitoring the plateau pressure (Pplateau), auto-PEEP, and its hemodynamic effects are required to avoid complications.
[†] Direct way of setting the I : E ratio (i.e., Siemens Servo Ventilator).

(a) Because Palv, Ppl, and lung volumes are difficult to determine at the bedside, monitoring the *plateau pressure (end-inflation hold pressure)* is recommended as the best approximation of the peak alveolar pressure.

(b) A plateau pressure of 35 cm H_2O or more, in the absence of significantly decreased chest wall compliance, should be avoided.

(c) Peak airway pressure (Ppeak) reflects not only the elastic, but also the flow-resistive pressures of the respiratory system, and it should be used only as a gross estimate for the risk of baro-trauma (i.e., high Ppeak may be due to a small endotracheal tube, bron-chospasm, secretions, high inspiratory peak flow, or worsening of lung or chest wall compliance) that may or may not mean alveolar overinflation.

(d) Determining the tidal volume (VT): ARDS is a nonhomogeneous process with collapsed and flooded areas mixed with relatively normal aerated lung, resulting in a reduction in the TLC. Thus, it makes sense to ventilate ARDS patients with smaller than conventional VT. The VT chosen should be one that prevents lung overinflation (i.e., plateau pressure < 35 cm H_2O) and alveolar derecruitment at the end of expiration (inadequate oxygenation). This usually means an initial VT of 7 to 8 mL/kg, which may need to be reduced to 5 mL/kg.

(e) Setting the respiratory rate: The machine rate should be determined considering the patient's metabolic demands, intrinsic rate, and desired I:E ratio. It is usually set between 25 and 40 breaths per minute. Even with these rates (plus the low VT used), minute ventilation may not be high enough for ARDS patients. Allowing CO_2 retention (i.e., 60 mm Hg) and respiratory acidemia (i.e., pH 7.2 to 7.25) in an effort to limit barotrauma is referred as *permissive hypercapnia*.

(3) *Controlling the hemodynamic effects of mechanical ventilation*: The increase in end-expiratory lung volume and mean alveolar pressure produced by the ventilatory strategies described above can have deleterious hemodynamics consequences. It is important to document that a ventilator change aimed at increasing O_2 saturation does not reduce the total amount of O_2 delivered to the tissues via a reduction in cardiac index. In severe cases, the cardiac index should be maintained >2.5 L/min/m^2 with the use of inotropic agents (dobutamine or dopamine if hypotension is present).

2. Hypercapnic Respiratory Failure

The main goal in treating patients with hypercapnic respiratory failure is to improve alveolar ventilation through the use of mechanical ventilation. This is most commonly done through an endotracheal tube using a volume-controlled ventilator (usual initial settings are VT 5 to 9 mL/kg, A/C mode, rate 8 to 10 breaths per minute, and FiO$_2$ 1.0). ABGs are checked 10 to 20 minutes later to detect inadverted and potentially life-threatening acute alkalosis secondary to overcorrection of the hypercapnia and to adjust the FiO$_2$. Noninvasive mechanical ventilation has been effective in patients with neuromuscular conditions. The management of hypercapnic respiratory failure in asthma and COPD is discussed above.

■ VI. BAROTRAUMA

A. Definition

Barotrauma is lung injury that is related to high *alveolar* pressures (and volumes). In the intensive care unit (ICU) setting, *barotrauma* specifically refers to positive-pressure ventilator-induced lung damage. Occasionally, a patient may be admitted to the ICU after a diving accident (sudden decompression) or foreign body aspiration (ball-valve mechanism).

B. Clinical Manifestations

1. *Classic mechanical ventilator-induced barotrauma* is manifested by *extra-alveolar air* in the form of

      a. Pulmonary interstitial emphysema (PIE)
      b. Subpleural air cysts
      c. Pneumomediastinum
      d. Pneumothorax (PTX)
      e. Subcutaneous emphysema
      f. Pneumopericardium
      g. Pneumoretroperitoneum
      h. Pneumoperitoneum
      i. Gas emboli (main clinical manifestation in diving accidents)

2. *Tension PTX* occurs in 30% to 97% of all PTXs in mechanically ventilated patients and is characterized by worsening hypoxemia, hypotension, or even cardiovascular collapse with pulseless electrical activity (PEA). Chest x-ray shows lung collapse with hemithorax expansion and contralateral mediastinal shift.

3. Physical examination reveals
      a. Absent breath sounds, hyperresonance to percussion, and decreased chest excursion on the affected side in cases of PTX.
      b. Crepitation on palpation or auscultation is found in cases of subcutaneous emphysema.
      c. Mediastinal "crunch" in pneumomediastinum.
      d. Changes in mental status or neurologic deficits are usually found in patients with gas embolism.

4. Development or worsening of *diffuse lung injury* (in the form of noncardiogenic pulmonary edema) also has been associated with positive-pressure ventilation.

C. Pathophysiology
  1. Alveolar rupture occurs at the site where alveoli attach to the bronchovascular sheath. From there, extra-alveolar air may dissect the peribronchovascular tissues into different planes to produce the clinical manifestations listed above. Alternatively, direct rupture of a subpleural cyst into the pleural cavity may also cause PTX.
  2. Positive-pressure mechanical ventilation has also shown to produce
      a. Increased lung microvascular permeability and filtration pressure
      b. Alveolar epithelial injury
      c. Alteration of surfactant function and turnover

D. Diagnosis
  1. A high index of suspicion should be maintained in those patients at risk for barotrauma (i.e., use of high VT, high plateau pressure, peak pressure, PEEP, dynamic hyperin-

flation, extensive lung damage, and prolonged mechanical ventilation).

2. Chest x-ray will usually confirm a diagnosis of extra-alveolar air. PIE (seen as linear radiolucent streaks) is the first radiologic sign and should alert the physician for the risk of progression to PTX

3. The classic radiologic sign of PTX (pleural line separated from the apicolateral chest wall) may not be present in ICU patients when an antero-posterior (AP)portable chest x-ray is taken in the supine or semirecumbent position. In those patients, attention should also be paid to the mediastinal and subpulmonic recesses where air accumulates.

E. Management

1. *Extra-alveolar air without PTX* is managed conservatively. Observation and avoidance of risk factors if possible, is indicated (see "Avoiding Barotrauma," above).

2. In general, all PTXs in a mechanically ventilated patient should be treated with *tube thoracotomy* (see Chapter 15, "Special Techniques").

3. The use of *"prophylactic" tube thoracotomy* for high-risk mechanically ventilated patients is controversial and not recommended. Instead, it is advised to follow these patients closely and be prepared for immediate placement of a chest tube should PTX develop.

4. Persistent *bronchopleural fistula(s)* despite chest tube suction should be managed with the lowest VT, Ppeak, and Pplateau that permit adequate ventilation. High-frequency jet ventilation (HFJV), independent lung ventilation, or surgery should be considered if the air leak is massive and does not respond to the usual management.

5. Recompression in a hyperbaric chamber is indicated for diving accidents resulting in *air embolism.*

■ VII. MASSIVE HEMOPTYSIS

A. Definition

Hemoptysis is the expectoration of blood that originates from below the larynx. It is considered massive when the rate of bleeding is at least 400 mL in 6 hours or 600 mL in a 24-hour period.

B. Etiology

The most common causes of massive hemoptysis are

1. Tuberculosis (rupture of Rasmussen's aneurysm)
2. Bronchiectasis (erosion of bronchial vasculature)
3. Bronchogenic carcinoma (invasion of pulmonary vessels)
4. Lung abscess (destruction of fairly normal vessels due to inflammation)

Other etiologies include bronchial carcinoids, cystic fibrosis, broncholithiasis, aspergilloma, trauma, bronchovascular and arteriovenous (A-V)fistulas, mitral stenosis, and the pulmonary-renal syndrome.

C. Evaluation
   1. Differentiate Hemoptysis From Hematemesis

      Hemoptysis is usually bright red blood, frothy, with an alkaline pH. In contrast, hematemesis is usually darker with an acidic pH. At times this differentiation cannot be made easily, because hematemesis may produce blood aspiration into the tracheobronchial tree, which in turn causes "hemoptysis," and, on the other hand, patients with hemoptysis may swallow blood and vomit it after coughing.

   2. Localize the Bleeding Site

      Localization of the bleeding site is important to adequately plan any interventional procedure. Bleeding coming from the upper airways can be excluded by performing an ear, nose, and throat (ENT) examination.

      a. Chest x-ray may suggest the bleeding site
         (1) Lung masses, apical cavitary lesions, or infiltrates in the chest x-ray should point to these sites as the source of bleeding.
         (2) A normal chest x-ray is consistent with bleeding arising from the airways.
         (3) Roentgenograms showing bilateral or diffuse disease are not helpful in pointing out the origin of bleeding.

      b. *Bronchoscopy* should be performed to further identify the site and cause of bleeding and to achieve temporary control. The type and timing of the procedure depend on the rate of bleeding.
         (1) When *flexible fiberoptic bronchoscopy (FFB)* is done, the patient must be intubated with a large endotracheal tube that may be used to tamponade the affected lung if necessary.
         (2) *Rigid bronchoscopy* is the preferred temporizing method to evaluate and control a massive bleeding. This procedure should be done under general anesthesia in the operating room by trained physicians.

   c. *Angiography* of the bronchial and pulmonary circulation is recommended when bronchoscopy cannot determine the bleeding site in more peripheral lesions.

  3. Laboratory Determinations

   Obtain ABGs to determine if acidosis exists and to confirm level of oxygenation. The obtain a complete blood cell count, PT, partial thromboplastin time (PTT), bleeding time, creatinine, serum urea nitrogen (BUN), and request blood type and cross-matching.

D. Management

  1. Ensure Adequate Ventilation and Oxygenation

   This should be the main priority if we consider that the mode of death in massive hemoptysis is asphyxiation (as little as 150 cc of blood are needed to fill the airways).

   a. Depending on the rate of bleeding, it may only be necessary to administer supplemental O_2 through nasal cannula or face mask or, on the other extreme, it may be necessary to perform endotracheal intubation (single- or double-lumen [Carlen's tube]) to aspirate the blood and ventilate the patient while definitive therapy is being prepared.

   b. Position the patient in *the lateral decubitus position with the bleeding site down.*

  2. Ensure Stable Hemodynamic Conditions

   a. Obtain adequate venous access.

   b. Administer fluids as needed (normal saline or blood).

  3. Suppress Cough

   a. Codeine 60 mg PO q6h.

   b. Sedatives may be added (i.e., midazolam 2 mg or lorazepam 1 mg, IV q2h prn).

  4. Control the Bleeding Site

   a. *Bronchoscopic procedures* include

    (1) Bronchial packing through a rigid bronchoscope

    (2) Tamponade of airway with a balloon-tipped (Fogarty) catheter through a rigid bronchoscope or alongside a flexible bronchoscope

    (3) Bronchial lavage with cold saline through a rigid bronchoscope

    (4) Coagulation of visible lesions with a Neodynium-YAG laser (not helpful in very active, brisk bleeding)

   b. *Bronchial artery embolization* is the method of choice for patients with massive or submassive hemoptysis and contraindications for surgery. Given its high success rate (90%), embolization has become a first-line treatment for all patients with massive or recurrent hemoptysis.

c. *Surgical resection* is recommended for localized lesions that can be removed. It should not be offered to patients with
(1) Metastatic lung cancer
(2) Severe pulmonary or cardiovascular status

d. *Correct coagulopathy* if present (i.e., administer FFP and vitamin K if PT is prolonged, transfuse platelets in severe thrombocytopenia).

E. Prognosis
1. Although the underlying medical condition(s) affect the prognosis in massive hemoptysis, the best estimator of mortality is the rate of bleeding. A study by Cracco showed that hemoptysis of 600 cc occurring over
a. 4 hours has 71% mortality
b. 4 to 16 hours has 45% mortality
c. 16 to 48 hours has 5% mortality
2. Median operative mortality in massive hemoptysis is 17%. Actively bleeding patients at the time of the surgery have a higher mortality when compared with nonactively bleeding patients.

■ VIII. USEFUL FACTS AND FORMULAS

A. Lung Volumes
Normal values for pulmonary volumes and capacities in humans are depicted in Table 13.7.
The *vital capacity* (VC) is calculated as follows:

Table 13.7. Normal Values for Lung Volumes in Upright Subjects

Volume or capacity	Approximate value in upright subjects
Total lung capacity (TLC)	6 L
Vital capacity (VC)	4.5 L
Residual volume (RV)	1.5 L
Inspiratory capacity (IC)	3 L
Functional residual capacity (FRC)	3 L
Inspiratory reserve volume (IRV)	2.5 L
Expiratory reserve volume (ERV)	1.5 L
Tidal volume (V_T)	0.5 L

$$VC = IRV + ERV + V_T$$

The *residual volume* (RV) is calculated as the difference between the functional residual capacity (FRC) and the expiratory reserve volume (ERV):

$$RV = FRC - EV$$

Alternatively, if the total lung capacity (TLC) and vital capacity (VC) are known, the following formula can be utilized:

$$RV = TLC - VC$$

The oldest method to measure *FRC* is the *equilibration technique*, utilizing the following formula:

$$FRC = [(C_1 \times V_1)/C_2] - V_1$$

where C_1 = known concentration of a test gas in the spirometer; V_1 = volume of gas in the spirometer; C_2 = the fractional value of the gas after the subject breathes in the spirometer until the concentration of the test gas equals that in the spirometer.

Another way to measure FRC is by utilizing the *nitrogen washout procedure* and the following formula:

$$FRC = (V_B \times C_B)/C_X$$

where V_B = amount of exhaled nitrogen volume in the bag; C_B = fractional concentration of nitrogen in the bag; C_X = subject initial fractional concentration of nitrogen (0.80).

Alternatively, FRC can be calculated using body plethysmography as follows:

$$FRC = (\Delta/\Delta P)(P_B + \Delta P)$$

where ΔV = change in volume; ΔP = change in pressure; P_B = atmospheric pressure minus water vapor pressure (P_{H2O}).

The *tidal volume* (V_T) is the sum of the dead space volume (V_D) and the alveolar volume (V_A):

$$V_T = V_D + V_A$$

The average *dead space volume* (V_D) is estimated as $1\,mL/lb$ body weight. For an average 70-kg man:

$$V_D = 70 \times 2.2 \times 1 = 154\,mL$$

B. Pulmonary Ventilation

The easiest way of estimating *minute ventilation* (V_E) is by using the following formula:

$$V_E = V_T \times RR = mL/min$$

where V_T = tidal volume; RR = respiratory rate.

Minute ventilation is also the sum of dead space (V_D) and alveolar ventilation (V_A):

$$V_E = V_A + V_D$$

The *alveolar ventilation* (V_A) can be calculated as:

$$V_A = (V_T - V_D) \times N$$

where N = frequency of breathing in breaths per minute; V_D = dead space ventilation.

An alternative method requires knowledge of the CO_2 production by the patient. The *production of CO_2* ($\dot{V}CO_2$) can be calculated as follows:

$$\dot{V}CO_2 = V_A \times F_{ACO2}$$

where F_{ACO2} = fractional concentration of CO_2 in the alveolar gas; and $V_A = \dot{V}CO_2/F_{ACO2}$.

Dead space ventilation (V_D) can be calculated if the minute ventilation (V_E) is known:

$$V_D = V_E ([PaCO_2 - PECO_2])/PaCO_2$$

The *partial pressure of alveolar CO_2* ($PACO_2$) is more convenient for these calculations and practical purposes:

$$PACO_2 = F_{ACO2} \times (P_B - 47)$$

In normal lungs, the *arterial CO_2* ($PaCO_2$) approximates the $PACO_2$. Therefore, the V_A formula can be rewritten as

$$V_A = K (\dot{V}CO_2/PaCO_2)$$

where K = a factor (0.863) that converts CO_2 concentrations to pressure (mm Hg).

C. Gas Transport in Blood

The difference between the inspired and expired fractional concentration of O_2 represents the *oxygen uptake* ($\dot{V}O_2$):

$$\dot{V}O_2 = (V_I \times FiO2) - (V_E \times F_EO_2)$$

where V_I = volume of gas inhaled; FiO2 = fractional concentration of inspired oxygen; V_E = volume of gas exhaled; F_EO_2 = fractional concentration of expired oxygen.

The amount of *O_2 in solution in 100 mL of blood* is calculated as (assuming a partial O_2 pressure of 70 mm Hg):

$$(PO_2/760) \times \alpha O_2 = 70/760 \times 2.3 = 0.21\, mL/100\, mL$$

The PaO_2 at which hemoglobin is 50% saturated (P_{50}) can be calculated from the venous pH and arterial blood gases as

$$P_{50} = \text{antilog}\frac{\text{Log}(1/k)}{n} = \text{normal } 22 - 30\text{mm Hg}$$

where

$$(1/k) = (\text{antilog}\,[n \times \log \text{PaO2}_{7.4}]) \times (100 - \text{SaO}_2/\text{SaO}_2)$$

$$\text{antilog}\,[n \times \log \text{PaO2}_{7.4}] = \log \text{PaO}_2 - 0.5\,(7.4 - \text{venous pH})$$

n = Hill constant = 2.7 for hemoglobin A

The *Fick equation* for *oxygen consumption* (VO_2) is calculated as follows:

$$VO_2 = Q(CaO_2 - C\bar{v}O_2)$$

where Q = cardiac output (L/min); CaO_2 = arterial oxygen content; CvO_2 = mixed venous oxygen content.

The volume of carbon dioxide exhaled per unit time (*CO_2 production* or $\dot{V}CO_2$) is calculated as follows:

$$\dot{V}CO_2 = (V_E \times F_ECO_2) - (V_I \times F_ICO_2)$$

where V_E = volume of gas exhaled per unit time; F_ECO_2 = fractional concentration of carbon dioxide in the exhaled gas; V_I = volume of gas inhaled per unit time; F_ICO_2 = fractional concentration of inspired carbon dioxide.

Since the inspired gas usually contains negligible amounts of carbon dioxide, another representation of this formula is

$$\dot{V}CO_2 = V_E \times F_ECO_2$$

D. Pulmonary Circulation

The *mean pulmonary artery pressure* (PAP) can be calculated utilizing the following formula:

$$PAP = (PVR \times PBF) + PAOP$$

where PVR = pulmonary vascular resistance; PBF = pulmonary blood flow (which typically equals the cardiac output). Reorganizing the above formula, the *pulmonary vascular resistance* (PVR) is then calculated as

$$PVR = (\text{Mean PAP} - PAOP)/CO$$

where PAOP = pulmonary artery occlusion pressure; CO = cardiac output.

The pressures that surround the vessels in the pulmonary circulation contribute to the *transmural pressure* (Ptm) represented as

$$Ptm = Pvas - Pis$$

where Pvas = vascular pressure; Pis = perivascular interstitial pressure.

When the left atrial pressure (Pla) is available, the *driving pressure* responsible for producing *pulmonary blood flow* is then calculated as

$$(Ppa - Pla) = Q \times Rvas$$

where Ppa = mean pulmonary arterial pressure; Pla = mean left atrial pressure; Q = pulmonary blood flow; Rvas = pulmonary vascular resistance.

The *pulmonary vascular compliance* (Cvas) can be calculated utilizing the following formula:

$$Cvas = \Delta Vvas / \Delta Pvas$$

where $\Delta Vvas$ = change in blood volume; $\Delta Pvas$ = change in vascular pressure.

The *blood flow zones* in an idealized upright lung with normal pressure differences are depicted in Table 13.8.

E. Mechanics and Gas Flow

The pressure inside the lungs relative to the pressure outside is known as the *transpulmonary pressure* (TP) and is calculated as

$$TP = P_{alv} - P_{pl}$$

where P_{alv} = alveolar pressure; P_{pl} = pleural pressure.

The change in volume (ΔV) for a unit pressure (ΔP) under conditions of no flow is the *static compliance*:

$$\text{Static compliance } (C_s) = \frac{\Delta V}{\Delta P}$$

Clinically, this formula can be simplified as follows:

Table 13.8. Pulmonary Blood Flow Zones

Blood flow zones	Pressures
I	Palv > Ppa > Ppv
II	Ppa > Palv > Ppv
III	Ppa > Ppv > Palv
IV	Ppa > Ppv > Palv

Abbreviations: Palv = pressure surrounding the alveolar vessels; Ppa = mean pulmonary arterial pressure; Ppv = mean venous (left atrial) pressure.

$$C_s = \frac{V_T}{\text{Plateau airway pressure} - (\text{PEEP} + \text{autoPEEP})}$$

where V_T = tidal volume. Normal C_s value is 100 mL/cm H_2O.

The *dynamic compliance* (C_{dyn}) can be calculated utilizing the following formula:

$$C_{dyn} = \frac{V_T}{\text{Peak airway pressure} - (\text{PEEP} + \text{autoPEEP})}$$

Normal C_{dyn} value is 100 mL/cm H_2O.

The specific compliance (C_{spec}) is calculated utilizing the following formula:

$$C_{spec} = C_{stat}/\text{FRC}$$

The *chest wall compliance* (C_W) can be calculated as

$$C_W = \frac{V_T}{\text{Airway pressure} - \text{Atmospheric pressure}}$$

Another formula that can be used under special circumstances (i.e., lung transplantation) is the *separate lung compliance* (C_X) and is calculated as

$$C_x = \frac{V_T}{\text{Airway pressure} - \text{Intrapleural pressure}}$$

The type of gas flow in the lung is *laminar flow* and is described mathematically by the *Poiseuille equation*:

$$\Delta P = \frac{8\mu l V}{\pi r^4}$$

where ΔP = hydrostatic pressure drop; V = gas flow; μ = gas viscosity; l = path length; r = radius of the tube. From this equation, resistance ($R = \Delta P/V$) can be calculated:

$$R = \frac{8\mu l}{\pi r^4}$$

On the other hand, *the pressure drop during turbulent flow* can be calculated utilizing the following formula:

$$\Delta P = \frac{\mu l^- \rho^-}{r^{19/4}}$$

where ΔP = pressure drop during turbulent flow; μ = viscosity; ρ = density.

The *Reynolds number* (Re) is the ratio of the pressure loss due to density-dependent or inertial flow vs. the pressure loss due to viscous flow. This number is used to predict the nature of a particular flow and is calculated as follows:

$$Re = \frac{2\rho r V}{\mu A}$$

The *airway resistance* (Raw) using body plethysmography can be calculated utilizing the following formula:

$$Raw = \frac{\Delta Vbox}{V} \times \frac{Palv}{V} = \frac{Palv}{\Delta Vbox}$$

where $\Delta Vbox$ = volume changes in the box; V = flow; Palv = alveolar pressure.

The *work of the respiratory system* (W) can be calculated as

$$W = P \times V$$

where P = pressure; V = volume.

F. Ventilation/Perfusion

The physiological *dead space* can be calculated utilizing the classic *Bohr equation*:

$$V_D/V_T = \frac{P_ACO_2 - P_ECO_2}{P_ACO_2}$$

where P_ACO_2 = partial pressure of carbon dioxide in the alveolar gas; P_ECO_2 = partial pressure of carbon dioxide in mixed expired gas.

The above formula with the *Enghoff modification* is used in clinical practice:

$$V_D/V_T = \frac{PaCO_2 - P_ECO_2}{PaCO_2} = 0.30 \text{ in healthy subjects}$$

The quantity of blood passing through pulmonary right-to-left *shunts* (Qs/Q) is calculated as

$$Qs/Q = \frac{Cc'O_2 - CaO_2}{Cc'O_2 - C\overline{v}O_2}$$

where

$$Cc'O_2 = (Hb \times 1.38) + P_AO_2 \times \frac{\alpha}{760}$$

Therefore, the Qs/Q formula can be rearranged as

$$Qs/Q = \frac{(P_AO_2 - PaO_2) \times 0.0031}{(P_AO_2 - PaO_2) \times 0.0031 + (CaO_2 - C\overline{v}O_2)}$$

G. Alveolar Gas Equation

The *alveolar air equation* is based firmly on Dalton's law but is expressed in terms that emphasize alveolar O_2 and CO_2:

$$P_AO_2 = (P_{ATM} - P_{H2O})FiO_2 - PCO_2/RQ$$

where P_AO_2 = partial pressure of O_2 in the alveolus under present conditions; P_{ATM} = current, local atmospheric pressure. P_{H2O} = vapor pressure of water at body temperature and 100% relative humidity; FiO_2 = fraction of inspired O_2; PCO_2 = partial pressure of CO_2 in arterial blood; RQ = respiratory quotient.

At *sea level*, this equation can be simplified to

$$P_AO_2 = 150 - 1.25 \times PaCO_2$$

The *arterial oxygen tension (PaO₂) corrected for age* is calculated as

$$PaO_2 \text{ age-corrected} = 100 - 1/3 \text{ age (in years)}$$

The *alveolar-arterial O_2 gradient* is *age-corrected* according to the following formula:

$$\text{Age correction} = 2.5 + (0.25 \times [\text{age in years}])$$

14

Renal and Fluid-Electrolyte Disorders

■ I. ACID-BASE DISTURBANCES

An *acidosis* is any process that tends (in the absence of buffering or compensation) to cause the accumulation of hydrogen ions (H^+). If the pH of the blood is lower than normal (<7.35), *acidemia* is present. Similarly, any process that tends to cause the accumulation of bicarbonate (HCO_3) is an *alkalosis*. An elevated blood pH (>7.45) is referred to as *alkalemia*. When the acid-base disturbance arises as a result of changes in the carbon dioxide tension (PCO_2) of the blood, a respiratory process is present. Conversely, when the acid-base disturbance occurs as a result of accumulation of nonvolatile acids or loss of HCO_3 (or substances metabolized to HCO_3), a metabolic process is present. Acidosis and alkalosis can be either primary or compensatory for a different acid-base problem.

A. Approach to Acid-Base Disturbances
1. The initial evaluation of acid-base disorders requires the simultaneous examination of arterial blood gases (ABGs) and serum electrolytes.
2. The typical patterns of blood pH, PCO_2, and HCO_3 in various acid-base problems are listed in Table 14.1.
3. The adequacy of compensation for a primary acid-base abnormality can also be assessed.
    a. For patients with metabolic acidosis, the expected PCO_2 can be calculated as

$$PCO_2 = ([HCO_3] \times 1.5) + 8 \, (\pm 2)$$

   (1) If the actual PCO_2 is greater than expected, a simultaneous respiratory acidosis is present.

Table 14.1. Systematic Evaluation of Acid-Base Disorders

Compensated process	
Metabolic acidosis	pH ↓ PCO$_2$ ↓ HCO$_3$ ↓
Respiratory acidosis	pH ↓ PCO$_2$ ↑ HCO$_3$ ↑
Metabolic alkalosis	pH ↑ PCO$_2$ ↑ HCO$_3$ ↑
Respiratory alkalosis	pH ↑ PCO$_2$ ↓ HCO$_3$ ↓
Uncompensated process	
Metabolic acidosis	pH ↓ PCO$_2$—HCO$_3$ ↓
Respiratory acidosis	pH ↓ PCO$_2$ ↑ HCO$_3$—
Metabolic alkalosis	pH ↑ PCO$_2$—HCO3 ↑
Respiratory alkalosis	pH ↑ PCO$_2$ ↓ HCO$_3$—
Mixed process	
Metabolic/Respiratory Acidosis	pH ↓ PCO$_2$ ↑ HCO$_3$ ↓
Metabolic/Respiratory Alkalosis	pH ↑ PCO$_2$ ↓ HCO$_3$ ↑

(2) If the measured PCO$_2$ is less than expected, a simultaneous respiratory alkalosis is present.

b. For patients with metabolic alkalosis, the expected PCO$_2$ can be calculated as

$$PCO_2 = \{([HCO_3] - 25) \times 0.7\} + 40\,(\pm 2)$$

(1) Respiratory compensation for a primary metabolic alkalosis is limited to a PCO$_2$ of about 55 mm Hg. Even this limit may not be attained in patients with chronic pulmonary or hepatic disease or congestive heart failure.

c. Metabolic compensation for respiratory acid-base disturbances depends in part on the duration of the problem.

(1) For patients with chronic respiratory acidosis, the expected [HCO$_3$] can be calculated as

$$[HCO_3] = (PCO_2 - 40) \times 0.35 + 25(\pm 2)$$

(a) The upper limit for this process is [HCO$_3$] = 55 mEq/L.

(b) If the degree of compensation is inadequate, the possibility of a mixed acid-base disturbance or a superimposed acute process should be entertained.

(2) The expected degree of compensation for acute respiratory acidosis is calculated as

$$[HCO_3] = (PCO_2 - 40) \times 0.10 + 25(\pm 2)$$

The upper limit of compensation for acute respiratory acidosis is [HCO$_3$] = 30 mEq/L.

(3) The expected metabolic response to chronic respiratory alkalosis can be estimated by

$$[HCO_3] = 25 - (40 - PCO_2) \times 0.5 \, (\pm 2)$$

Inadequate compensation for chronic respiratory alkalosis should raise the possibility of a superimposed acute respiratory alkalosis, or a mixed acid-base problem.

(4) The expected metabolic response to acute respiratory alkalosis can be calculated as

$$[HCO_3] = 25 - (40 - PCO_2) \times 0.25 \, (\pm 2)$$

B. Metabolic Acidosis

The clinical consequences of metabolic acidosis are due to abnormalities of intracellular pH, transcellular ionic shifts, or both.

1. Signs and symptoms include tachypnea, depressed cardiac function, fatigue, weakness, and altered mental status.
2. Laboratory findings: hyperkalemia, calciuresis, and changes in carbohydrate and lipid metabolism.
3. Other specific findings may occur due to the etiology of the underlying cause of the acidosis.
4. Metabolic acidoses are classified based on whether the plasma anion gap (AG) is normal or elevated. Its value is calculated as

$$AG = [Na^+] - ([Cl^-] + [HCO_3]) \quad (nl = 10 - 15 \, mEq/L)$$

5. The differential diagnosis of primary metabolic acidosis is listed in Table 14.2.
   a. In general, high AG metabolic acidoses are caused by the accumulation of an acid in the plasma whose anion is something other than Cl⁻. These acids can be endogenous (i.e., lactic acid, ketoacids, uremic acids), exogenous (i.e., salicylates), or the endogenous meta-

Table 14.2. Causes of Metabolic Acidosis

Elevated Anion Gap	Normal Anion Gap
Methanol	Urinary-enteric fistula
Uremia	Saline volume expansion
Ketoacidosis	Endocrinopathies
Paraldehyde	Diarrhea
Lactic acidosis	Carbonic anhydrase inhibition
Ethylene glycol	Acid-chloride administration
Salicylates	Renal tubular acidosis
	Mineralocorticoid antagonists

bolic products of exogenous toxins (i.e., paraldehyde, methanol, ethylene glycol).
  b. The accumulation of these unmeasured acid anions should be stoichiometrically equal to the observed decrease in $[HCO_3]$.
  c. This equality will be preserved when the normal difference is maintained. Thus, if a normal anion gap = $12\,mEq/L$, and a normal $[HCO_3] = 25\,mEq/L$, in a pure high AG metabolic acidosis:

$$[Na^+] - ([Cl^-] + 25) = 12; \quad or$$
$$[Na^+] - ([Cl^-]) = 37 \pm 3.$$

  If $([Na^+] - [Cl^-])$ is significantly >37, then a coexistent metabolic alkalosis should be suspected.
  If the difference is significantly <37, then a coexistent normal anion gap acidosis is probably present.
  d. The causes of metabolic acidosis with a normal anion gap are listed in Table 14.2. These so-called hyperchloremic acidoses occur either due to the administration of exogenous acids whose anion is chloride (e.g., HCl, NH_4Cl, $CaCl_2$) or the loss of a body fluid that is relatively low in chloride but high in bicarbonate or its metabolic equivalent.
    (1) In cases of normal AG metabolic acidosis, measurement of the urinary AG can be diagnostically useful. It is calculated as

$$AG_U = U_{Na} + U_K - U_{Cl}$$

    The AG_U is inversely related to urinary ammonium (NH_4) excretion. Its value should be less than zero in acidotic patients with gastrointestinal (GI) bicarbonate losses, since renal ammoniagenesis ought to be well preserved. In patients with acidosis due to urinary bicarbonate losses, especially if caused by renal tubular acidosis (RTA), the AG_U should be greater than zero.
6. The primary therapy of metabolic acidosis is to treat the underlying disease.
7. The use of exogenous $NaHCO_3$ in the therapy of metabolic acidosis (especially lactic acidosis) is somewhat controversial, since evidence exists that such treatment can actually accelerate lactate production. However, it is generally accepted that severe acidemia (pH < 7.20) of metabolic origin should be corrected with $NaHCO_3$. The amount of bicarbonate required can be calculated by

HCO_3 deficit
$$= \text{body wt(kg)} \times 0.5 \times (\text{target} - \text{actual } [HCO_3])$$

  a. Administration of $NaHCO_3$ as an isotonic solution (i.e., 3 ampules of $NaHCO_3$ per liter of sterile water or 5% dextrose in water) will reduce the risk of hypernatremia in patients at particular risk.

8. Dialysis is sometimes indicated not only for the correction of acidosis but also for the rapid elimination of certain toxins that cause acidosis, such as methanol and ethylene glycol, even if the serum urea nitrogen (BUN) and creatinine are normal.

9. Treatment of chronic metabolic acidosis, especially if caused by RTA, includes oral alkali replacement as well as therapy of any associated electrolyte abnormalities.

C. Respiratory Acidosis

1. The clinical effects of respiratory acidosis include findings compatible with intracellular acidosis in addition to syndromes caused by abnormal pulmonary gas exchange. Of these, the most important is hypoxemic encephalopathy. Signs of chronic pulmonary disease, including cor pulmonale, may be present.

2. Some common causes of respiratory acidosis are listed in Table 14.3.

3. Chronic respiratory acidosis is seldom associated with severe acidemia (pH < 7.20) even if marked hypercapnia (PCO_2 > 100 mm Hg) is present. A superimposed acute metabolic or respiratory acidosis should be suspected if arterial pH is outside of this expected range.

4. The most important aspect of treatment of acute respiratory acidosis is the immediate restoration of effective alveolar gas exchange.

  a. This usually requires mechanical ventilation.
  b. If intubation is not immediately available, supplemental oxygen and $NaHCO_3$ should be cautiously administered.

5. Treatment of chronic respiratory acidosis depends mainly on the prevention and prompt recognition and therapy of intercurrent complications such as infections and congestive heart failure.

D. Metabolic Alkalosis

1. The clinical features of metabolic alkalosis are nonspecific.

  a. Evidence of neuromuscular irritability or latent tetany may be present.
  b. Cardiac dysrhythmias can occur.

2. Hypokalemia and hypochloremia are usually present.

3. The plasma AG is frequently elevated, due partly to a slight increase in lactate levels but mainly due to release

Table 14.3. Causes of Respiratory Acidosis

Central Nervous System Disorders
  Drugs (narcotics, anesthetics, tranquilizers)
  Brain stem injury
  Primary hypoventilation

Peripheral Nervous System Disorders
  Infectious diseases (botulism, tetanus, polio)
  Amyotrophic lateral sclerosis
  Guillain-Barré syndrome
  Spinal cord/phrenic nerve injury
  Organophosphates

Primary Muscular Disease
  Muscular dystrophy
  Myasthenia gravis
  Severe hypokalemia

Pulmonary Disease
  Chronic obstructive lung disease
  Pneumonia
  Pulmonary edema
  Smoke inhalation
  Pulmonary embolism

Thoracic/Upper Airway Disorders
  Chest wall (flail chest, pneumothorax, kyphoscoliosis)
  Airway Obstruction (laryngospasm, foreign body)

Failure of Mechanical Ventilator

of H^+ ions from plasma proteins (especially albumin) as part of the buffering process.
4. Urine pH measurements are not helpful.
5. The most useful biochemical determination is the level of urinary chloride (U_{Cl}), which forms the basis for classification of metabolic alkalosis.
    a. Metabolic alkalosis associated with a $U_{Cl} < 10\,mEq/L$ are termed *chloride responsive*, whereas those with a $U_{Cl} > 20\,mEq/L$ are termed *chloride resistant.*
    b. In some cases, U_{Cl} falls between these levels, in which case, no definite classification is possible.
6. Causes of metabolic alkalosis are listed in Table 14.4.
7. Since the kidney can ordinarily excrete a vast amount of HCO_3, acid loss (or base accumulation) alone does not usually result in a sustained alkalosis.
    a. If coexistent volume depletion is present, alkalosis can be persistent. This is by far the most common pathogenesis for metabolic alkalosis. This combination occurs when body fluids rich in NaCl and poor

Table 14.4. Causes of Metabolic Alkalosis

Chloride Responsive
  Gastrointestinal disorders
    Gastric: vomiting, nasogastric suction
    Colonic: villous adenoma, chloride diarrhea
  Renal disorders
    Diuretic therapy
    Posthypercapnic alkalosis
  Cystic fibrosis

Chloride Resistant
  Hypermineralocorticoid states
  Severe potassium depletion
  Bartter's syndrome

Miscellaneous
  Alkali administration (antacids, transfusions)
  Hypercalcemia
  Poorly absorbable anion administration (antibiotics)

    in $NaHCO_3$ are lost, usually from the intestinal tract
    or kidneys. Rarely, other sites of NaCl loss (e.g., skin
    losses in cystic fibrosis) may be present.

b. Extracellular fluid volume contraction causes avid
    NaCl and $NaHCO_3$ reabsorption in all nephron sites
    with attendant decreases in U_{Cl} and perpetuation of
    the alkalosis.

c. Hypokalemia occurs due to intracellular K^+ shifts and
    mineralocorticoid-induced urinary K^+ losses.

d. Much less commonly, metabolic alkalosis occurs in
    the absence of significant volume depletion. This sit-
    uation is most often associated with hypermineralo-
    corticoidism as a primary feature. The excessive
    mineralocorticoid activity can be either endogenous
    (e.g., Conn's syndrome, Cushing's syndrome) or
    exogenous (e.g., licorice, chewing tobacco). In
    these cases, excessive renal reabsorption of $NaHCO_3$
    and NaCl occurs in the absence of significant chlo-
    ride deficits. Therefore, U_{Cl} levels remain relatively
    high.

e. Severe total body potassium deficits exceeding
    1000 mEq may result in the inability to correct meta-
    bolic alkalosis but probably does not cause the dis-
    order in humans. Metabolic alkalosis with high U_{Cl}
    occurs in Bartter's syndrome, which is characterized
    by renal wasting of K^+ and Cl^-, normal blood pres-
    sure, and partial response to prostaglandin inhibition.

8. Some patients present with intermediate levels of chloride excretion (U_{Cl} 10 to 20 mEq/L). Many of these patients will be found to have excessive alkali administration, especially in the form of antacids or citrate anticoagulation of blood products.
9. The treatment of metabolic alkalosis depends on its cause.
   a. The underlying source of acid loss or base accumulation should be identified and corrected if possible.
   b. Administration of NaCl (and usually KCl as well) is mandatory in patients with chloride-responsive alkalosis.
   c. In some situations, urinary HCO_3 excretion can be hastened with the use of the carbonic anhydrase inhibitor acetazolamide. This may be of particular benefit in patients with diuretic-dependent congestive heart failure and associated alkalosis.
   d. In rare cases, infusion of HCl or NH_4Cl may be necessary.
      (1) This therapy requires an intensive care unit (ICU) setting and use of a central venous catheter.
      (2) It should be considered only in cases where the arterial pH exceeds 7.60.
      (3) The target pH for treatment with intravenous acid is 7.55.
      (4) The amount of acid required can be calculated by

      mEq HCl

      $$= \text{body wt(kg)} \times 0.5 \times (\text{actual} - \text{target } [HCO_3])$$

      (5) This solution should be infused over a period of 12 to 24 hours with frequent monitoring of blood chemistries and ABGs during therapy.
   e. In patients with severe alkalemia complicating acute or chronic renal failure, hemodialysis with an acid bath solution can be employed.

E. Respiratory Alkalosis
   1. Symptoms and signs of respiratory alkalosis include
      a. Neuromuscular irritability
      b. Cardiac dysrhythmias and electrocardiographic changes of ischemia
   2. Laboratory findings include
      a. Mild hyponatremia, hypokalemia, and hyperchloremia
   3. Some causes of respiratory alkalosis are listed in Table 14.5.
   4. Treatment of respiratory alkalosis depends on the cause.

Table 14.5. Causes of Respiratory Alkalosis

Iatrogenic (hemodialysis, mechanical ventilation)

Central Stimulation of Respiration
    Anxiety/pain
    Trauma
    Infections (meningitis, encephalitis)
    Intracranial tumors
    Cerebrovascular accidents
    Drugs (salicylates, exogenous catecholamines)
    Miscellaneous (fever, cirrhosis)

Hypoxemic Stimulation of Respiration
    Pneumonia
    Volume overload/pulmonary edema
    Pulmonary emboli
    Decreased lung compliance
    High altitude
    Carbon monoxide intoxication

        a. Supplemental O_2 is beneficial in hypoxemic patients.
        b. Rebreathing techniques are effective in patients with hyperventilation due to anxiety.
            (1) Patients with respiratory alkalosis due to underlying central nervous system (CNS) disease may require a period of intubation with paralysis and mechanical ventilation if the primary process is not directly treatable.
        c. Drug-induced hyperventilation can sometimes be treated with dialysis and other measures designed to accelerate drug elimination.

■ II. ACUTE RENAL FAILURE

Acute renal failure (ARF) is defined as a relatively sudden (over hours to days) decrease in renal function leading to serious derangements of body fluid homeostasis. It is usually classified as being due to prerenal, postrenal, or intrinsic renal disorders. Prerenal ARF is caused by renal perfusion defects. Postrenal ARF is caused by obstruction of the urinary tract. Intrinsic ARF is due to parenchymal disease of the kidneys.

    A. Prerenal ARF
        1. The causes of prerenal ARF are listed in Table 14.6.
            a. Prerenal ARF also occurs in situations characterized by renal hypoperfusion despite adequate or even

Table 14.6. Causes of Prerenal ARF

Absolute ECF Volume Depletion
  Extrarenal volume losses
    GI losses
    Third-space losses
    Inadequate fluid intake
    Hemorrhage
  Renal volume losses (diuretics)

Relative ECF Volume Depletion
  Congestive heart failure
  Decreased peripheral vascular resistance

Changes in Renal Vascular Tone
  Nonsteroidal anti-inflammatory drugs
  Angiotensin-converting enzyme inhibitors
  Hepatorenal syndrome

Abbreviation: ECF, extracellular fluid.

expanded extracellular fluid (ECF) volume. This is due to global or local abnormalities in circulation leading to renal insufficiency. Frequent examples include congestive heart failure and decreased peripheral vascular resistance as may accompany the sepsis.

  b. Renal blood flow may be selectively impaired by certain drugs (especially nonsteroidal anti-inflammatory drugs [NSAIDs] and angiotensin inhibitors) or in the hepatorenal syndrome.

  c. Whenever renal blood flow is severely curtailed, ischemic acute renal failure is a possibility.

2. The diagnosis of prerenal ARF can often be made on clinical grounds.

  a. The history and physical examination are crucial.

  b. Assessment of serial weights and intake/output records are valuable if available.

  c. Oliguria is a customary finding.

  d. The urinalysis reveals urinary concentration (specific gravity >1.020) but is typically otherwise benign.

  e. A ratio of BUN/creatinine >20:1 is suggestive *but not diagnostic* of prerenal ARF.

  f. The most helpful feature is evidence of avid sodium reabsorption in an oliguric patient.

    (1) Sodium avidity can be assessed by determining the fractional excretion of sodium (FE_{Na}), calculated as

Table 14.7. Causes of Postrenal ARF

Urethral Obstruction
  Urethral valves
  Prostatic hypertrophy

Bladder Obstruction
  Neurogenic bladder
  Bladder tumors
  Cystitis

Ureteral Obstruction

Intrinsic
  Ureteral stones
  Papillary necrosis

Extrinsic
  Tumors
  Retroperitoneal fibrosis
  Aortic aneurysm
  Pregnancy

$$FE_{Na} = (U_{Na} \times P_{creat})/(P_{Na} \times U_{creat}) \times 100$$

    (2) Values <1% suggest prerenal azotemia in the appropriate clinical setting.
  g. In occasional cases when doubt remains, measurement of central venous pressure or pulmonary capillary wedge pressure may be useful in guiding therapy.
  3. Treatment of prerenal ARF depends on correction of the underlying cause and replacement of any volume deficits.
    a. The cause of fluid losses should be identified and treated if possible.
    b. Left ventricular function should be maximized if congestive heart failure (CHF) is playing a role.
    c. Offending drugs should be discontinued.
    d. Hepatic transplantation may restore renal function to normal in patients with hepatorenal syndrome.
    e. In addition to treatment of the underlying disease, volume expansion with appropriate intravenous fluids (usually normal saline or blood products) is required in patients unable to ingest sufficient sodium and water.

B. Postrenal ARF
  1. Some causes of postrenal ARF are listed in Table 14.7.
  2. The diagnosis of postrenal ARF can be suspected on history and physical examination.

       a. Alternating polyuria and oligoanuria is suggestive of subtotal urinary obstruction, as is a very large postvoiding residual urine volume.

3. Laboratory tests are usually nonspecific.

       a. The urinalysis may be normal or disclose evidence of hematuria, pyuria, or crystalluria.

       b. The best screening test for obstruction is renal ultrasound, which has a specificity of >90%.

       c. In cases in which obstruction is still suspected despite a negative ultrasound, retrograde pyelography can be performed.

4. Therapy of postrenal ARF largely depends on the site of obstruction.

       a. The coexistence of obstruction and urinary tract infection is a urologic emergency mandating broad-spectrum antibiotic coverage and immediate decompression of the urinary tract.

           (1) Upper tract disease can be effectively approached with indwelling stents or percutaneous nephrostomy.

           (2) Lower urinary obstruction can be relieved with urethral or suprapubic catheterization.

       b. After the patient's medical condition has stabilized, it is often possible to undertake definitive repair of the obstructing lesion. Relief of even long-standing obstruction is generally indicated, since some functional recovery may occur, even weeks or months later.

C. Intrinsic ARF

1. Some causes of intrinsic ARF are listed in Table 14.8.

2. Acute tubular necrosis (ATN) is by far the most common cause of intrinsic ARF among hospitalized patients.

       a. Multiple drugs and toxins can cause ATN, including aminoglycoside antibiotics, certain chemotherapeutic agents (i.e., cis-platinum, mithramycin), and radiographic contrast materials.

       b. Ischemia is another major factor causing ATN.

       c. ATN is especially common in patients with major trauma, recent major surgery (particularly vascular operations), sepsis, or crush injury.

3. Acute interstitial nephritis (AIN) is usually caused by exposure to a drug or allergen. Rare idiopathic cases are encountered.

       a. Probably the most common drugs causing AIN are NSAIDs.

Table 14.8. Causes of Intrinsic ARF

Glomerular Diseases
  Acute glomerulonephritis
  Rapidly progressive glomerulonephritis

Tubulointerstitial Diseases
  Acute tubular necrosis
    Drug-induced
    Ischemic
  Acute interstitial nephritis
    Allergic/drug induced
    Idiopathic

Vascular Diseases
  Renal artery
    Thrombosis/embolus
    Dissection
    Trauma
  Renal microcirculation
    Vasculitis
    Malignant hypertension
    Disseminated intravascular coagulation (DIC)
    Thrombotic Thrombocytopenic purpura (TTP)
    Cholesterol atheroemboli
  Renal vein thrombosis

     b. Other frequent agents include antibiotics (particularly penicillins, cephalosporins, and sulfa derivatives), loop and thiazide diuretics, and cimetidine.
     c. Recognition of this entity is especially important, since effective therapy depends on withdrawal of the offending drug.
  4. The diagnosis of intrinsic ARF depends heavily on the history and physical examination with subsequent directed laboratory and radiographic evaluation.
     a. Medications in particular should be carefully reviewed.
     b. The urine sediment should be examined; it is valuable to note that intrinsic ARF is almost invariably accompanied by abnormalities on urinalysis, and their absence should raise the suspicion of pre- or postrenal causes.
     c. The presence of urinary eosinophils can be used to support a diagnosis of AIN or cholesterol microemboli.
     d. The FE_{Na} is typically >3% in intrinsic ARF.
     e. Serologic evaluation of patients with suspected vasculitis should include antinuclear antibodies

(ANA), complements, hepatitis B surface antigen, cryoglobulins, and rheumatoid factor.

  f. More invasive studies (e.g., angiography, renal biopsy) may be appropriate depending on the clinical circumstances.

 5. Therapy of intrinsic ARF is largely supportive.

  a. Offending drugs should be identified and withdrawn or substituted if possible.

  b. Control of fluid and electrolyte balance, modification of drug dosages, and dialysis should be entertained.

  c. Specific therapy directed at a particular disease process is possible in occasional circumstances. A major aspect of the management of ARF is a recognition of the situations in which it is likely to occur with appropriate measures to reduce its probability.

   (1) Medications with the least risk of nephrotoxicity should be chosen in patients liable to ARF.

   (2) Volume depletion should be avoided or corrected.

   (3) Calcium channel blockers may be helpful in ameliorating ARF if given prophylactically (i.e., before angiography or renovascular surgery).

 6. Despite many advances in the diagnosis and treatment of ARF, mortality remains at least 50% in critically ill patients.

■ III. ELECTROLYTE ABNORMALITIES

Certain electrolyte abnormalities that occur frequently pose a serious risk to ICU patients, even if the disorder has been present for a long time.

 A. Calcium

  Calcium exists in three forms in the circulation: free ionized calcium (iCa^{++}); in soluble complexes with phosphate, citrate, and bicarbonate; and bound to plasma proteins (principally albumin). Of these, the iCa^{++} is physiologically most important. The normal value for iCa^{++} is 4.0 to 4.9 mg/dL, 2.4 to 2.6 mEq/L, or 1.2 to 1.3 mmol/L (note difference in units).

  Maintenance of normal iCa^{++} levels depends on the interaction between GI absorption, bone fluxes, and renal excretion, governed by parathyroid hormone (PTH), 1,25-dihydroxyvitamin D ($1,25\text{-}D_3$), and calcitonin.

1. Hypercalcemia
   a. Most patients with hypercalcemia are asymptomatic at the time of diagnosis. However, numerous signs and symptoms may occur depending on the severity and rate of development of hypercalcemia. These include
      (1) Nausea
      (2) Constipation
      (3) Anorexia
      (4) Pancreatitis
      (5) Peptic ulcers
      (6) Renal insufficiency
      (7) Polyuria
      (8) Urolithiasis
      (9) Bone pain
      (10) Weakness
      (11) Confusion and coma
   b. Symptomatic patients require urgent treatment.
   c. Some causes of hypercalcemia are listed in Table 14.9.
   d. Hypercalcemia is a medical emergency whose acute treatment is largely independent of the cause.
   e. Therapy is outlined in Table 14.10.
      (1) Intravenous (IV) normal saline should be administered at a rate of 150 to 250 mL/h.
      (2) Furosemide is indicated to prevent volume overload and to decrease calcium reabsorption (a minor effect).
      (3) Calcitonin's effectiveness is limited by the phenomenon of osteoclast escape, which develops within a few days of beginning treatment.
      (4) Diphosphonates such as etidronate will reduce calcium levels to normal within 5 days in 75% of patients.

Table 14.9. Disorders of Calcium Homeostasis

Hypercalcemia	Hypocalcemia
Hyperparathyroidism	Hypoparathyroidism
Hyperthyroidism	Pseudohypoparathyroidism
Acute renal failure	Vitamin D deficiency
Malignancy	Malignancy
Excessive Vitamin A or D	Hyperphosphatemia
Granulomatous diseases	Pancreatitis
Thiazide diuretics	Neonatal tetany
Immobilization	Calcium complex formation

Table 14.10. Treatment of Hypercalcemia

IV Fluids: Normal saline 150–250 mL/h
(± furosemide 40–80 mg IV q4–6 h)
Corticosteroids: Prednisone (or equivalent) 1 mg/kg/d
Calcitonin: 4 U/kg SQ q12 h
Etidronate: 7.5 mg/kg/d IV q day × 1–4 days
Mithramycin: 25 μg/kg IV q day × 3–4 days
Indomethacin: 25–50 mg PO q8 h
Dialysis

      (5) Mithramycin is the most potent hypocalcemic agent available, but its use is limited by serious renal, hepatic, and bone marrow side effects.

      (6) In hypercalcemia patients, oral NSAIDs are indicated only in patients with prostaglandin-mediated hypercalcemia.

      (7) Dialysis with low calcium dialysate may be necessary in patients with refractory hypercalcemia, particularly if renal function is impaired.

  2. Hypocalcemia

    a. The clinical manifestations of hypocalcemia are usually related to effects on excitable tissues.

      (1) Neurologic findings include overt or latent tetany and mental status changes.

      (2) Cardiovascular manifestations include dysrhythmias, hypotension, and decreased myocardial contractility.

    b. Some causes of hypocalcemia are listed in Table 14.9.

    c. Hypoalbuminemia can cause a lowering of the total calcium but normal iCa^{++}.

    d. Treatment of hypocalcemia is summarized in Table 14.11.

      (1) Patients with latent or overt tetany require immediate parenteral replacement. IV calcium should be administered through a central catheter if possible to avoid the risk of extravasation and skin necrosis.

      (2) Correction of aggravating electrolyte abnormalities (hyperphosphatemia, hypomagnesemia) should take place simultaneously.

Table 14.11. Treatment of Hypocalcemia

Calcium Bolus: 10–30 mL 10% Ca-gluconate or $CaCl_2$ slow IV push over 15–30 min

Calcium Infusion: 40 mL 10% Ca-gluconate in 500 mL D_5W IV at 20 mL/h, titrate to desired iCa^{++}

Hyperphosphatemia: $CaCO_3$ 650 mg 1–3 tabs PO tid with meals $Al(OH)_3$ gels 30–60 mL PO tid with meals

Hypomagnesemia: 2 mL 50% $MgSO_4$ IV or IM q4–6 h

Oral Calcium: $CaCO_3$, Ca-acetate, or Ca-lactate 1–3 tabs qid on an empty stomach

Vitamin D: Calcitriol 0.25–0.5 µg q12–24 h

---

   (3) Oral calcium and vitamin D supplements are satisfactory for milder, asymptomatic cases.

B. Magnesium

Magnesium is the second most common intracellular cation (after potassium). Most of its biologic effects depend on its role as a cofactor for intracellular enzymes, particularly adenosine triphosphate (ATP)-dependent systems. Magnesium balance is determined by the relationship between dietary ingestion and renal excretion. Urinary magnesium excretion is increased by sodium and calcium loading, diuretics, and PTH. It is decreased by volume depletion.

1. Hypomagnesemia

 a. Since most magnesium is intracellular, it can be difficult to estimate the magnitude of magnesium depletion from serum levels. However, hypomagnesemia and simultaneous hypomagnesiuria ($U_{Mg} < 1$ mEq/d) strongly suggest depleted body stores.

 b. Symptoms of hypomagnesemia include weakness, anorexia, and nausea. Some physical signs are latent tetany, hyperreflexia, tremors, dysrhythmias, delirium, and coma.

 c. Important associated laboratory abnormalities include hypokalemia and hypocalcemia that may be refractory to treatment until magnesium stores are repleted.

 d. Some common causes of hypomagnesemia are listed in Table 14.12.

  (1) Gastrointestinal causes include steatorrheic malabsorption, pancreatitis, dietary deficiency, and prolonged diarrhea or vomiting.

Table 14.12. Disorders of Magnesium Homeostasis

Hypomagnesemia	Hypermagnesemia
GI disorders	Renal failure
Endocrinopathies	Massive Mg ingestion
Renal Mg losses	
Alcoholism	

      (2) Several endocrinopathies, including diabetes mellitus, hyperparathyroidism, primary hyperaldosteronism, and hyperthyroidism can lead to hypomagnesemia.

      (3) Excessive renal magnesium losses can occur in patients with congenital magnesium wasting, ketoacidosis, Bartter's syndrome, hyperaldosteronism, and the syndrome of inappropriate antidiuretic hormone secretion (SIADH).

      (4) Multiple drugs cause renal magnesium loss, including diuretics (except acetazolamide), cis-platinum, and cyclosporine.

      (5) Hypomagnesemia associated with alcoholism has been attributed to urinary magnesium losses, decreased dietary intake, and alcoholic or starvation ketoacidosis.

  e. Many cases of hypomagnesemia can be prevented and treated by the inclusion of magnesium supplements in patients receiving parenteral nutrition and treatment for diabetic ketoacidosis.

      (1) Mild cases of magnesium depletion ($[Mg^{++}]$ 1.3 to 1.6 mg/dL) can be corrected by intake of a high-magnesium diet. Food sources of magnesium include meats and green vegetables.

  f. Pharmacologic replacement is indicated in more severe cases.

      (1) Oral supplementation can be provided with MgO 400 to 3200 mg/d. Diarrhea is a potential side effect of this treatment.

      (2) Parenteral therapy with 1 to 2 g (2 to 4 mL) of 50% $MgSO_4$ repeated q4–6h as needed is sufficient therapy for most patients.

      (3) Serum magnesium levels and deep tendon reflexes must be monitored closely during treatment, since life-threatening hypermagnesemia can occur.

2. Hypermagnesemia
   a. The clinical features of magnesium excess are frequently confused with those of hypercalcemia. They include
      (1) Nausea
      (2) Altered mental status
      (3) Weakness and diminished tendon reflexes
      (4) Hypotension
      (5) Dysrhythmias
      (6) Respiratory paralysis
   b. The most frequent condition predisposing patients to hypermagnesemia is chronic renal failure. Sustained hypermagnesemia only occurs in the setting of renal insufficiency, although acute magnesium excess can occur in the setting of overzealous replacement of magnesium deficiency.
   c. Therapy of hypermagnesemia involves discontinuing magnesium intake, infusion of Ca-gluconate 15 mg/kg over 4 hours (which acts as a direct magnesium antagonist), and dialysis with a magnesium-free bath in severe cases.

C. Phosphate

Phosphate is an abundant intracellular anion, critically important in energy metabolism and structural integrity of literally all cells. The overwhelming majority of dietary phosphate is normally absorbed, but a significant amount (approximately 200 mg/d) is secreted in the stool. Renal excretion eliminates the remainder, about 400 to 1500 mg/d depending on intake. Urinary phosphorus excretion is increased by PTH, volume expansion, corticosteroids, and calcitonin and is decreased by insulin, thyroid hormone, and vitamin D. Movement of phosphate into cells is enhanced during alkalemia, by glucose and some other carbohydrates, and by hormones including insulin, epinephrine, and corticosteroids.

1. Hypophosphatemia
   a. Hypophosphatemia is characterized by altered mental status, weakness or myopathy progressing to rhabdomyolysis, osteomalacia, dysfunction of all blood cell types, anorexia, respiratory failure, and decreased cardiac contractility. However, most cases of phosphate depletion are asymptomatic unless severe.
   b. Some causes of hypophosphatemia are listed in Table 14.13.
      (1) Respiratory and metabolic alkalosis are associated with intracellular uptake of phosphate.

Table 14.13. Disorders of Phosphate Homeostasis

Hypophosphatemia	Hyperphosphatemia
Intracellular shifts	Massive cell lysis
Inadequate ingestion	Increased ingestion
GI losses	Renal failure
Renal losses	

    (2) Refeeding after prolonged starvation precipitates hypophosphatemia largely due to intracellular shifts mediated by glucose and insulin.

    (3) Administration or excessive activity of other hormones (epinephrine, growth hormone, steroids, gastrin, and glucagon) can cause hypophosphatemia by similar mechanisms.

    (4) Malnutrition alone does not typically cause severe hypophosphatemia. However, GI losses due to malabsorption of phosphate or use of phosphorus-binding antacids can lead to marked phosphate depletion.

    (5) Excessive renal losses of phosphate are present in Fanconi's syndrome, after renal transplantation in some patients, following recovery from urinary obstruction or ATN, and with vitamin D-resistant rickets.

  c. The best treatment of hypophosphatemia is often prevention.

    (1) Phosphate deficiency can be avoided by preventive supplementation in patients with malnutrition undergoing hyperalimentation or refeeding, or who are chronic alcoholics, on long-term antacids, or who have uncontrolled diabetes mellitus or ketoacidosis.

    (2) Treatment of established hypophosphatemia depends on its severity and cause.

      (a) Patients with mild hypophosphatemia due to intracellular shifts can be followed closely without active intervention unless the serum phosphorus drops <1.5 mg/dL.

      (b) Dietary supplementation in the form of increased intake of dairy products is adequate in most asymptomatic patients.

      (c) Oral supplementation can be provided with sodium and/or potassium phosphate, although diarrhea is often a dose-limiting side effect.

(d) Severe symptomatic hypophosphatemia is treated with elemental phosphorus (as sodium or potassium phosphate) 2 mg/kg IV q6h until oral repletion can begin, usually at a phosphorus level of 2.0 mg/dL.

(e) Use of parenteral phosphate is relatively contraindicated in patients with oliguric renal failure.

(f) Possible complications of IV phosphorus include dysrhythmias, hyperphosphatemia, hypocalcemia, hyperkalemia, and volume overload.

2. Hyperphosphatemia

a. Many of the symptoms of hyperphosphatemia can be attributed to the reciprocal fall in iCa^{++} that generally occurs (see above).

b. Severe hyperphosphatemia can also cause ARF, particularly in the setting of massive cell lysis. Metastatic calcifications caused by precipitation of $Ca-PO_4$ crystals in essentially any tissue or organ can lead to widespread symptoms and signs.

c. The causes of hyperphosphatemia are summarized in Table 14.13.

d. Treatment of hyperphosphatemia involves decreasing ingestion with phosphorus-restricted diets as well as increasing elimination via the GI tract and kidneys.

(1) Phosphate binders containing magnesium, calcium, or aluminum will accelerate stool phosphorus losses even in patients who are NPO.

(2) Magnesium-containing agents should be avoided in patients with renal failure.

(3) Renal excretion of phosphate is enhanced by acetazolamide, volume expansion, and alkaline diuresis. Unfortunately, the frequent coexistence of renal failure with hyperphosphatemia often makes this route unreliable.

(4) Hemodialysis or peritoneal dialysis is effective for acute or chronic hyperphosphatemia.

D. Potassium

Potassium is the most abundant intracellular cation. Only about 2% of total body potassium is in the ECF. Intracellular

Table 14.14. Factors Affecting Cellular Potassium Distribution

Increasing K^+	Decreasing K^+
Alkalosis	
Insulin	Acidosis
Beta$_2$-agonists	Glucagon
	Alpha-agonists
	Hyperosmolarity

Table 14.15. Disorders of Potassium Homeostasis

Hypokalemia	Hyperkalemia
Pseudohypokalemia	
Cellular K^+ uptake	Pseudohyperkalemia
Poor dietary K^+ intake	Cellular K^+ loss
GI losses	Excessive K^+ intake
Renal losses	Inadequate renal excretion
	Cell lysis

potassium is responsible for maintaining cell volume and resting membrane potential. A number of factors regulate potassium movement into cells. These are summarized in Table 14.14.

1. Hypokalemia
   a. Abnormally low ECF [K^+] can have widespread pathophysiologic effects. Dominant among these are neuromuscular and cardiac events.
      (1) Neuromuscular problems include GI hypomotility, skeletal muscle weakness or paralysis, and rhabdomyolysis.
      (2) Cardiac manifestations include the appearance of a U wave on the electrocardiogram, ventricular and atrial dysrhythmias, predisposition to digoxin toxicity, and cardiac necrosis.
      (3) Cellular metabolism and renal function can also be impaired.
   b. The causes of hypokalemia are listed in Table 14.15.
      (1) Pseudohypokalemia reflects in vitro potassium uptake by leukemic cells in patients with severe leukocytosis (white blood cell [WBC] counts >10^5/mm^3).
      (2) Intracellular shifts of potassium occur in alkalosis, insulin overdose, use of beta$_2$-agonists, hypokalemic periodic paralysis, and barium poisoning.

   (3) Patients with anorexia nervosa, alcoholism, or severe dietary restrictions may develop significant hypokalemia.

   (4) Excessive GI potassium losses occur in patients with protracted vomiting, diarrhea, and laxative abuse.

   (5) Renal losses occur in patients with renal tubular acidosis, hyperaldosteronism, treatment of diabetic ketoacidosis, hypomagnesemia, and metabolic alkalosis. In addition, numerous drugs cause renal potassium wasting including diuretics and antibiotics (penicillins, cephalosporins, aminoglycosides, amphotericin).

c. Treatment of hypokalemia is imprecise, since the degree of total body K^+ depletion is usually impossible to calculate.

   (1) Ongoing potassium losses should be halted if possible, and aggravating abnormalities (alkalosis, hypomagnesemia) corrected.

   (2) The particular potassium salt employed depends on the specific clinical problem. KCl is preferred in patients with concomitant metabolic alkalosis and is effective in all forms of hypokalemia. Bicarbonate or phosphate salts of potassium may be preferred if acidosis or hypophosphatemia is present.

   (3) Oral potassium preparations are effective but can have an unpalatable taste and cause GI irritation.

   (4) Potassium can be given by slow IV infusion (10 to 20 mEq/h) through a central or peripheral line; concentrations above 40 mEq/L should be avoided in peripheral IVs to decrease the risk of phlebitis.

   (5) Frequent monitoring of serum $[K^+]$ is essential during parenteral potassium repletion.

   (6) Potassium-sparing diuretics are occasionally useful but should be used with caution in patients receiving potassium supplements.

2. Hyperkalemia

   a. The principal clinical abnormalities of hyperkalemia are neuromuscular and cardiac. Weakness, paresthesias, and paralysis can occur but are usually overshadowed by cardiac disturbances. These include

    (1) Progressive electrocardiogram (ECG) appearance of peaked T waves.
    (2) Flattened P waves.
    (3) Prolonged PR interval.
    (4) Widening of the QRS complex.
    (5) The development of a sine wave pattern presages the onset of ventricular fibrillation or asystole.

  b. Some causes of hyperkalemia are presented in Table 14.15.

    (1) Pseudohyperkalemia is due to in vitro release of potassium from red blood cells, leukocytes, or platelets.
    (2) Release of potassium from cells contributes to hyperkalemia in acidosis, poorly controlled diabetes mellitus, beta-blockade, hyperkalemic periodic paralysis, hyperosmolar states, and digitalis toxicity.
    (3) Potassium ingestion seldom results in hyperkalemia if renal function is normal except when excessive parenteral potassium supplements have been administered.
    (4) Inadequate renal excretion occurs in patients with advanced renal failure, deficiencies of adrenal hormones, and numerous drugs. These include potassium-sparing diuretics, NSAIDs, angiotensin-converting enzyme inhibitors, and cyclosporine.
    (5) Severe hyperkalemia is a frequent finding in patients with massive in vivo hemolysis or tumor lysis syndrome.

  c. The treatment of hyperkalemia is outlined in Table 14.16.

Table 14.16. Therapy of Hyperkalemia

10% Calcium gluconate: 10–30 mL IV   Onset <5 min
50% dextrose 50 mL + regular insulin 5 U IV q30 min   Onset 15–30 min
$NaHCO_3$ 50 mL (50 mEq) IV q30 min × 4 doses   Onset 15–30 min
Kayexalate in sorbitol 30–60 g PO/enema q4–6 h   Onset 1–2 h
Dialysis

(1) Calcium does not affect the serum potassium but rather antagonizes the cardiac toxicity of hyperkalemia.

(2) Glucose/insulin and bicarbonate infusions lower serum $[K^+]$ by stimulating cellular potassium entry.

(3) Kayexalate is used to augment fecal potassium excretion; it is relatively ineffective unless the patient develops diarrhea or loose stools.

(4) Dialysis is extremely effective for life-threatening hyperkalemia.

(5) Diuretics and aldosterone analogues are occasionally useful adjunctive measures.

(6) The use of beta-adrenergic agents (i.e., albuterol) via nebulizations has received considerable attention in recent years for the acute management of hyperkalemia in endstage renal disease patients.

E. Sodium

Hyponatremia and hypernatremia are disorders of water balance. The osmolarity of a solution depends on the number of dissolved particles per liter. In clinical practice, this can be measured, or calculated, as follows:

$$P_{osm} = 2 \times [Na^+] + [glucose]/18 + [BUN]/2.8$$

Solutes restricted to one side of the plasma membrane are termed *effective osmoles;* changes in the quantity of effective osmoles in a body fluid obligate transmembrane water movement to maintain balance. Freely membrane-permeable substances such as urea do not cause water movement and are hence termed *ineffective osmoles*. The tonicity, or effective osmolarity, of a solution can be calculated by the following:

$$E_{osm} = 2 \times [Na^+] + [glucose]/18$$

Regulation of plasma osmolarity depends on the interplay between water ingestion and renal water excretion. Renal mechanisms of water balance require the adequate delivery of salt and water to distal nephron sites as well as manipulation of tubular water permeability under the influence of antidiuretic hormone (ADH). ADH is secreted by the posterior pituitary in response to hypertonicity as well as other nonosmotic stimuli, including hypovolemia, nausea, pain, and several drugs (i.e., nicotine, narcotics, vincristine, cyclophosphamide, chlorpropamide, and clofibrate). ADH increases renal water permeability, leading to increased water reabsorption and hypertonic urine. Normal thirst is even more responsive to changes in osmolarity than ADH is; consequently, thirst should be considered the primary guardian of plasma tonicity.

1. Hyponatremia

   a. Symptoms of hyponatremia are caused by osmotic movement of water from the ECF into cells.

      (1) Conditions characterized by hyponatremia with normal or elevated osmolarity (due to accumulation of unmeasured osmotically active solutes) are not symptomatic.

      (2) Brain cells are most sensitive to changes in volume; hence, most symptoms of hyponatremia are neurologic. They include nausea, neuromuscular irritability, altered mental status, and seizures.

      (3) The likelihood of symptomatic hyponatremia depends on its severity and the rapidity with which it develops.

   b. Some causes of hyponatremia are listed in Table 14.17.

      (1) Pseudohyponatremia is defined as a low measured serum sodium despite a normal or elevated plasma osmolarity. Causes include hyperlipidemia, hyperproteinemia, hyperglycemia, mannitol infusion, and radiographic contrast agents. Measurement of plasma osmolarity before initiation of therapy

Table 14.17. Causes of Hyponatremia

Pseudohyponatremia

Pure water intoxication

Hyponatremia with appropriate ADH secretion
  Hypovolemia
  Congestive heart failure
  Endocrinopathies
  Renal disease
  Cirrhosis

Syndrome of inappropriate antidiuretic hormone secretion
  Idiopathic
  Drug-induced
  Pulmonary diseases
  CNS diseases
  Malignancy

Combination of factors
  Marathon runner syndrome (Varon-Ayus syndrome)

for hyponatremia is vital to exclude pseudo-hyponatremia.

(2) Hyponatremia due to pure water intoxication is extremely rare due to the efficiency with which the kidneys can excrete even massive water loads.

(3) Most cases of true hyponatremia are associated with elevated ADH activity that is provoked by some nonosmotic stimulus.

(4) Volume depletion of any cause is a major stimulus for ADH release. This includes states of relative volume depletion such as CHF.

(5) Hypothyroidism and adrenal insufficiency are also causes of hyponatremia.

(6) Many renal diseases including nephrotic syndrome predispose to hyponatremia due to inadequate delivery of solute to the distal nephron.

(7) Hyponatremia in untreated cirrhosis is caused by excessive ADH secretion and impaired distal sodium delivery.

(8) SIADH has multiple causes including drugs, pulmonary diseases, CNS diseases, and cancer. See also Chapter 4, "Endocrinologic Disorders."

(9) Hyponatremia in marathon runners (Varon-Ayus Syndrome).

c. Symptomatic hyponatremia is a medical emergency regardless of duration.

d. After the plasma osmolarity has been determined, therapy with 3% NaCl should be instituted. The amount of NaCl required to correct hyponatremia to a specified target level is

mEq NaCl
$$= 0.6 \times (\text{weight [kg]}) \times (\text{target Na}^+ - \text{plasma Na}^+)$$

The amount of 3% saline required to achieve this goal is

$$3\% \text{ NaCl (mL)} = (1000) \times (\text{mEq NaCl})/513$$

The target [Na$^+$] should be an increase of 20 mEq/L above the actual [Na$^+$] or 130 mEq/L, whichever is lower. The rate of correction is 1.0 to 1.5 mEq/L/h. These calculations often underestimate the actual rate of correction due to ongoing urinary sodium losses.

e. In addition to hypertonic saline infusion, all IV fluids including medications should be given in 0.9% NaCl, and a fluid restriction of 1000 to 1500 mL/d instituted if possible.

f. Demeclocycline 150 to 300 mg PO q12h has been used successfully in the treatment of SIADH but is contraindicated in cirrhosis.

g. *Central pontine myelinolysis* is a rare complication occurring after correction of chronic (but not acute) hyponatremia if the serum [Na⁺] is raised by >25 mEq/L during the first 48 hours of therapy.

2. Hypernatremia

a. Symptoms of hypernatremia are caused by cellular dehydration, particularly of neurons. They include altered mental status, nausea, seizures, and intracranial hemorrhage. Myoclonus, metabolic acidosis, and hyperglycemia due to peripheral insulin resistance are also common.

b. Most hypernatremic patients are volume depleted; the finding of volume overload should suggest the possibility of acute salt poisoning.

c. Causes of hypernatremia are listed in Table 14.18.

(1) Diabetes insipidus (DI) can be of central or nephrogenic origin (see Chapter 4, "Endocrinologic Disorders").

(2) The most common cause of hypernatremia is excessive water loss.

(a) Excessive renal water loss with hypernatremia has been reported in patients with renal failure, hypercalcemia, hypokalemia, sickle cell disease, osmotic diuresis, postobstructive diuresis, sickle cell disease, and drugs (including alcohol, lithium, demeclocycline, oral hypoglycemics, and others).

Table 14.18. Causes of Hypernatremia

Diabetes insipidus
H₂O losses
Renal
GI
Insensible
Salt poisoning
H₂O deprivation
Primary hypodipsia
Mineralocorticoid excess

    (b) GI water losses due to gastroenteritis are an especially common cause of hypernatremia in children.

    (c) Insensible water losses via the skin or respiratory tract occur with prolonged exposure to hot climates, thermal burns, and fever.

(3) Salt poisoning is a rare cause of outpatient hypernatremia but is more common in hospitalized patients as a complication of hypertonic $NaHCO_3$ therapy for severe acidosis.

(4) Water deprivation is a fundamental feature of practically all cases of hypernatremia but is rarely the sole cause of the problem.

(5) Entities characterized by increased mineralocorticoid activity (Conn's syndrome and Cushing's syndrome) are sometimes accompanied by mild-to-moderate hypernatremia.

d. The treatment of hypernatremia is replacement of free water deficits and correction of contributing electrolyte problems and hypovolemia if present.

(1) The water deficit is calculated as

H_2O deficit (L)

$= 0.6 \times$ weight (kg) $\times$

$[(\text{target Na}^+)/(\text{actual Na}^+) - 1]$

The target sodium is either 148 mEq/L or a decrease of 20 to 25 mEq/L in the plasma $[\text{Na}^+]$ from its initial value, whichever is higher. The goal of therapy is to reduce the plasma $[\text{Na}^+]$ by 1.0 to 1.5 mEq/L/h.

(2) Faster rates of correction of chronic hypernatremia may precipitate rehydration seizures.

(3) The choice of fluid and route of administration depend on the clinical circumstances. Distilled or tap water given PO or via nasogastric (NG) tube is preferred when feasible. If the enteral route is unavailable, 0.45% NaCl can be administered by peripheral vein without significant risk of hemolysis.

(4) Patients with clinical evidence of volume overload who cannot tolerate the sodium load of 0.45% NaCl should be given distilled water IV through a central catheter.

(5) D_5W is at least relatively contraindicated in many patients because of the coexistence of insulin resistance and the consequent risk of worsening hyperosmolarity due to unmetabolized dextrose.

(6) Diuretics or dialysis can be employed for patients with salt poisoning.

(7) Vasopressin analogues are useful in the long-term management of central DI.

■ IV. FLUID AND ELECTROLYTE THERAPY

In addition to the more specific treatments outlined above, some general guidelines regarding fluid and electrolyte therapy are useful. Administration of fluids and nutrition are essential but frequently overlooked considerations in the care of the ICU patient. Special care must be exercised in the selection and administration of IV fluids to the critically ill with ongoing renal or extrarenal fluid and electrolyte losses. IV fluids are potentially the most dangerous drugs used in the hospital; constant vigilance is required.

A. For essentially all ICU patients, some IV access is necessary.

B. Whenever possible, the GI tract should be employed for maintenance fluids, nutrition, and medications.

C. The type of fluid used depends on the clinical situation. Some general comments can be made:

1. For routine maintenance, crystalloid solutions are employed.

   a. In an otherwise well NPO patient, obligatory water losses amount to about 1000 mL/d.

   b. Sodium losses are minimized by virtually complete renal sodium reclamation, but some urinary potassium excretion continues (30 to 60 mEq/d) and must be replaced.

   c. Excessive protein catabolism and starvation ketosis can be prevented by inclusion of glucose 150 to 200 g daily in maintenance fluids.

   d. Supplements of other vitamins and minerals may be necessary if parenteral therapy lasts a week or more.

2. Colloid solutions such as blood products, albumin, and plasma are indicated for the rapid expansion of intravascular volume with minimal effects on other components of the ECF.

■ V. DIALYSIS

ICU patients frequently develop homeostatic abnormalities that cannot be managed conservatively. In such a case, dialysis or a related modality becomes necessary.

A. Dialysis is indicated in many different situations.
   1. Volume overload manifested by pulmonary edema or severe hypertension unresponsive to diuretics can be effectively treated with dialysis or ultrafiltration.
   2. Dialysis is useful for the treatment of several electrolyte abnormalities, including severe acidosis or alkalosis, hyperkalemia, hypo- or hypernatremia, hypercalcemia, hyperphosphatemia, and hypermagnesemia.
   3. Symptoms caused by accumulation of uremic toxins are best treated with dialysis.
   4. Poisonings with ethylene glycol, methanol, salicylates, and others can be effectively treated with dialysis.

B. The most frequently used dialysis modality in the ICU is hemodialysis (HD) or one of its variants. The choice between HD and peritoneal dialysis (PD) is usually a matter of the physician's preference, but in some cases a clear preference is evident.
   1. HD is the therapy of choice in severely catabolic patients due to more efficient removal of urea and other low molecular weight nitrogenous wastes.
      a. A large-bore dual-lumen central venous catheter is required for vascular access.
      b. For standard hemodialysis orders, the physician specifies the type of membrane to be used (more biocompatible membranes such as cellulose acetate are preferred in the ICU), the duration of therapy, blood flow speed, type of anticoagulation, composition of the dialysate with respect to Na^+, K^+, Ca^{++}, and HCO_3, the desired amount of fluid removal, and any additional medications or treatments required (e.g., blood products, antibiotics, or erythropoietin).
      c. The most common complication of HD is hypotension, generally treated with fluid boluses of normal saline or albumin. In some cases, alternate treatments must be considered if hypotension is severe. Other serious potential complications of dialysis include dysrhythmias (presumably due to acute electrolyte fluxes) and hypoxemia (caused by membrane-induced complement activation and leukocyte sequestration in pulmonary capillaries as well as a

decrease in minute ventilation due to removal of CO_2 by dialysis).

2. To accomplish fluid and solute removal in hypotensive patients, several variants of hemodialysis have been developed.

   a. Continuous arteriovenous hemofiltration (CAVH) with or without dialysis is used in many ICUs. It has the specific advantage of allowing removal of large amounts of fluid even in patients with serious hemodynamic compromise. The patient's own arterial pressure is used to drive ultrafiltration across a highly permeable membrane. Fluid removal may exceed 500 mL/h with CAVH, so provision must be made for a pump to limit ultrafiltration or replacement with an adequate amount of a balanced salt solution. Solute removal can be accelerated by the passing peritoneal dialysate across the ultrafiltrate side of the membrane. CAVH generally requires a femoral arterial access and thus may not be possible in patients with severe vascular disease.

   b. A modification of this technique, known as continuous venovenous hemofiltration (CVVH), has recently been introduced and is gaining favor. Vascular access is simplified, since an arterial access is not required, but CVVH does require additional equipment in the form of pumps and alarms.

3. PD has less efficient clearance of low molecular weight solutes than HD, so PD is generally not first-line therapy in hypercatabolic ICU patients.

   a. PD is much better tolerated from a hemodynamic standpoint and may be preferred in unstable patients.

   b. It is technically easier than HD in small children. Access to the peritoneal cavity is obtained with a flexible catheter that can be placed at the bedside.

   c. PD can be done continuously or intermittently with a minimum of equipment and staff. Ultrafiltration is controlled by changing the glucose concentration (and hence osmolarity) of the dialysate.

   d. PD orders should include the number and duration of exchanges, the composition of the dialysate with respect to glucose, sodium, and calcium, and whether any additives such as antibiotics, heparin, insulin, or potassium are to be included.

   e. The most common complication of PD is peritonitis. Parenteral or intraperitoneal antibiotics should result in clinical improvement within 24 to 48 h; if not, consideration should be given to catheter removal.

    f. Hyperglycemia resulting from absorption of dialysate glucose can be managed by intraperitoneal or subcutaneous insulin administration.

■ VI. RHABDOMYOLYSIS

Rhabdomyolysis is a condition characterized by release of muscle cell contents into the circulation caused by skeletal muscle necrosis.

A. Signs and symptoms occur due to toxicity of pigment globin proteins and accompanying fluid and electrolyte shifts.

B. Some causes of rhabdomyolysis are listed in Table 14.19.

    1. Trauma causes muscle injury both by direct pressure and muscle hypoperfusion due to shock and vasospasm.

    2. Ischemic events such as arterial thrombosis and compartment syndromes can lead to muscle necrosis.

    3. Numerous drugs and toxins including heroin, phencyclidine, cocaine, succinylcholine, and lipid-lowering agents have also been associated with rhabdomyolysis.

    4. Infections due to coxsackie, influenza, and measles viruses as well as bacterial infections with *Clostridium*, *Staphylococcus*, and *Legionella* spp. can cause skeletal muscle injury.

    5. Excessive muscle activity (seizures, status asthmaticus, marathon running) have been reported as infrequent causes of rhabdomyolysis. In cases of heat stroke, some degree of muscle injury is invariably present.

C. The diagnosis of rhabdomyolysis depends on a thorough history and physical examination.

    1. Muscle pain is present in about half the cases.

    2. Symptoms or signs related to various electrolyte abnormalities may be present.

    3. Fever and evidence of ECF volume depletion can frequently be documented.

Table 14.19. Causes of Rhabdomyolysis

Trauma
Ischemia
Drugs/toxins
Infections
Excessive muscle activity
Heat stroke

4. Urinalysis reveals bloody-appearing urine with a positive dipstick test for blood *in the absence* of apparent red blood cells on microscopic examination of the sediment.
5. Common early electrolyte abnormalities include hyponatremia, hyperkalemia, hypocalcemia, hyperphosphatemia, hypermagnesemia, hyperuricemia, and metabolic acidosis. Hypercalcemia may be a later finding.
6. ARF occurs in about 30% of patients.
7. Intracellular muscle enzymes (creatine kinase and aldolase) are invariably elevated, often to astronomic levels.
8. Low-grade DIC is present in the overwhelming majority of cases; its absence should prompt a consideration of other diagnoses.
9. As muscle groups swell in response to injury, persistent or recurrent muscle injury can occur leading to clinical exacerbation 48 to 72 hours after the initial injury ("second-wave phenomenon").

D. Principles of treatment are outlined in Table 14.20.
1. Vigorous volume expansion is essential, especially in the initial stages, when 2 to 3 L/h are frequently necessary. After the patient has stabilized, fluid administration is reduced to 300 to 500 mL/h to maintain brisk urine output (>200 mL/h).
2. Producing an alkaline diuresis (urine pH > 8) by IV infusion of isotonic $NaHCO_3$ (3 amps $NaHCO_3$ per liter D_5W) has been suggested as a possible means of increasing urine myoglobin solubility, but this has not been tested in well-controlled clinical trials.
   (a) The use of diuretics to prevent tubular obstruction has some experimental support but has not been validated in practice.
3. Treatment of electrolyte abnormalities as discussed in previous sections is of paramount importance.

Table 14.20. Treatment of Rhabdomyolysis

IV fluids
Normal saline volume expansion
Bicarbonate infusions
Diuretics
Mannitol
Furosemide
Treatment of electrolyte disorders
Dialysis

    4. Dialysis is indicated for the treatment of severe ARF and resistant electrolyte problems.

E. Survival of patients with rhabdomyolysis given appropriate intensive care is 80% to 90%.

■ VII. USEFUL FACTS AND FORMULAS

A. Acid-Base Equations/Facts

The normal relationship between bicarbonate (HCO_3^-), hydrogen ions (H^+), and carbon dioxide is expressed in the *Henderson equation*:

$$[H^+] = 24 \times \left(PCO_2 / [HCO_3^-] \right)$$

where PCO_2 = partial pressure of carbon dioxide.

This interaction can also be represented by the *Henderson-Hasselbalch equation*:

$$pH = 6.10 + \log\left([HCO_3^-] / 0.03 \times PCO_2 \right)$$

The mean response equations for simple acid-base disturbances are depicted in Table 14.21.

The amount of *NaHCO₃ needed* to raise the serum $[HCO_3^-]$ can be calculated as follows:

$$\begin{aligned}
&NaHCO_3 \text{ required (mEq)}\\
&= \text{Body weight (kg)} \times 0.7 \times\\
&\quad \left(\text{Desired} \left[HCO_3^- \right] - \text{Current} \left[HCO_3^- \right] \right)
\end{aligned}$$

Table 14.21. Selected Response Equations for Simple Acid-Base Disturbances

Acid-base disturbance	Equation
Metabolic acidosis	$\Delta PaCO_2 \approx 1.2\Delta[HCO_3^-]$
Metabolic alkalosis	$\Delta PaCO_2 \approx 0.7\Delta[HCO_3^-]$
Respiratory acidosis	
Acute	$\Delta[HCO_3^-] \approx 0.1\Delta PaCO_2$
	$\Delta[H^+] \approx 0.75\Delta PaCO_2$
Chronic	$\Delta[HCO_3^-] \approx 0.3\Delta PaCO_2$
	$\Delta[H^+] \approx 0.3\Delta PaCO_2$
Respiratory alkalosis	
Acute	$\Delta[HCO_3^-] \approx 0.2\Delta PaCO_2$
	$\Delta[H^-] \approx 0.75\Delta PaCO_2$
Chronic	$\Delta[HCO_3^-] \approx 0.5\Delta PaCO_2$
	$\Delta[H^+] \approx 0.5\Delta PaCO_2$

Alternatively, the following formula can be utilized to calculate the *base deficit* in metabolic acidosis:

HCO_3^- deficit
$$= (\text{desired } HCO_3 - \text{observed } HCO_3) \times 0.4 (\text{body weight (kg)})$$

The *chloride deficit* in the treatment of metabolic alkalosis can be calculated utilizing the following formula:

Cl^- Deficit (mEq)
$$= 0.5 \,(\text{weight in Kg}) \left(103 - \text{measured } Cl^-\right)$$

B. Renal Function Formulas

The *glomerular filtration rate* (GFR) can be approximated, adjusted to age based on the following formulas:

< 45 years: GFR = 12.49 − 0.37 (age)

≥45 years: GFR = 153 − 1.07 (age)

A formula derived by *Cockcroft and Gault* is commonly used to estimate *creatinine clearance*:

Creatinine clearance (mL/min)
$$= \frac{140 - \text{age}}{\text{Serum creatinine (mg/dL)}} \times \frac{\text{Body weight (kg)}}{72}$$

In women the value obtained from this equation is multiplied by a factor of 0.85.

This formula can also be adjusted for lean body weight (LBW) calculated from the following

LBW (male) = 50kg + 2.3kg/inch > 5 feet

LBW (female) = 45.5kg + 2.3kg/inch > 5 feet

Alternatively, the creatinine clearance (C_{cr}) can be calculated as follows:

$$C_{cr} = \frac{(U_{cr} \cdot V)}{P_{cr}}$$

where U_{cr} = concentration of creatinine in a timed collection of urine; P_{cr} = concentration of creatinine in the plasma; V = urine flow rate (volume divided by period of collection).

Another commonly employed formula to calculate the creatinine clearance is *Jelliffe's formula*:

$$C_{cr} = \frac{98 - 0.8(\text{age} - 20)}{P_{cr}}$$

Table 14.22. Creatinine Clearance Values Under Selected Conditions

Condition	Value
Normal	>100 mL/min
Mild renal failure	40–60 mL/min
Moderate renal failure	10–40 mL/min
Severe renal failure	<10 mL/min

In this formula, age is rounded to nearest decade. In females, the above result is multiplied by a factor of 0.9.

A more complicated and potentially more accurate way to calculate creatinine clearance is *Mawer's formula:*

$$C_{cr}(\text{males}) = \frac{\text{LBW}\,[29.3 - (0.203 \times \text{age})]\,[1 - (0.03 \times P_{cr})]}{14.4\,(P_{cr})}$$

$$C_{cr}(\text{females}) = \frac{\text{LBW}\,[25.3 - (0.174 \times \text{age})]\,[1 - (0.03 \times P_{cr})]}{14.4\,(P_{cr})}$$

Hull's formula for creatinine clearance is calculated as

$$C_{cr} = [(145 - \text{age})/P_{cr}] - 3$$

In females the result is multiplied by a factor of 0.85.

Ranges for *creatinine clearance* under selected conditions are depicted in Table 14.22.

C. Selected Electrolytes

The *transtubular potassium gradient* (TTKG) allows one to estimate the potassium secretory response in the cortical collecting duct. This index corrects for water reabsorption in the cortical and medullary collecting ducts:

$$\text{TTKG} = \text{Corrected urine } K^+ / \text{Serum } K^+$$

$$\text{Corrected urine } K^+ = \frac{\text{Urine } K^+}{\text{Uosm/Posm}}$$

The normal renal conservation of potassium is reflected by a TTKG < 2.

The percentage of *magnesium retention* (MR) can be calculated by the following formula:

$$\text{MR}(\%) = 1 - \frac{\substack{\text{Postinfusion} \\ 24-\text{hour} \\ \text{urine Mg}^{++}} - (\text{Preinusion} \times \text{Postinfusion})}{\text{Total elemental magnesium infused}} \times 1$$

The *fractional tubular reabsorption of phosphate* (TRP) allows for quantification of renal phosphate wasting and is calculated as

$$TRP = 1 - C_{po4}/C_{cr}$$

where C_{PO4}/C_{cr} = fractional excretion of phosphate.

In conditions such as proximal renal tubular acidosis, the *fractional excretion of HCO_3^-* ($FEHCO_3^-$) can be calculated as

$$FEHCO_3^- = \frac{Urine\,[HCO_3^-]\,(mEq/L)}{Serum\,[HCO_3^-]\,(mEq/L)} \times \frac{Serum\,creatinine\,(mg/dL)}{Urine\,creatinine\,(mg/dL)} \times 100$$

The *correction of calcium* based on the serum albumin/globulin levels is calculated as

$$\%\,Ca\,bound = 8(albumin) + 2(globulin) + 3$$

Another formula to correct *calcium based on the total protein* is

$$Corrected\,Ca = measured\,Ca/(0.6 + (total\,protein/8.5)$$

A quick bedside formula for calculation of the corrected calcium is

$$Corrected\,Ca = Calcium - albumin + 4$$

D. Osmolality Formulas

To calculate the *serum osmolality* (Osm), the following formula is employed:

$$Osm = 2Na^+ + BUN\,(mg/dL)/2.8 + glucose\,(mg/dL)/18$$

The *osmolar gap* (OG) is calculated as the difference between the measured osmolality and the calculated osmolality:

$$OG = Measured\,osmolality - Calculated\,osmolality$$

The approximate *urine osmolality* can be calculated from the following formula:

$$mOsm \sim (Urine\,specific\,gravity - 1) \times 40,000$$

E. Water Balance

To estimate the amount of *total body water* (TBW), the following formula is frequently employed:

$$TBW = Body\,weight\,(kg) \times 60\%$$

The *water deficit* of a patient can be estimated by the following equation:

Water deficit $= 0.6 \times$ Body weight in kg $\times (PNa/140 - 1)$

where PNa = plasma sodium concentration.

Alternatively, the *free water deficit* from the osmolality can be calculated as

H_2O deficit (L)

$$= \text{Total body weight (kg)} \times 0.6 \left(1 - \frac{\text{normal osm}}{\text{observed osm}} \right)$$

To calculate the *free water clearance* based on the osmolar clearance, the following formula can be utilized:

Free water clearance = Urine volume − Osmolar clearance
where the *osmolar clearance* is calculated as

$$\text{Osmolar clearance} = \frac{\text{Urine osmolarity} \times \text{urine volume}}{\text{Plasma osmolality}}$$

The *excess water* (EW) of a patient is calculated as

EW

$$= \text{TBW} - [\text{Actual plasma Na/Desired plasma Na}] \times \text{TBW}$$

F. Urinary/Renal Indices

The most common *urinary indices* used in the differential diagnosis of acute renal failure are depicted in Table 14.23.

To calculate the *renal failure index* (RFI), the following formula is commonly employed:

Table 14.23. Commonly Used Urinary Indices in Acute Renal Failure

Index	Prerenal	Acute tubular necrosis
Specific gravity	>1.020	<1.010
Urinary osmolality (mOsm/kg H_2O)	>500	<350
U_{osm}/P_{osm}	>1.3	<1.1
Urinary Na^+ (mEq/L)	<20	>40
U/P Cr	>40	<20
RFI	<1	>1
FENa (%)	<1	>1

Abbreviations: Cr, creatinine; P, plasma; RFI, renal failure index; U, urine; FENa, fractional excretion of sodium.

$$RFI = \frac{U\, Na^+}{U/P\, Cr}$$

The *fractional excretion of sodium* (FENa) is calculated as

$$FENa\,(\%) = \frac{\text{Quantity of } Na^+ \text{ excreted}}{\text{Quantity of } Na^+ \text{ filtered}} \times 100$$

or

$$FENa\,(\%) = \frac{U/P\, Na^+ \times 100}{U/P\, Cr}$$

or

$$FENa\,(\%) = \frac{U_{Na} \times V}{P_{Na} \times (U_{Cr} \times V/P_{Cr})} \times 100$$

or

$$FENa\,(\%) = \frac{U_{Na} \times P_{Cr}}{P_{Na} \times U_{Cr}} \times 100$$

where U_{Na} = urine sodium concentration; V = urine flow rate; P_{Na} = plasma sodium concentration; U_{Cr} = urine creatinine concentration; P_{Cr} = plasma creatinine concentration.

G. Hemodialysis Formulas

The following are useful equations in the management of the chronic hemodialysis patient.

The *protein catabolic rate* (PCR) is calculated as:

$$PCR\,(g/kg/d) = 0.22 + \frac{0.036 \times ID\, BUN \times 24}{ID\, interval}$$

where ID BUN = interdialytic rise in blood urea nitrogen (BUN) in mg/dL; ID interval = interdialytic interval in hours.

Alternatively, if blood urea is measured, the PCR can be calculated utilizing the following formula:

$$PCR\,(g/kg/d) = 0.22 + \frac{0.1 \times ID\, urea \times 24}{ID\, interval}$$

where ID urea = interdialytic rise in blood urea in mmol/L.

If the patient has a significant urine output, the contribution of the urinary urea excretion must be added to the PCR calculation and is calculated as follows:

Urine contribution to PCR

$$= \frac{\text{Urine urea N (g)} \times 150}{\text{ID interval (h)} \times \text{Body weight (kg)}}$$

Alternatively, if urine urea is measured:

Urine contribution to PCR

$$= \frac{\text{Urine urea (mmol)} \times 4.2}{\text{ID interval (h)} \times \text{Body weight (kg)}}$$

To calculate the *percentage of recirculation* during hemodialysis, the following formula is utilized:

$$\% \text{ Recirculation} = \frac{A2 - A1}{A2 - V} \times 100$$

where A2 = blood urea or creatinine concentration in arterial blood line after blood pump is stopped; A1 = arterial line blood urea or creatinine concentration; V = venous line urea or creatinine concentration.

The *volume of distribution of urea* can be calculated as follows:

Males: V = 2.447 − 0.09516A + 0.1074H + 0.3362W
Females: V = −2.097 + 0.1069H + 0.2466W

where V = volume in liters; A = age in years; H = height in centimeters; W = weight in kilograms.

The calculation of *residual renal function* for dialysis 3 times per week:

$$\text{GFR} = \frac{V \times U}{t \times (0.25 \, U_1 + 0.75 \, U_2)}$$

where V = urine volume in interdialytic period; U = urine urea nitrogen or urea concentration; t = interdialytic period in minutes; U_1 = postdialysis BUN or blood urea on first dialysis of the week; U_2 = predialysis BUN or blood urea on second dialysis of the week.

The *percent reduction of urea* (PRU) can be calculated utilizing the following formula:

$$\text{PRU} = \frac{\text{Pre urea} - \text{Post urea}}{\text{Pre urea}} \times 100$$

The *urea reduction ratio* (URR) is calculated as

$$\text{URR} = 100 \times \left(1 - \frac{\text{Postrurea}}{\text{Preurea}}\right)$$

Table 14.24. Urinalysis in Different Conditions

Condition	Findings	
Prerenal failure	SG:	>1.015
	pH:	<6
	Prot:	trace to 1+
	Sed:	sparse hyaline, fine granular cases or bland
Postrenal failure	SG:	1.010
	pH:	>6
	Prot:	trace to 1+
	Hb:	+
	Sed:	RBCs, WBCs
Acute tubular necrosis (ATN)	"Muddy" brown urine	
	SG:	1.010
	pH:	6–7
	Prot:	trace to 1+
	Blood:	+
	Sed:	RBCs, WBCs, RTE cells, RTE casts, pigmented casts
Glomerular diseases	SG:	>1.020
	pH:	>6
	Prot:	1 to 4+
	Sed:	RBCs, RBC casts, WBC, oval fat bodies, free fat droplets, fatty casts
Vascular diseases	SG:	>1.020 if proglomerular
	pH:	<6
	Prot:	trace to 2+
	Sed:	RBCs and RBC casts with glomerular involvement
Interstitial diseases	SG:	1.010
	pH:	6–7
	Prot:	trace to 1+
	Sed:	WBCs, WBC casts, eosinophils, RBCs, RTE cells

Abbreviations: RBC, red blood cells; RTE, renal tubular epithelial cells; WBC, white blood cells; SG, urine specific gravity; Prot, protein; Sed, urinary sediment.

H. Urinalysis

Please refer also to Chapter 20 for additional laboratory values. The most common *urinalysis* manifestations of renal diseases are depicted in Table 14.24.

Some elements and substances can modify the color of urine in humans, as depicted in Table 14.25.

Table 14.25. Urine Color Based on the Presence of Elements or Substances

Elements/substances	Characteristic color
White blood cells Precipitated phosphates Chyle	Milky white
Bilirubin Chloroquine Sulfasalazine Nitrofurantoin Urobilin	Yellow/amber
Phenazopyridine Hemoglobin myoglobin Red blood cells Phenothiazines Phenytoin Prophyrins Beets Red-colored candies	Brown/red
Melanin Phenol Methyldopa Metronidazole Quinine	Brown/black
Pseudomonas infection Amitriptyline Methylene blue Biliverdin Propofol	Blue/green

Table 14.26. Normal Urinary Excretion of Selected Amino acids

Amino acid	Normal excretion (mg/g of creatinine)
Cystine	18
Lysine	130
Arginine	16
Ornithine	22

I. Other Formulas/Facts

To determine whether a patient has aminoaciduria or not, the *fractional reabsorption of an amino acid* (FR_A) is determined utilizing the following formula:

$$FR_A = 1 - [Urine]_A / [Plasma]_A \div [Urine]_{Cr} / [Plasm]_{Cr} \times 100\%$$

The normal *urinary excretion of amino acids* in patients older than 2 years is depicted in Table 14.26.

When acute renal failure (ARF) is due to *uric acid nephropathy (UAN)*, the following equation is generally > 1:

$$\text{Index} = \frac{\text{spot urine uric acid (mg/dL)}}{\text{spot urine creatinine (mg/dL)}} = > 1.0$$

15

Special Techniques

■ I. AIRWAY MANAGEMENT

A. The first technique in the management of patients with airway problems is manual opening of the airway (i.e., head-tilt, chin-lift). See Chapter 2, "The Basics of Critical Care."

B. Adjuncts for Artificial Airway
   1. Oropharyngeal Airways
      a. Oropharyngeal airways are available in a number of different sizes and styles.
      b. These devices routinely should be sized from the angle of the jaw to the central incisors.
      c. Techniques for insertion include the following:
         (1) The Inverted Technique: The oral airway is placed upside down and rotated to the appropriate position after negotiating the tongue.
         (2) Tongue Depressors Technique: A tongue depressor is used to manipulate the base of the tongue to prevent occlusion of the airway by impeachment of the tongue on the end of the oral airway.
   2. Nasopharyngeal Airways
      a. Nasopharyngeal airways are also available in a number of sizes, which should be measured from the tragus of the ear to the tip of the nose.
         (1) Great care should be exercised to ensure that the angled opening of the distal portion of the airway does not traumatize nasal passages, resulting in epistaxis.

Table 15.1. Indications for Intubation

1. Ventilation of the patient
2. Airway obstruction
3. Tracheal bronchial toilet
4. Airway protection
5. Impending respiratory failure

        (2) Well-lubricated nasopharyngeal airways appear to be better tolerated in the alert patient as compared to oropharyngeal airways.

C. Endotracheal Intubation
    1. Common indications for endotracheal intubation are depicted in Table 15.1.
    2. Orotracheal Intubation
        a. The oral route is the most common and easily mastered approach for tracheal intubation.
        b. Routinely, this technique involves visualization of the glottis, the use of a laryngoscope, and passage of the endotracheal tube into the trachea under direct vision. Table 15.2 lists the essential equipment that should be available for orotracheal intubation.
        c. Intubation Technique
            (1) Positioning of the Patient: It is important to align the axis of the trachea, pharynx, and the oral cavity to effect endotracheal intubation. This requires that the axis be aligned by placing the patient's head in the "sniffing" position. A small pad or folded towel may be used to raise the occiput for proper alignment (see Figure 15.1A).
            (2) After proper positioning and ensuring that all the necessary equipment is available, laryngoscopy may be performed by inserting the laryngoscope into the oropharyngeal airway and examining the airway. Two types of blades are commonly used:
                (a) The Miller blade is used to lift the epiglottis to obtain visualization of the tracheal opening.
                (b) The Mackintosh blade fits into the vallecula, resulting in adherence of the

Table 15.2. Equipment Necessary for Endotracheal Intubation

Oxygenation Equipment
— Oxygen source
— Regulators and tubing

Endotracheal Tubes
— Appropriate numbers and sizes of endotracheal tubes should be available.
— A malleable stylet to stiffen the tube for insertion.
— Silicon jelly as a lubricant.
— Appropriate volume syringe(s) for cuff inflation.

Laryngoscope
— Laryngoscope handle with functioning batteries.
— Straight and curved blades of the sizes necessary for the proposed intubation with functioning lightbulbs or fiberoptic tracks.

Fixation Device for the Endotracheal Tube
— Adhesive tape or commercially available tube-fixation devices.

Means of Assessment for Appropriate Position of Endotracheal Tube
— Stethoscope
— End-tidal CO_2 monitoring device
— Pulse oximeter

epiglottis to the back of the blade (see Figure 15.1A). The tongue and other oral contents are displaced to the left side (see Figure 15.1B). The Miller blade is inserted more midline, elevating the tongue upward.

(c) Care should be exercised in the use of the laryngoscope. Proper technique is to lift the laryngoscope upward and not to use it as a fulcrum (see Figures 15.1A and 15.1B).

(d) A Sellick maneuver (pressure on the cricoid to help occlude the epiglottis during manipulation of the airway) is commonly performed to help prevent aspiration and to stabilize the glottis during the intubation procedure.

(3) After identifying the laryngeal opening (see Figure 15.1B), the trachea is entered under direct visualization by placing the endotracheal tube through the vocal cords.

(a) This can be most easily accomplished by placing the endotracheal tube in the right corner of the mouth, directing the

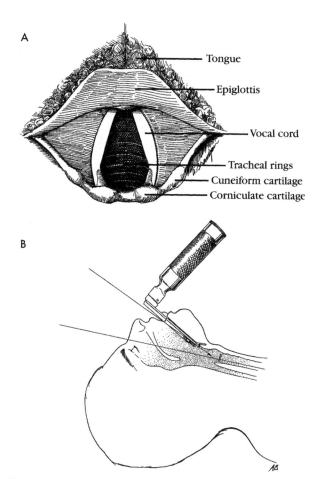

Figure 15.1. Endotracheal intubation. *(A)* Proper use of the laryngoscope during intubation. *(B)* View of the larynx during direct laryngoscopy. (From Allison EJ Jr: *Advanced life support skills,* St. Louis, 1994, Mosby-Year Book.)

tip into the glottic opening. This technique does not require interruption of the view of the vocal cords during intubation.
- (b) Insertion should be stopped when the cuff is displaced 2 cm from the glottic opening (external markings are typically at 21 or 23 cm from the central incisors of average size women and men, respectively).
- (c) The cuff is blown up to a moderate tension of the pilot balloon and ventilation with 100% oxygen begun.
- (4) Tube placement is ascertained by auscultation of chest and abdomen, examination of the rise and fall of the chest, condensation of the respiratory gas mixture in the endotracheal tube, maintenance of adequate saturation on pulse oximetry, and when available end-tidal CO_2 indicators.
3. Nasotracheal Intubation
   a. Nasotracheal intubation can be performed under direct visualization using the laryngoscope.
      - (1) The tube is placed through the nares, and the tip is visualized in the pharynx.
      - (2) McGill forceps can be used to manipulate the end of the endotracheal tube through the vocal cords to achieve proper positioning.
   b. Blind nasal insertion.
      - (1) The location of the endotracheal tube is ascertained through auscultation.
      - (2) This technique is reserved for those patients who have spontaneous ventilations.
      - (3) An endotracheal tube of appropriate size is inserted through the naris and advanced to the pharynx.
      - (4) Auscultation using the unaided ear and listening at the nasal end is used as the endotracheal tube is advanced.
      - (5) The tube is inserted through the glottic opening during inspiration, and appropriate position is confirmed as noted above.
      - (6) Nasal intubation may result in severe epistaxis in patients with coagulopathy or if performed with excessive force.
      - (7) Patients with mid-face fractures *should not* be nasally intubated.

(8) Sinusitis is a recognized complication of nasal intubation and should be considered when determining the route of intubation.

4. No matter the route of intubation of the trachea, all endotracheal tubes should be secured with adhesive tape or other securing devices to prevent dislodgment.

5. Common Complications of Endotracheal Intubation
   a. During Laryngoscopy and Intubation
      (1) Dental and oral soft tissue trauma
      (2) Dysrhythmias, hypertension/hypotension
      (3) Aspiration of gastric contents
   b. While Endotracheal Tube Is in Place
      (1) Tube obstruction
      (2) Esophageal intubation
      (3) Accidental extubation
      (4) Tracheal mucosa ischemia
   c. Delayed Complications
      (1) Tracheal stenosis
      (2) Vocal cord paralysis
      (3) Laryngeal edema

D. Cricothyroidotomy
   1. The cricothyroid membrane can be identified by palpation below thyroid cartilage.
   2. A large-bore (14- or 16-gauge) catheter may be placed through the cricothyroid membrane into the trachea and used to ventilate and oxygenate patients in whom other airway maneuvers are unsuccessful.
   3. Free release of air from the catheter will confirm tracheal position.
   4. The tip of the catheter should be angled inferiorly, and after tracheal penetration with the plastic cannula, it should be advanced.
   5. The cannula may be adapted to fit the 15-mm opening of a standard *Ambu* bag, or alternatively, a portable high-frequency jet ventilator device may be used to provide oxygenation to the patient.
   6. Surgical cricothyroidotomy
      a. Percutaneous technique: A needle is used, passing into the trachea, and a guide wire is positioned in the trachea through the needle. A dilator is then passed, and a cricothyroidotomy tube with an internal obturator is inserted.
      b. Surgical technique: A small midline incision is made over the cricothyroid membrane, which is then

opened, and an appropriate cannula is placed in the trachea.

■ II. CARDIOVERSION/DEFIBRILLATION

A. The major indications for the utilization of these techniques are covered in Chapter 2 ("The Basics of Critical Care") and Chapter 3 ("Cardiovascular Disorders").

B. Preparation
   An appropriately functioning monitor/defibrillator and conductive pads or gel must be available.

C. Procedure for Defibrillation
   1. Institute basic life support if not already begun.
   2. Determine cardiac rhythm. If the patient is not already placed on a cardiac monitor, then the *"quick-look"* capabilities of the monitor/defibrillator may be used.
   3. Turn on the monitor section of the monitor/defibrillator.
   4. Select the paddle lead for the monitor/defibrillator.
   5. Place the paddles on the right upper sternal and left lateral position or anteroposteriorly (see Figure 15.2).
   6. Observe rhythm.
      a. If ventricular fibrillation is observed,
         (1) Turn on the power to the defibrillator unit and make sure that the unit is in the defibrillation (*"defib"*) mode.
         (2) Select the appropriate energy level. See Chapter 2 ("The Basics of Critical Care") and Chapter 3 ("Cardiovascular Disorders").
         (3) Place electrode gel or other conductive media, and position the paddles as mentioned above. Firm pressure should be applied.
         (4) Perform discharge of the defibrillator by simultaneously depressing both discharge buttons located on the defibrillator paddles.

D. Procedure for Synchronized Cardioversion
   After determining cardioversion is appropriate,
   1. Turn on the power to the defibrillator unit.
   2. Make sure that the defibrillator unit is in the synchronized (*"sync"*) mode.
   3. Apply conductive gel or other material to the paddles, and position them as noted above.

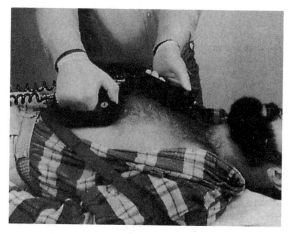

Figure 15.2. Standard positioning of cardioversion/defibrillation electrodes on the anterior portion of the thorax. (From Allison EJ Jr: *Advanced life support skills,* St. Louis, 1994, Mosby-Year Book.)

       4. Confirm that an acceptable electrocardiogram (ECG) signal is being received from the monitor/defibrillator unit.

       5. Discharge the energy by depressing both discharge buttons located on the defibrillator paddles and by observing the unit to ensure that the shock is delivered.

  E. Avoid administering countershocks directly over implanted pacemakers or defibrillators and over nitroglycerin patches on the surface of the patient's skin. The potential for serious injury with this device exists. You need to make sure that other rescuers/health-care providers are clear of the victim, before delivering shocks.

  F. Complications

       1. An adverse rhythm may be produced by administering electrical countershocks.

       2. Burns of the skin may result, particularly when poor electrical conduction has been established. The use of gel or other conductive material is mandatory, and firm pressure (approximately 25 pounds) should be applied to the paddles.

       3. Myocardial injury.

       4. Systemic embolization.

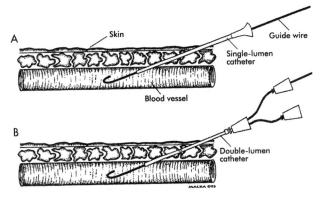

Figure 15.3. Modified Seldinger technique for vascular access. *(A)* Single-lumen catheter. *(B)* Double-lumen catheter.

■ III. VASCULAR ACCESS

A. Modified Seldinger Technique

This technique is a simple method of obtaining access to vascular spaces.

1. After appropriate preparation, draping, and positioning, a needle is percutaneously placed into the vascular structure. A guide wire with a flexible end (either J or straight) is inserted through the needle and into the lumen of the vessel (see Figure 15.3).

2. The needle is subsequently removed, and the catheter is inserted over the extraluminal end of the guide wire and subsequently passed over the wire into the vessel.

3. The catheter is advanced and the guide wire removed. When appropriately positioned, the catheter is secured with suture or tape.

B. Central Venous Access

1. The major indications for central venous access are depicted in Table 15.3.

2. No absolute contraindications to central venous access exist. Relative contraindications may include bleeding diathesis and central venous thrombosis.

3. Choice of Central Cannulation Route

Table 15.3. Indications for Central Venous Cannulation

Difficult peripheral venous cannulation
Drug administration
Emergency dialysis
Total parental nutrition
Hemodynamic monitoring

Table 15.4. Equipment Necessary for Central Venous Cannulation

Appropriate intravenous fluid with administration tubing
Prep solution (routinely Iodophor)
Sterile towels
10-ml syringe with Luer-lok
25-gauge needle for local anesthesia
1% lidocaine
Appropriate size and gauge introducer needle
Spring guide wire
Number 11 blade
Vessel dilator
Selected catheter
Suture material

  a. Subclavian, internal jugular, and femoral routes have all been used extensively for central cannulation.
  b. The specific site chosen is dependent upon the clinical circumstances and the skill of the operator.
  c. Subclavian insertion has a higher risk of pneumothorax. It also presents a noncompressible vascular puncture site.
  d. There is a small but significant incidence of carotid puncture during internal jugular cannulation.
4. Table 15.4 displays the equipment necessary for central venous cannulation.
5. Internal Jugular Catheterization (Anterior Approach)
  a. In the nonemergent setting, informed consent should be obtained.
  b. Position the patient in a 15- to 20-degree Trendelenburg position, and remove the headboard of the bed.
  c. Wash, gown, and glove.
  d. Prepare the operative site gently with Iodophor solution, and drape the region with sterile towels.
  e. The internal jugular vein lies beneath the sternocleidomastoid muscle and slightly in front of the carotid artery, as shown in Figure 15.4.

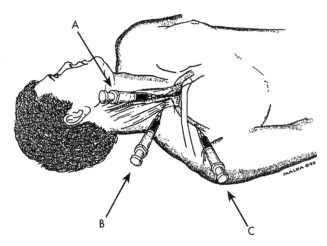

Figure 15.4. Central venous cannulation. (See text for details.)

    f. In the anterior approach, the carotid artery is palpated (left index and middle finger), the puncture site is infiltrated with 1% lidocaine, and a finding needle is passed immediately lateral to the carotid pulsation beneath the medial edge of the sternocleidomastoid muscle at the level of the thyroid cartilage. The needle is advanced at an angle of approximately 30 degrees to the skin (directed toward the ipsilateral nipple). The vessel should be encountered within 3 cm. When gentle suction on the syringe produces a rush of venous blood, the needle is removed, and the procedure is repeated with the larger gauge introducer needle on a 5- or 10-mm Luer-lok syringe. Once the venous puncture has been achieved, a guide wire is passed into the vessel (a vessel dilator can be used), and the venous catheter is inserted over the wire through a very small skin incision made over the wire. The wire subsequently is removed, and intravenous (IV) extension tubing is attached.

6. Internal Jugular Catheterization (Middle Approach)

    a. With the patient supine in the 20-degree Trendelenburg position and the patient's head slightly turned to the contralateral side, local anesthetic is infiltrated at the junction of the sternal and clavicular heads of the sternocleidomastoid muscle. The needle is inserted with an angle of approximately 30 degrees to the skin and again directed toward the ipsilateral nipple. The vessel should be entered within 2 to 3 cm of insertion (see Figure 15.4A). Once vascular access has been obtained, the procedure is repeated with the introducer needle, the guide wire is passed through the needle, and cannulation is completed as noted above.

7. Internal Jugular Catheterization (Posterior Approach)

   a. The patient is again positioned in the 20-degree Trendelenburg position with the head facing the contralateral shoulder. After preparation of the skin and local anesthesia as noted above, the needle is inserted through the skin at the posterolateral margin of the sternocleidomastoid muscle (approximately 4 cm above the sternoclavicular junction). This is the approximate point where the external jugular vein crosses the posterior margin of the sternocleidomastoid muscle, a commonly used landmark. The needle is advanced in a caudal and medial direction, aiming at the contralateral nipple (see Figure 15.4B). Once venous access with the introducer needle has been obtained, a guide wire is placed into the catheter and cannulation proceeds as noted above.

C. Subclavian Vein Cannulation

   1. The patient is prepped and positioned in a manner analogous to that for internal jugular vein cannulation; however, a rolled-up towel should be placed longitudinal between the scapula to allow the shoulders to drop back.

   2. The patient's head is turned 45 degrees away from the side of intended placement.

   3. The puncture site is identified approximately 1 cm below the inferior margin of the clavicle at the junction of the medial and middle two thirds (see Figure 15.4C).

   4. Infiltration with 1% lidocaine of the region is accomplished. In addition, lidocaine is also injected into the periosteum of the clavicle.

   5. The anesthesia needle is removed, and the introducer needle is inserted into the skin at this point. The tip is aimed at the suprasternal notch, passing just beneath the clavicle. The bevel of the needle should be pointed toward the head (cephalad). When free flow of blood is obtained from the introducer needle, the bevel can be rotated 180 degrees, helping to facilitate thoracic placement of the

guide wire. The catheter is threaded, the wire is removed, fluid flow is established, and the catheter is then secured.

D. Femoral Vein
   1. This approach is easily performed in most patients.
   2. The patient is placed supine, knees extended, and the foot of the anticipated cannulation site is rotated outward 15 to 30 degrees.
   3. The site of insertion is cleaned and prepped, as noted previously, and the region is draped.
   4. The insertion point is identified, lying 2 to 3 cm inferior to the inguinal ligament (1 to 2 cm medial to the femoral pulse. (The reader is reminded of the *navl* mnemonic of the structures in this region: nerve, artery, vein, lymphatics.)
   5. As for internal jugular cannulation, a 22-gauge finder needle is commonly used for local anesthesia infiltration as well as localization of the vessel.
   6. After the femoral vein has been found, the introducer needle is placed on a syringe and inserted into the femoral vein.
   7. Next, a flexible guide wire is placed, and the needle is exchanged for the vascular cannula. The catheter is then secured.

E. Complications of Central Venous Access
   Infection, pneumothorax (more common with subclavian approach), hemothorax, chylothorax, intrapleural infusion of IV fluids, dysrhythmias, thrombosis, air embolism, pericardial tamponade, neurological injuries, and hematomas.

■ IV. ARTERIAL LINE

1. The common sites for arterial cannulation include the radial, femoral, dorsalis pedis, and axillary, with the radial artery being most frequently used.
2. For radial artery cannulation, many authorities believe the "Allen test" should be performed first. This test is done by occluding both radial and ulnar arteries immediately proximal to the palmar crest. Opening and closing of the hands produces blanching of the hands and digits. The tester removes pressure over the ulnar artery and notes the time to return of normal color. Seven seconds are reported as normal, from 7 to 14 seconds is indeterminate, and >14 seconds is abnormal. However, this may be quite difficult to perform in the intensive care unit

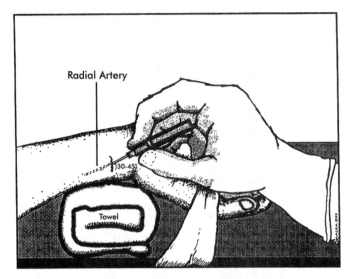

Figure 15.5. Radial arterial cannulation.

(ICU) with an uncooperative patient, and a normal Allen test does not ensure that a vascular complication will not occur.

3. Preparation after informed consent is obtained.
   a. The patient's arm should be extended with the volar side upward on an arm board or bedside table.
   b. A small towel is placed at the level of the wrist. Placing the hand in dorsiflexion will facilitate cannulation (see Figure 15.5).
   c. The region of insertion is cleansed as noted above, sterile drapes are placed, and a fine-gauge needle is used to infiltrate a small quantity of 1% lidocaine at the site of insertion.

4. We find a typical 20- or 22-gauge catheter-over-needle technique to be acceptable for radial artery cannulation. Catheter-over-needle with guide-wire devices are also available, and a traditional Seldinger technique may also be used.
   a. The overneedle catheter (usually without syringe) is inserted parallel to the projected course of the radial artery at an angle of 30 to 45 degrees to the skin.
   b. The needle is advanced slowly until pulsatile blood is obtained.

   c. The plastic catheter is then advanced into the artery, where, if a guide wire is being used, this is placed through the needle into the vessel. The catheter is then advanced.

   d. The needle is removed, and appropriate tubing is attached. The catheter is then secured in place.

5. Complications include thrombosis, infection, aneurysm formation (especially in femoral arterial lines).

■ V. PULMONARY ARTERY CATHETERIZATION

A. Intravenous access must be obtained using one of the techniques described above. The introducer sheath is then placed into the desired vessel.

B. The appropriate monitoring system must be in place, including pressure transducers for all ports that will be monitored.

   1. High-pressure tubing must be flushed with appropriate solution.

   2. The clinician should observe and test the dynamic response by watching the pressure wave on the bedside monitor while activating the flush device and quickly releasing it.

   3. Each lumen of the catheter should be flushed and connected to the appropriate monitoring line, and the balloon inflated to ensure an intact symmetrical balloon.

   4. Rapid whipping of the catheter tip will convince the operator that the monitoring system is functioning properly when the catheter is inserted into the introducer.

C. Continuous recording of distal port should be instituted.

D. The catheter is advanced approximately 20 cm (in the adult patient) for either subclavian or internal jugular insertions, at which point a central venous pressure wave form should be seen (see Figure 15.6).

E. The balloon is inflated with 1 to 1.5 cc of air, and the catheter is further advanced into the vascular system.

F. Within 30 or 40 cm of catheter insertion, the right ventricular (RV) pressure wave form is usually seen (see Figure 15.6). This is easily identified by the steep upstroke, typically 2 to 3 times larger than the right atrial (RA) pressure.

G. Passage in the PA generally occurs at 40 to 50 cm of catheter and may be identified by the dicrotic notch of the downslope.

H. A pulmonary artery wedge pressure is usually noted at 50 to 60 cm of catheter and looks much like a RA wave form (see Figure 15.6).

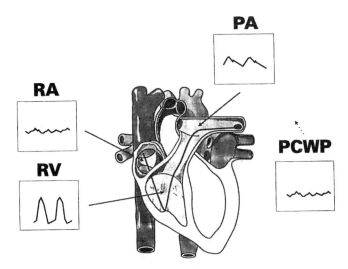

Figure 15.6. Pulmonary artery catheterization and waveforms. (See text for details.)

I. Complications include dysrhythmias, valvular damage, knotting of the catheter, atrial or ventricular perforation, air embolism, pulmonary embolism, pulmonary arterial injury, and catheter-related sepsis.

■ VI. TUBE THORACOSTOMY

A. The drainage system should be prepared before the chest tube is placed.
1. All the couplings and tubing should be inspected, and appropriate fluid levels should be maintained.
2. A "three-bottle system" (all of which may be maintained in a single commercial thoracostomy drainage system) is depicted in Figure 15.7E. The first bottle is the trap bottle, which collects the fluid emanating from the chest tube itself. The second bottle represents the water-seal bottle. Air is precluded from entering the pleural space through the system by the water in the water-seal bottle. The third

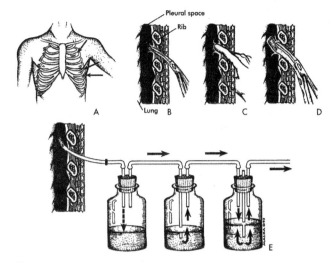

Figure 15.7. Tube thoracostomy. (See text for details.)

bottle represents the manometer bottle. Suction applied to the manometer bottle is regulated by the distance that the center tube lies below the surface of the water. For example, if the central tube lies 20 cm below the surface of the water, suction levels producing pressure in excess of − 20 cm of water simply result in bubbling of ambient air in the manometer bottle, thus, maintaining the −20-cm water pressure limit.

B. Surgical Technique
  1. The contents of a chest tube tray are depicted in Table 15.5.
  2. The patient should be positioned with the side for tube insertion uppermost.
  3. The operator should be gowned and gloved.
  4. The chest tube is usually inserted in the anterior axillary line in the fifth or sixth intercostal space.
  5. The incision site should be prepped and draped, and lidocaine should be infiltrated one intercostal space below the rib of the selected intercostal space of insertion. The periosteum, subcutaneous tissue, and pleural space should be infiltrated. Aspiration of fluid or air will confirm infiltrated pleural space.

Table 15.5. Contents of the Chest Tube Tray

— Sterile towels and drapes

— 1% or 2% lidocaine

— 10-mL syringe

— 22- and 25-gauge needles

— 1-0 silk suture with cutting needle (2 packages)

— 2 large *Kelly* clamps

— 2 medium *Kelly* clamps

— Suture scissors

— 4-inch-square gauze pads

— Chest drainage, suction system, and appropriate chest tube

6. A small skin incision, appropriate to the size of the chest tube, is made with a scalpel over the anesthetized rib (see Figure 15.7A).
7. Extend the incision into the subcutaneous tissue and muscle at the intercostal space, preferably using the blunt side of the scalpel or trocar.
8. A large clamp with an open end using spreading maneuvers is used until the pleural space is reached (see Figure 15.7B).
9. The index finger of the operator is used to explore the pleural space to ensure that the lung, diaphragm, or another structure is not adherent (see Figure 15.7C).
10. The tube is inserted, generally toward the apex of the pleural space for treatment of pneumothoraces, by grasping the tube with a medium clamp, maneuvering it through the dissected tunnel (see Figure 15.7D), and ensuring that the last hole of the thoracostomy tube lies within the pleural space. The tube is fixed at the insertion site with 1-0 silk suture.
    a. A number of techniques are used, but commonly the suture ends are not cut but wrapped around the tube and secured with tape. These may be used to close the wound when the tube is pulled out.
11. The external end of the chest tube is then attached to the system, and the connections are taped over.
12. A sterile dressing with tape is applied to the skin.
C. Complications include tube malposition, empyema or wound infection, blockage of tube by blood or fibrin clot, and lung injuries.

■ VII. INTRA-AORTIC BALLOON PUMP (IABP)

A. Indications for the Use of IABP
   1. Pump failure
      a. After acute myocardial ischemic event
      b. Cardiogenic shock
      c. Postcardiac transplant patient
      d. In the pre- or postoperative period of cardiac surgery
   2. Acute mitral valvular regurgitation
   3. Unstable angina pectoris
   4. Other

B. Insertion should normally be accomplished by those with experience. The technique is also dependent upon the particular catheter and approach to be used.
   1. Once the catheter is in place, its function is rather easy to visualize (see Figure 15.8).
   2. During ventricular systole, the balloon (present in the proximal aorta), deflates, decreasing afterload on the heart and improving ventricular performance.
   3. During diastole, the inflated balloon occludes 75% to 90% of the cross-sectional area of the descending aorta, thereby increasing coronary perfusion.
   4. Helium is most commonly used for inflation and deflation of the balloon.

C. Complications include balloon membrane rupture or perforation, limb ischemia, aortic dissection, renal failure, thrombocytopenia and infection.

■ VIII. PERICARDIOCENTESIS

A. Blind pericardiocentesis should be performed in life-threatening situations (i.e., decompensated cardiac tamponade).
   1. We prefer the subxiphoid approach.
      a. If possible, the patient is placed upright or if necessary in a semireclining position.
      b. Venous access, continuous ECG monitoring, and blood pressure monitoring should have been established. Personnel and equipment necessary for cardiac resuscitation must be on hand.
      c. Sedation and analgesia as appropriate to the setting should be provided.
      d. The region is prepped and draped.

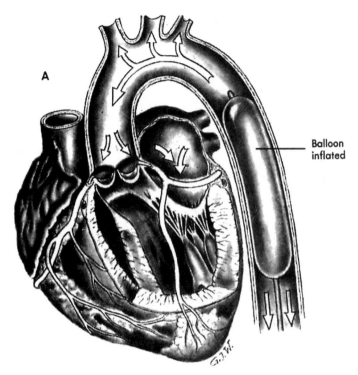

Figure 15.8. Intra-aortic balloon pump. From Thelan LA et al: *Critical care nursing,* ed 2. St. Louis, 1994, Mosby-Year Book.)

    e. 1% lidocaine local, and an 18- or a 20-gauge cardiac or spinal needle attached to a syringe with local anesthetic is prepared.

    f. For ECG monitoring, an alligator clip connected to the V lead of an ECG monitor may be placed on the needle (see Figure 15.9).

    g. The needle tip is introduced between the xiphoid and left costal margin and directed to the left shoulder.

    h. Continuous gentle suction is applied to the syringe. Intermittently, local anesthetic may be injected, which helps to clear the needle and anesthetize the deeper tissues.

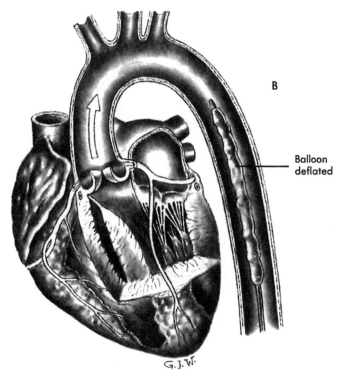

Balloon deflated

Figure 15.8. *Continued*

      i. The sensation of pericardial passage will usually be felt by the operator.

      j. Epicardial contact will be recognized by the ECG tracing, showing injury current. If this should occur, the needle should be withdrawn slightly.

2. After entrance into the pericardial cavity, removal of 50 mL of pericardial fluid is usually enough.

3. A pliable soft catheter may be inserted into the pericardial space using a guide wire, allowing the needle to be withdrawn. Real-time transthoracic echocardiography

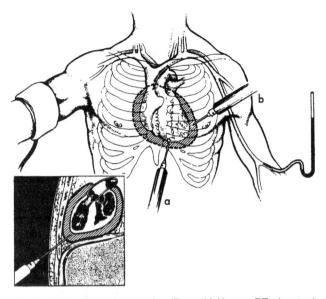

Figure 15.9. Pericardiocentesis. (From McKenna RE Jr et al: Pleural and pericardial effusions in cancer patients. *Curr Prob Cancer* 1985;9:1.)

    allows tracking of the needle tip to ensure correct location throughout the aspiration procedure.

    4. In an alternative approach, the needle is angled toward the right shoulder rather than the left shoulder.

B. Complications include cardiac chamber puncture, dysrhythmias, pneumothorax, vasovagal reactions, and cardiac arrest.

16

Toxicology

■ I. GENERAL MANAGEMENT

A. History
   Obtain as accurate a history as possible, including the substance ingested or inhaled and the amount and time of ingestion. Always consider possible ingestion or inhalation of multiple substances.

B. Cardiorespiratory Care
   The most important aspects of initial management are basic care of respiratory and cardiovascular function: Maintain a patent airway, ensure adequate respiration (support ventilation when necessary), and treat shock if present.
   1. Airway
      a. Loss of airway patency and reflexes may lead to obstruction, aspiration, or respiratory arrest.
      b. Maintain proper airway position; suction; use oropharyngeal or nasopharyngeal adjuncts as needed.
      c. Absent or depressed gag reflex in an unconscious or obtunded patient indicates an inability to protect the airway; endotracheal intubation is indicated.
   2. Respirations
      a. Respiratory failure is the most frequent cause of death in poisoned patients, and usually it is a result of (CNS) central nervous system depression.
      b. Assist ventilation, and perform endotracheal intubation as required.
      c. Obtain and follow arterial blood gases.

3. Circulation
    a. Monitor blood pressure, pulse, and cardiac rhythm.
    b. Initiate intravenous line.
    c. If hypotension is present, administer fluid challenge with normal saline 10 to 20 mL/kg.
    d. If hypotension persists, administer dopamine 5 to 15 µg/kg/min.
    e. With intractable hypotension, insert pulmonary artery catheter, if possible.
        (1) If central venous pressure or pulmonary artery occlusion (wedge) pressure is low, administer fluids.
        (2) If cardiac output is low, consider increasing the dose of dopamine or administering dobutamine (begin at 1 to 5 µg/kg/min IV, and adjust as required).
        (3) If systemic vascular resistance is low, administer intravenous (IV) norepinephrine. Begin at 0.1 µg/kg/min, and increase as required. Once norepinephrine is initiated, dopamine dosage should be decreased to 1 to 3 µg/kg/min.

C. Gastrointestinal Decontamination
    The traditional sequence for gastrointestinal decontamination is emptying of stomach by induced emesis or gastric lavage followed by administration of activated charcoal. However, there is controversy regarding this: Activated charcoal administration may be as effective as gastric emptying if 60 minutes or longer have elapsed since ingestion. This portion of treatment of the poisoned patient will generally be performed before admission to the intensive care unit. However, it will occasionally be necessary in the intensive care area, especially if the diagnosis of poisoning is delayed.
    1. Induced Emesis
        a. Useful in early management of oral poisoning and for removal of material poorly adsorbed by activated charcoal (alcohols, ethylene glycol, iron, lithium).
        b. Relatively rarely useful in the intensive care unit patient, who is likely to have diminished level of consciousness or decreased capacity to protect the airway.
        c. Administer syrup of ipecac (30 mL for adults, 15 mL for children <5 years old, 10 mL for children <1 year old). Repeat if no emesis in 20 minutes.
            (1) Not recommended in children <9 months old.
            (2) If the second dose does not produce vomiting, perform gastric lavage.

  d. Contraindications
    (1) Comatose or seizing patient
    (2) Ingestion of corrosive agents or petroleum distillates
    (3) Ingestion of substance likely to produce coma or seizures rapidly
2. Gastric Lavage

     Gastric lavage is contraindicated if the patient is obtunded or comatose until endotracheal intubation is performed to protect the airway. Performance in an obtunded patient may lead to vomiting and aspiration of gastric contents. Other complications include perforation of the nasal mucosa, production of epistaxis, tracheal intubation, and stimulation of ventricular dysrhythmias. Lavage is controversial in corrosive ingestion.

     Utilize a 36–40 Fr tube in adults, 24–26 Fr in children. Check for the position of the tube by injecting air and auscultating the stomach. Administer lavage fluid in aliquots of 200 to 300 mL, then allow return of fluid by gravity drainage. Continue until the lavage fluid is clear of ingested fragments or substance color (or longer if the circumstances of the ingestion dictate).
3. Activated Charcoal
    a. Limits absorption of virtually all ingested substances. Administer 1 g/kg orally or via gastric tube after emesis or lavage is completed.
    b. Repeat doses of 15 to 20 g at 1- or 2-hour intervals, or continuous activated charcoal instillation may be useful in some instances (i.e., theophylline overdose).
    c. Contraindicated in corrosive ingestion, ileus, or intestinal obstruction.
4. Cathartics
    a. Frequently used, but their effectiveness is not well established.
    b. Administer along with activated charcoal.
    c. Magnesium citrate 10% 3 to 4 mL/kg or sorbitol 70% 1 to 2 mL/kg. If no charcoal is present in stool after 6 hours, repeat half dose.
5. Whole Bowel Irrigation
    a. Effectiveness not fully studied. May be useful in substantial ingestion of substances poorly adsorbed by activated charcoal or enteric-coated tablets.
    b. Administer polyethylene glycol electrolyte solution (CoLyte or GoLYTELY) 2 L/h by gastric tube until stool is free of particulate material.
    c. Do not use in unconscious or obtunded patients.

D. Forced Diuresis and Control of Urine pH

May increase urinary excretion of some agents for which renal excretion is the major route of elimination. Do not use in patients with renal failure or congestive heart failure.

1. Alkalinization

a. May be useful in overdose with salicylates, phenobarbital.

b. Administer sodium bicarbonate 1 to 2 mEq/kg IV to achieve a urinary ph ≥ 7.0.

c. Monitor serum pH.

2. Acidification

a. May be useful in overdose with phencyclidine, amphetamines, quinine, quinidine, strychnine, cyclic antidepressants.

b. Administer ammonium chloride 75 mg/kg IV in 4 to 6 divided doses to achieve a urinary pH ≤ 6.0.

c. Do not use in the presence of rhabdomyolysis, myoglobinuria, or hepatic failure.

d. Monitor serum pH.

E. Hemodialysis

May be useful in severe intoxication with amphetamines, methanol, ethylene glycol, isopropyl alcohol, lithium, salicylates. If fluid or acid-base abnormalities are present, these can also be corrected.

F. Charcoal Hemoperfusion

1. Utilizes an extracorporeal circuit through an activated charcoal column.

2. May be useful in severe intoxication with barbiturates, some beta-blockers, ethchlorvinol, meprobamate, phenytoin, salicylates, and theophylline.

3. Potential complications: hypotension and thrombocytopenia.

G. Toxicology Screen

1. Should be used to confirm diagnosis in all cases.

2. Specific levels may be necessary in overdose with certain substances to guide therapy (i.e., acetaminophen, iron, lithium, methanol, salicylates, theophylline).

H. Poison Control Centers

Notify poison control centers with management questions or complicated or unusual poisonings. Telephone numbers for these centers are listed in Table 16.1.

Table 16.1. Telephone Numbers for U.S. Regional Poison Control Centers

State	City	800 Number (in state only)	Telephone number
Alabama	Birmingham	(800) 292-6678	(205) 939-9201
	Tuscaloosa	(800) 462-0800	(205) 345-0600
Arizona	Phoenix		(602) 253-3334
	Tucson	(800) 362-0101	(602) 626-6016
California	Fresno	(800) 346-5922	(209) 445-1222
	Los Angeles	(800) 825-2722	(213) 484-5151
	Sacramento	(800) 342-9293	(916) 453-3692
	San Diego	(800) 876-4766	(619) 543-6000
	San Francisco	(800) 523-2222	(415) 476-6600
Colorado	Denver	(800) 332-3073	(303) 629-1123
District of Columbia	Washington		(202) 625-3333
Florida	Tampa	(800) 282-3171	(813) 253-4444
Georgia	Atlanta	(800) 282-5846	(404) 589-4400
Kentucky	Louisville	(800) 722-5725	(502) 589-8222
Maryland	Baltimore	(800) 492-2414	(301) 528-7701
Massachusetts	Boston	(800) 682-9211	(617) 232-2120
Michigan	Detroit	(800) 462-6642	(313) 745-5711
	Grand Rapids	(800) 632-2727	(616) 774-7851
Minnesota	Minneapolis		(612) 347-3141
	St. Paul	(800) 222-1222	(612) 221-2113
Missouri	St. Louis	(800) 392-9111	(314) 772-5200
Montana		(800) 332-3073	
Nebraska	Omaha	(800) 642-9999	(402) 390-5400
New Jersey	Newark	(800) 962-1253	(201) 923-0764
New Mexico	Albuquerque	(800) 432-6866	(505) 843-2551
New York	New York City		(212) 340-4494
Ohio	Cincinnati	(800) 872-5111	(513) 558-5111
	Columbus	(800) 682-7625	(614) 228-1323
Oregon	Portland	(800) 452-7165	(503) 279-8968
Pennsylvania	Pittsburgh		(412) 681-6669
	Philadelphia		(215) 386-2100
Rhode Island	Providence		(401) 277-5727
Texas	Austin		(512) 478-4490
	Dallas	(800) 441-0040	(214) 590-5000
	Galveston		(409) 765-9728
	Houston	(800) 392-8548	(713) 654-1701
Utah	Salt Lake City	(800) 456-7707	(801) 581-2151
West Virginia	Charleston	(800) 642-3625	(304) 348-4211
Wyoming		(800) 332-3073	

■ II. ACETAMINOPHEN

Acetaminophen is a widely used analgesic and antipyretic. It is found in combination with other analgesics and in various cold remedies (i.e., Comtrex, Congesprin, Excedrin PM, 4-Way Cold Tablets). Toxicity of significant overdose lies in production of hepatic necrosis. This is probably related to overwhelming of hepatic glutathione capacity to detoxify acetaminophen metabolic products. The diagnosis may be overlooked, especially in patients with alcoholic liver disease.

A. Clinical Effects

1. In 16 to 24 hours following ingestion, there are minimal symptoms except gastrointestinal distress.

2. For the next 4 days, the patient may be asymptomatic. The peak of liver function abnormalities occurs 72 to 96 hours after ingestion.

3. Resolution or hepatic failure may result; renal failure occasionally occurs.

B. Diagnostic Studies

1. Obtain serum acetaminophen as soon as 4 hours and as late as 24 hours following ingestion, and plot the level on a nomogram (Figure 16.1). The nomogram is useful only in acute ingestion.

2. There is good correlation between timed serum and subsequent hepatotoxicity. If the level is in the hepatotoxic range, administer *n*-acetylcysteine.

3. Obtain prothrombin time and transaminase levels, serum urea nitrogen (BUN), creatinine.

C. Management

1. Induce emesis or perform gastric lavage.

2. Antidote: *n*-acetylcysteine.

   a. Prevents liver injury when administered early following intoxication.

   b. Is the only oral administration approved in the United States. However, the IV formulation may be available at participating study centers. Contact a poison control center or a toxicologic consultant if IV administration is necessary.

3. Cimetidine may be an adjunctive agent in treatment because of its ability to inhibit cytochrome P-450, preventing the formation of toxic metabolites. The dose is not determined; 300 mg q6h may be administered.

D. Adverse Effects

1. Nausea and vomiting. If the dose is vomited, repeat administration.

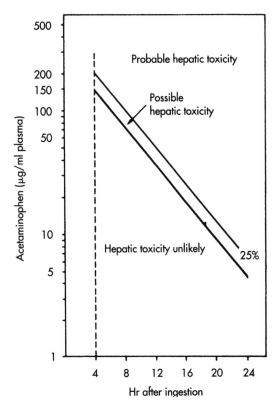

Figure 16.1. Rumack-Matthew nomogram for acetaminophen poisoning. (From Rumack BH, Mathew H: Acetaminophen poisoning and toxicity. *Pediatrics* 1975;55:871–876.)

2. Antiemetic medication (i.e., metoclopramide 10 to 20 mg IV q4h as needed) may be necessary for persistent vomiting.

E. Antidote Administration
1. Loading: 140 mg/kg (1.4 mL/kg of 10% solution or 0.7 mL/kg of 20% solution) diluted to 5% solution in grapefruit juice.

2. Maintenance: 70 mg/kg q4h for 17 doses or until the acetaminophen level is zero. May obtain levels every 12 hours.
3. Because activated charcoal adsorbs acetylcysteine, increase the acetylcysteine loading dose by 30% if this has
been administered.

■ III. ALCOHOL

Ethyl alcohol is found in beverages, as well as perfumes, mouthwashes,
and pharmaceutical preparations.

A. Overdose
1. Clinical Effects
   a. Variable depending on the individual: slurred speech,
   impaired judgment, behavior changes, combative-
   ness, ataxia.
   b. At very high levels, somnolence and respiratory
   depression occur. When death occurs as a result of
   intoxication, it is usually due to respiratory depression.
   c. Also occurring: cardiac dysrhythmias, hypertension,
   hypoglycemia, hypomagnesemia, hypophosphatemia, seizures, hypothermia, rhabdomyolysis,
   Wernicke's encephalopathy.
   d. Alcoholic ketoacidosis: metabolic acidosis with increased anion and osmolar gaps, and ketosis. Associated nausea, vomiting, abdominal pain.
2. Metabolism of Alcohol
   Rate is 12 to 50 mg/dL/h (average of 20 mg/dL/h).
3. Admission Criteria
   Admission to the intensive care unit may be required
   for trauma, seizures, hypothermia, and severe metabolic
   abnormalities.
4. Management
   a. Management is mainly supportive, with observation
   predominant. Intubate and ventilate if necessary.
   b. Administer IV glucose 50 g and thiamine 100 mg to
   all obtunded patients after serum glucose level is
   drawn.
   c. Correct volume depletion as needed.
   d. If the patient is violent or very agitated, use physical
   restraints as needed. Sedation with haloperidol may
   be necessary.
   e. Treatment of alcoholic ketoacidosis: Fluid replacement with D5%/normal saline. Observe for

Table 16.2. Appearance of Findings of Alcohol Withdrawal

Findings	Hours elapsed since cessation of alcohol intake
Tremor, agitation, sleep disturbance, hyperexcitability	6–8
Hallucinations	24–36
Seizures	7–48
Confusion, delusions, autonomic hyperreactivity, disorientation	72–120

appearance of hypoglycemia, hypophosphatemia, and hypokalemia.

B. Withdrawal
  1. Withdrawal following chronic use produces a number of signs and symptoms, including anxiety, insomnia, tremulousness, nausea, vomiting, tachycardia, hyperthermia, delirium, hallucinations, and seizures. The typical time of appearance of withdrawal findings are listed in Table 16.2.
  2. The hallmark of delirium tremens is significant alteration of the sensorium (global confusion, hallucinations, delusions, disorientation) accompanied by autonomic CNS hyperreactivity.
  3. Management
     a. Sedation
        (1) Benzodiazepines: Administer diazepam 2 to 5 mg IV, repeat q5min as needed, then 5 to 20 mg IV or PO q6h, or chlordiazepoxide 25 to 100 mg IV or PO q6h, or lorazepam 1 to 2 mg IV, IM or PO, or
        (2) Phenobarbital 260 mg slow IV, repeat as needed to produce light sedation, or
        (3) Haloperidol: Begin with 0.5 to 1.0 mg IV or IM q1–6h, but much larger doses may be required.
        (4) Propofol: 5 to 20 cc/h to achieve required sedation level.
     b. Thiamine 100 mg IV
     c. If severe hypertension or tachycardia is present, administer clonidine 0.1 to 0.2 mg q6h.

C. Other Alcohols
  1. Methanol
     a. Methanol (methyl alcohol) is widely used as a solvent, is found in windshield washer solution and antifreeze, and is used as a solid canned fuel.

  b. It produces CNS intoxication similar to that of ethanol. Other toxic effects include acidosis and retinal cell toxicity.

  c. Ethanol acts as a competitive substrate for alcohol dehydrogenase, the enzyme that produces toxic metabolites from methanol.

  d. Treatment

   (1) Hemodialysis.

   (2) Administration of IV ethanol (0.6 mg/kg initially and infusion of 66 mg/kg/h to maintain a blood alcohol level of 100 mg/dL. Administer as 10% ethanol diluted in D5%W.

   (3) Hemodialysis and treatment with ethyl alcohol are indicated with serum methanol levels >50 mg/dL.

 2. Isopropyl Alcohol

  a. Isopropyl alcohol is used as a solvent and medicinally as a rubbing alcohol and a sterilizing agent.

  b. It is more toxic than ethyl alcohol but less than methyl alcohol.

  c. Toxicity may be produced by ingestion of isopropyl alcohol or by inhalation of vapor.

  d. Signs and symptoms of intoxication are similar to methanol, but there is no retinal toxicity. Additional complications: dehydration and hemorrhagic gastritis.

  e. Treatment: gastric lavage, activated charcoal, maintenance of fluid balance and blood pressure. Hemodialysis may be used in severe cases.

◼ IV. ANGIOTENSIN-CONVERTING ENZYME (ACE) INHIBITORS

ACE inhibitors are antihypertensive agents that are in common use, either as individual agents or in combination with a diuretic (see Table 16.3).

 A. Toxic Effects

  The most common finding is hypotension. Fluid disturbances and electrolyte abnormalities may occur with agents combined with diuretics.

 B. Clinical Effects

  Dizziness, light-headedness, syncope, cough

Table 16.3. Angiotensin-Converting Enzyme Inhibitors

Benalepril (Lotensin)
Captopril (Capoten)
Enalapril (Vasotec)
Fesinopril (Monopril)
Lisinopril (Prinivil, Zestril)
Quinapril (Accupril)
Ramipril (Altace)
Combined with hydrochlorothiazide:
Captopril (Capozide)
Enalapril (Vaseretic)
Lisinopril (Prinzide, Zestoretic)

   C. Management
1. Perform gastric lavage or induce emesis.
2. Administer activated charcoal and cathartic.
3. Monitor blood pressure continuously.
4. Treatment is largely supportive. If hypotension is present, administer normal saline fluid infusion. Administer dopamine infusion if this does not correct hypotension. Naloxone has been reported to reverse hypotension.
5. In severe overdose, consider hemodialysis in overdose with captopril, enalapril, or lisinopril.

■ V. BETA-BLOCKERS

Common beta-blockers in use include propranolol, atenolol, metoprolol, pindolol, and nadolol. Agents are used for a variety of medical indications, including control of hypertension, cardiac dysrhythmias, angina pectoris, and glaucoma. Duration of toxicity varies greatly, depending on the agent ingested.

   A. Clinical Effects
1. Toxic effects include beta-adrenergic blockade, producing bradycardia, hypotension, bronchospasm.
2. Effects resulting from sodium-dependent membrane depression are seen primarily with lipid-soluble agents (i.e., propranolol, metoprolol) and include hypotension, Atrioventricular (A-V) block, QRS widening.
3. Seizures and coma may also occur.
4. Metabolic effects include hyperkalemia and hypoglycemia.

   B. Management
1. Perform gastric lavage; do not induce emesis.

2. Administer activated charcoal and cathartic.
3. Monitor cardiac rhythm.
4. If the patient is hypotensive, administer fluids, pressor agents, as required.
5. Administer atropine (0.01 to 0.03 mg/kg IV) and isoproterenol (start at 4 µg/min) for bradycardia.
6. In unresponsive hypotension and bradycardia, administer glucagon, 5 to 10 mg IV. Follow with 1- to 5-mg/min IV infusion.
7. Hemoperfusion may be useful for atenolol and nadolol overdose.
8. Monitor serum glucose and electrolytes, particularly potassium.

■ VI. COCAINE

Cocaine produces clinical symptoms on the basis of adrenergic stimulation, CNS stimulation, and increased metabolic rate. It is most commonly inhaled or injected parenterally. Use of free-base "crack" cocaine is very prevalent, as is the concomitant use of other drugs. Complications of cocaine abuse include hypertension with resulting intracerebral hemorrhage or aortic dissection, myocardial infarction, cerebrovascular accident, hyperthermia, and rhabdomyolysis.

A. Clinical Effects
1. The onset of toxic symptoms is within 30 to 60 minutes of injection or inhalation.
2. Patients present most often with hypertension, dysrhythmias, pupillary dilatation, agitation, anxiety, or psychosis.
3. Seizures, hyperthermia, and rhabdomyolysis may occur.
4. Hypertension may produce intracranial hemorrhage or thoracic aortic rupture.
5. Chest pain may occur and is sometimes of myocardial origin. Myocardial infarction may occur. Cocaine is dysrhythmogenic and may produce sinus tachycardia, premature ventricular contractions, ventricular tachycardia, and ventricular fibrillation.

B. Management
1. In oral ingestion, perform gastric lavage and administer activated charcoal.
2. Sedate with IV benzodiazepines or haloperidol.
3. For hypertension, treat with phentolamine 0.02 to 0.2 mg/kg or nitroprusside 2 to 10 µg/kg/min IV. If tachycardia is also present, administer esmolol (0.5 mg/kg loading, then

0.05 mg/kg/min) IV or labetalol 10 to 20 mg IV. May also use clonidine 0.1 to 0.2 mg q6h.
  a. Avoid the isolated use of beta-blockers.
  b. Consider obtaining computed tomograph (CT) of the head in cases of possible intracerebral hemorrhage.
4. Urine toxicology screen will confirm the diagnosis.

■ VII. CYANIDE

Cyanide is a chemical with a variety of industrial uses. Sodium nitroprusside contains cyanide, which is released into solution in increased quantity by exposure to light. The gas hydrogen cyanide is a product of combustion of plastics and a variety of other materials. A third of all smoke inhalation victims have increased cyanide levels.

A. Mechanism
  Toxicity is via chemical asphyxia, cyanide-blockade of cellular oxygen utilization. Exposure to small amounts of hydrogen cyanide gas or ingestion of a small quantity of cyanide salt can be rapidly fatal.

B. Clinical Effects
  1. Respiratory failure and cardiovascular collapse. Rapidly developing coma and severe lactic acidosis.
  2. Syncope, seizures, headache, nausea, confusion.
  3. Cyanide poisoning may occur with prolonged IV administration of sodium nitroprusside. Consider this if such patients develop CNS depression, seizures, lactic acidosis, or cardiovascular instability.
    a. May occur with an infusion rate >2 µg/kg/min.
    b. Infusion rates of >10 µg/kg/min should not be continued for prolonged periods of time because of this hazard.
    c. If cyanide intoxication is suspected, discontinue infusion and treat as below.
    d. Onset is usually at least several days after institution of sodium nitroprusside treatment, but it may occur within 6 hours of high-dose administration.

C. Management
  1. Administer oxygen, maintain airway, and assist respirations.
  2. Treat hypotension and seizures in standard fashion.
  3. Administer cyanide antidote kit.
    a. Have patient inhale amyl nitrite capsule.
    b. Administer sodium nitrite 300 mg IV.

c. These two produce methemoglobinemia, which may itself be toxic.

d. Administer sodium thiosulfate, which converts cyanide to thiocyanate, 150 mg/kg of a 25% solution IV (relatively contraindicated in renal failure).

4. If cyanide salt is ingested, lavage stomach and administer activated charcoal.

5. Hydroxycobalamin, a form of vitamin B12, is also used as an antidote.

   a. Administer 4 g intramuscularly (IM).

   b. The IV formulation is not available in the United States.

6. Other cyanide antidotes, dicobalt-EDTA and 4-dimethylamineophenol, are not currently available in the United States.

■ VIII. CYCLIC ANTIDEPRESSANTS

There is an estimated annual incidence of 500,000 cases of overdose with cyclic antidepressants. Many agents are in common use, including amitriptyline, desipramine, nortriptyline, doxepin, and imipramine (see Table 16.4). They may be found in medication combinations with other psychotropic agents.

Toxicity occurs via anticholinergic effects, alpha-adrenergic blockade, inhibition of norepinephrine reuptake, and inhibition of the fast sodium channel. Some drugs, such as haloperidol, morphine, and disulfiram, may prolong cyclic antidepressant toxicity by interfering with hydroxylation.

A. Clinical Effects

1. Tachycardia, myoclonus, delirium, coma, hyperthermia, pupillary dilatation, hypertension or hypotension, pro-

Table 16.4. Cyclic Antidepressants

Tricyclic
 Amitriptyline (Elavil, Endep, Etrafon, Limbitrol, Triavil)
 Amoxapine (Asendin)
 Desipramine (Norpramin)
 Doxepin (Sinequan)
 Imipramine (Tofranil)
 Nortriptyline (Pamelor)
 Protriptyline (Vivactil)
 Trimipramine (Surmontil)

Tetracyclic
 Maprotiline (Ludiomil)

longation of QRS and QT, A-V block, and myocardial depression.

2. The most important toxic effects are cardiovascular. A QRS duration >0.12 indicates serious toxicity. Sinus tachycardia is typical; supraventricular tachycardia, ventricular tachycardia, torsades des pointes, and ventricular fibrillation may occur. Bradycardia is a poor prognostic sign.

3. Rapid deterioration with the development of cardiovascular collapse, coma, or seizures may occur. Persistent seizures may produce hypothermia or rhabdomyolysis.

B. Management

1. Perform gastric lavage, and administer activated charcoal 100 g. Do not administer syrup of ipecac. Repeat doses of activated charcoal may be useful, and some have advocated continuous nasogastric instillation.

2. Continuous electrocardiographic monitoring is essential.

3. Treat hyperthermia (see Chapter 5, "Environmental Disorders") and seizures in usual fashion (diazepam 0.1 mg/kg IV per dose as needed, or phenytoin 15 mg/kg IV over 30 minutes).

4. Do not give physostigmine as an antidote, because it may produce seizures.

5. Administer sodium bicarbonate 50 to 100 mEq by IV bolus in widened QRS, hypotension, or metabolic acidosis. Monitor serum pH and electrolytes. Do not administer in metabolic alkalosis or pulmonary edema.

6. Beta-blockers have been used, but caution must be utilized, as patients may develop hypotension and cardiac arrest.

7. For ventricular dysrhythmias, administer lidocaine or phenytoin 15 mg/kg over 30 minutes.

8. For torsades des pointes, administer magnesium 2 to 4 g IV or isoproterenol. Do not use procainamide or quinidine.

9. In cardiovascular collapse, administer dopamine, phenylephrine, or norepinephrine.

■ IX. DIGOXIN

Digoxin is the most frequently used of the cardiac glycosides, being prescribed most commonly for congestive heart failure or dysrhythmias. The mechanism of digitalis toxicity involves interruption of potassium and calcium efflux from myocardial cells by inhibition of sodium, potassium-adenosine triphosphatase (potassium-ATP-ase). Intoxication may be the result of acute accidental or suicidal ingestion or chronic overdose. The clinical findings are different in these two settings.

A. Clinical Effects
    1. Acute Intoxication
        a. Nausea, vomiting, hyperkalemia
        b. Dysrhythmias
            (1) Bradycardia with sinus and atrioventricular block.
            (2) Ventricular dysrhythmias are uncommon.
    2. Chronic Intoxication
        a. Weakness, visual disturbances, hypomagnesemia. Potassium is normal or low.
        b. Dysrhythmias
            (1) Ventricular tachycardia and fibrillation are common.
            (2) Accelerated junctional rhythm and paroxysmal atrial tachycardia with block are common, especially in patients with chronic atrial fibrillation.

B. Diagnostic Studies
    1. Digoxin level: More useful in chronic intoxication. May be falsely high in acute overdose.
    2. Follow serum potassium, magnesium, BUN, creatinine.

C. Management
    1. Induce emesis, or perform gastric lavage if the patient has a history of significant ingestion. These may exacerbate bradycardia.
    2. Administer activated charcoal and cathartic.
    3. Digitoxin elimination is enhanced by repeat-dose activated charcoal.
    4. Monitor cardiac rhythm continuously.
    5. Hyperkalemia
        a. If >5.5 mEq/L, administer sodium bicarbonate 1 mEq/kg IV, glucose 0.5 g/kg, and regular insulin 0.1 U/kg IV, or polystyrene sulfonate (Kayexalate) 0.5 g/kg PO.
        b. Do not administer calcium.
    6. Bradycardia
        a. Atropine 0.5 to 2.0 mg IV as needed.
        b. Cardiac pacing may be required.
    7. Ventricular dysrhythmias
        a. Lidocaine 1 mg/kg IV bolus followed by 1 to 4 mg/min infusion, or
        b. Phenytoin 15 to 20 mg/kg IV no faster than 50 mg/min or

c. Magnesium sulfate 10%, 2 g IV over 20 minutes, and continuous infusion of 1 to 2 g/h.

D. Antidote: Digoxin-Specific Antibody Fragments (Digibind)
   1. Digoxin-specific antibodies a high affinity for digoxin, a lower affinity for digitoxin and other cardiac glycosides.
   2. Administer for life-threatening dysrhythmias due to digitalis intoxication, especially if hyperkalemia is present.
   3. Dosage: Each 40-mg vial of digoxin-specific antibodies absorbs 0.6 mg of digoxin. Dosage of antibodies to be administered to be calculated as follows:
      a. Calculate body load of digoxin: dose ingested/0.8 or serum drug concentration in ng/mL by mean volume of distribution of digoxin (5.6 L/kg × patient weight) or digitoxin (0.56 L/kg × patient weight) and divided by 1000 to obtain the load in milligrams.
      b. Number of vials required: body load (mg)/0.6 mg.
   4. Administer IV over 30 minutes.
   5. There are no known contraindications. In patients with preexisting heart disease, withdrawal of inotropic effect by removal of digitalis from the circulation. Monitor for development of heart failure.
   6. Reversal of signs of digitalis intoxication occur within 30 to 60 minutes of administration. Complete removal of digoxin occurs by 3 hours.

■ X. NARCOTICS

Narcotics include naturally occurring or synthetic derivatives of opiates. These are used both medically and as drugs of abuse. Commonly used narcotics are found in Table 16.5.

Table 16.5. Commonly Used Narcotic and Related Agents

Butorphanol (Stadol)
Codeine
Fentanyl
Hydrocodone (Anexsia, Vicodin)
Hydromorphone (Dilaudid)
Meperidine (Demerol)
Methadone
Morphine
Nalbuphine (Nubain)
Oxycodone (Percocet, Percodan, Tylox)
Pentazocine (Talwin)
Propoxyphene (Darvon)

Extremely potent synthetic "designer" opioids are derivatives of meperidine and fentanyl (i.e., "China white") and are also included in this group. Narcotics may be ingested, injected parenterally, or inhaled.

A. Clinical Effects
    1. Sedation; miosis; respiratory depression; decreased heart rate, respiratory rate, and blood pressure; diminished bowel sounds; and signs of transcutaneous injection (i.e., "track marks") may be present. Urine toxicology may confirm diagnosis, but a negative result does not exclude it.
    2. In significant overdose: coma, pinpoint pupils, severe respiratory depression, apnea.
    3. Complications of overdose include rhabdomyolysis and noncardiogenic pulmonary edema.
    4. Death is typically due to respiratory failure.

B. Management
    1. Maintain and assist ventilation as necessary.
    2. In oral ingestion, perform gastric lavage and administer activated charcoal and cathartic.
    3. Antidote: Naloxone (Narcan)
        a. Opioid antagonist, competitively blocks CNS opiate receptors.
        b. Administer 0.4 to 2.0 mg IV (may also be given IM, subcutaneously, intratracheally). Repeat as needed. No response to total of 10 mg is evidence against narcotic overdose.
        c. Duration of action is 1 to 4 hours. Repeated administration may be required, or administer as an infusion of 0.4 to 0.8 mg/h in 5% dextrose.
        d. Use in opiate-dependent patients may produce narcotic withdrawal syndrome.
        e. Higher doses are frequently required with pentazocine and designer opioids: Begin with an initial dose of 4 mg.
    4. If respiratory distress continues, monitor with chest radiograph and arterial blood gases (ABGs).
    5. If noncardiogenic pulmonary edema (which may also be produced by naloxone) is present, treat according to the guidelines for treating adult respiratory distress syndrome (ARDS) (see Chapter 13).

■ XI. PHENCYCLIDINE

Phencyclidine (PCP), formerly used as a legal anesthetic agent, is now an illicit drug.

A. Clinical Effects
   1. PCP produces hallucinations, alteration of mental status, and bizarre or violent behavior. Clinical status tends to wax and wane, and severe symptoms may persist for as long as 2 weeks.
   2. The patient's level of consciousness ranges from fully alert to comatose.
   3. The most common physical findings are nystagmus and hypertension. Pupils may be dilated or miotic.

B. Medical Complications
   1. Complications may be due to direct effect of the drug or injury sustained during intoxication.
   2. Major complications are indications for intensive care unit admission: seizures, hyperthermia, rhabdomyolysis, and acute renal failure.

C. Diagnostic Studies
   1. Serum and urine PCP levels correlate poorly with clinical effects.
   2. Check urine for myoglobin, which may indicate rhabdomyolysis.

D. Management
   1. Management is largely supportive.
   2. PCP is frequently smoked, so gastric decontamination is not useful in these cases. However, gastric lavage and activated charcoal may be indicated if large amounts have been ingested. Do not induce emesis.
   3. Hemodialysis and charcoal hemoperfusion are not effective in eliminating PCP.
   4. Acid diuresis may speed elimination but is rarely indicated.
   5. Severe agitation or violence: Utilize physical restraints. May administer haloperidol 10 mg IM or IV or benzodiazepines.
   6. Hypertension is usually mild and does not require treatment.
   7. Seizures: If persistent, treat with IV benzodiazepines or propofol.

■ XII. PHENYTOIN

Phenytoin toxicity may be due to acute overdose or chronic overingestion.

A. Clinical Effects
  1. Nausea, vomiting, lethargy, ataxia, agitation, irritability, hallucinations, and seizures.
  2. Horizontal nystagmus is characteristic of overdose.
  3. At very high levels: coma, respiratory arrest.
  4. Cardiac toxicity occurs only with iatrogenic IV overdose, not with oral ingestion.

B. Diagnostic Studies
  1. Phenytoin levels
      a. Therapeutic: 10 to 20 mg/L.
      b. Levels >20 mg/L: nystagmus.
      c. Levels >30 mg/L: ataxia.
      d. Levels >40 mg/L: lethargy is common.
  2. Serum Glucose: Hyperglycemia may occur.

C. Management
  1. Induce emesis or perform gastric lavage.
  2. Administer activated charcoal. Multiple doses of charcoal may enhance elimination.
  3. Some recommend the use of charcoal hemoperfusion for severe intoxication.
  3. Remainder of treatment is supportive.
  4. Monitor cardiac rhythm in IV overdose.

■ XIII. SALICYLATES

Salicylates are used for analgesic, antipyretic, and anti-inflammatory properties and are found in a variety of both prescription and over-the-counter preparations (i.e., Alka-Seltzer, Ascriptin, Bufferin, Excedrin Extra Strength). Poisoning may be the result of acute ingestion or chronic overdose.

A. Clinical Effects
  1. The clinical effects result from CNS respiratory stimulation, uncoupling of oxidative phosphorylation, and interference with platelet function and bleeding time.
  2. Cerebral and pulmonary edema occur by uncertain mechanisms.

3. Acute overdose
    a. Tachypnea, tinnitus, vomiting, lethargy, respiratory alkalosis, metabolic acidosis
    b. Severe: hypoglycemia, hyperthermia, seizures, coma, pulmonary edema
4. Chronic overdose
    a. Confusion, dehydration, metabolic acidosis. This presentation may mimic sepsis.
    b. Pulmonary edema is more common than in acute overdose.

B. Diagnostic Studies
    1. In acute ingestion, obtain the salicylate level, and plot it on a Done nomogram (Figure 16.2).
        a. Multiple determinations may be necessary with sustained-release preparations. Obtain every 2 to 3 hours for 12 hours following ingestion.
        b. Usual therapeutic levels in arthritis patients: 100 to 300 mg/L (10 to 30 mg/dL).
        c. A nomogram is not as useful in chronic intoxication.
    2. Follow ABGs, serum glucose and electrolytes, and chest radiographs.

C. Management
    1. Induce vomiting or perform gastric lavage if acute ingestion is suspected.
    2. Administer activated charcoal and cathartic.
    3. Monitor for development of pulmonary edema.
    4. Treat metabolic acidosis with IV sodium bicarbonate 1 mEq/kg to maintain pH at 7.40 to 7.50.
    5. Rehydrate with IV crystalloid solution if dehydration has resulted from vomiting or hyperventilation.
    6. Urinary alkalinization enhances excretion:
        a. Administer D5W containing sodium bicarbonate 100 mEq/L at 200 to 300 mL/h. Use care in chronic intoxication: Observe for development of pulmonary edema.
        b. Check urinary pH frequently; maintain at 6.0 to 7.0.
        c. Add 30 to 40 mEq KCl to each liter of IV solution (except in presence of renal failure).
    7. Hemodialysis and hemoperfusion are effective in removing salicylates (hemodialysis also corrects fluid and acid-base disturbance). Indications follow:
        a. Acute ingestion with serum levels >1200 mg/L (120 mg/dL) or severe acidosis.
        b. Chronic intoxication with serum levels >600 mg/L (60 mg/dL).

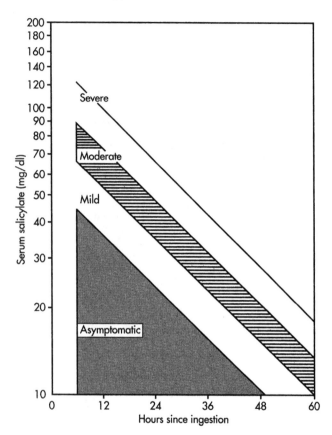

Figure 16.2. A Done nomogram for acute salicylate poisoning. (From Done AK: Salicylate intoxication: significance of measurements of salicylate in blood in cases of acute ingestion. *Pediatrics* 1960;26:800–807.)

■ XIV. SEDATIVES/HYPNOTICS

A large number of sedatives are in medical use. The most common are the barbiturates, nonbarbiturate sedative/hypnotics (i.e., chloral hydrate, meprobamate, paraldehyde), and benzodiazepines (see Table

Table 16.6. Commonly Used Sedative/Hypnotic Agents

Barbiturates
  Short-acting
    Secobarbital (Seconal)
    Pentobarbital (Nembutal)
  Intermediate-acting
    Amobarbital (Amytal)
    Apobarbital (Alurate)
    Butabarbital (Butisol)
  Long-acting
    Phenobarbital

Nonbarbiturates
  Chloral hydrate
  Ethchlorvinol (Placidyl)
  Meprobamate (Equagesic, Equanil, Miltown)
  Paraldehyde

Benzodiazepines
  Ultrashort-acting
    Midazolam (Versed)
    Temazepam (Restoril)
    Triazolam (Halcion)
  Short-acting
    Alprazolam (Xanax)
    Lorazepam (Ativan)
    Oxazepam (Serax)
  Long-acting
    Chlordiazepoxide (Librium)
    Chlorazepate (Tranxene)
    Diazepam (Valium)
    Flurazepam (Dalmane)
    Prazepam (Centrax)

16.6). The toxic/therapeutic ratio is very high for most benzodiazepines. Oral overdose with 20 times the therapeutic dose of diazepam may occur without significant CNS depression.

A. Clinical Effects
    1. The most prominent effect is CNS depression: lethargy, ataxia, slurred speech, progressing to coma and respiratory depression.
    2. Severe hypothermia, hypotension, and bradycardia may accompany deep coma due to barbiturates.
    3. Chloral hydrate may have cardiac effects, including dysrhythmias, hypotension, and myocardial depression.

B. Diagnostic Studies
    1. Barbiturates
        Serum levels >60 to 80 mg/L usually produce coma (>20 to 30 mg/L in short-acting barbiturates).

2. Benzodiazepines and Others
   Serum drug levels are of limited value.

C. Management
   1. Airway protection and ventilatory support are paramount.
   2. Induce emesis (if the patient is awake), or perform gastric lavage. Lavage is preferred for very short-acting agents, such as triazolam.
   3. Administer activated charcoal and a cathartic. Repeat-dose activated charcoal decreases the half-life of phenobarbital and meprobamate.
   4. Urinary alkalinization increases elimination of phenobarbital (but not other barbiturates) and meprobamate.
   5. Charcoal hemoperfusion may be indicated for severe barbiturate overdose.
   6. Benzodiazepine Antidote
      a. Flumazenil (Romazicon): Selective benzodiazepine CNS receptor competitive inhibitor. Use to reverse benzodiazepine-induced coma.
      b. Initial recommended dose is 0.2 mg IV over 30 seconds. Repeat 0.3 mg after 30 seconds, then 0.5 mg at 1-minute intervals.
      c. Most patients respond to cumulative doses of 1 to 2 mg. Reversal of CNS depression is unlikely if a dose of 5 mg has been given without effect.
      d. Adverse effects
         (1) Nausea and vomiting are most common.
         (2) In patients dependent on benzodiazepines, flumazenil may induce withdrawal syndrome (agitation, tachycardia, seizures).
      e. The duration of action of a single dose is 1 to 2 hours. If prolonged reversal is needed, give repeated doses, or administer as an IV infusion of 0.1 to 0.5 mg/h.

■ XV. THEOPHYLLINE

The mechanism of theophylline toxicity is via release of endogenous catecholamines, stimulation of beta$_2$-receptors, and inhibition of adenosine receptors. Clinical effects may be delayed for several hours following acute ingestion if a sustained-release formulation is involved. Toxicity may be acute or chronic.

A. Clinical Effects
   1. Common toxic effects include nausea, vomiting, tremor, tachycardia, and hypotension.

    2. Hypokalemia, hyperglycemia, and metabolic acidosis may occur (only in acute intoxication).

    3. Seizures and ventricular dysrhythmias may occur, especially with very high serum levels and with chronic intoxication.

B. Diagnostic Studies

    1. Serum theophylline level.

        a. Therapeutic: 15 to 20 mg/L

        b. In acute overdose with level >100 mg/L, seizures, hypotension, and ventricular dysrhythmias are common.

        c. Seizures may occur at levels of 40 to 60 mg/L in chronic overdose.

        d. Repeat levels q2–4h during treatment, and monitor for 12 to 16 hours.

    2. Monitor serum pH, glucose, and potassium levels.

C. Management

    1. Perform gastric lavage.

    2. Administer activated charcoal 100 g, and readminister 20 to 30 g q2–3h. Continuous infusion of activated charcoal has been recommended. Dilute charcoal in normal saline, and infuse at 0.25 to 0.5 g/kg/h up to a maximum rate of 50 g/h.

    3. Whole bowel irrigation has been recommended in the presence of undissolved sustained-release tablets that cannot be removed with gastric lavage.

    4. Treat seizures and ventricular dysrhythmias in standard fashion as required. Magnesium has been successful in some cases.

    5. For supraventricular tachycardia or rapid sinus tachycardia, ventricular dysrhythmias, or hypotension, administer esmolol 0.05 mg/kg/min or propranolol 0.01 to 0.03 mg/kg IV. Use with caution if wheezing is present.

    6. If theophylline level >100 mg/L or seizures or dysrhythmias do not respond to treatment, institute charcoal hemoperfusion.

    7. Hypokalemia usually resolves spontaneously.

■ XVI. USEFUL FACTS AND FORMULAS

A. Basic Formulas

The *therapeutic index* (TI) of a drug can be calculated as follows:

$$TI = \frac{LD_{50}}{ED_{50}}$$

where LD_{50} = median lethal dose; ED_{50} = median effective dose.

The *margin of safety* (MS) of a drug uses the ED_{99} for the desired effect and the LD_1 for the undesired effect:

$$MS = \frac{LD_1}{ED_{99}}$$

The *apparent volume of distribution* (V_d) can be calculated by the following equation:

$$V_d = \frac{Dose_{iv}}{C_0}$$

where $Dose_{iv}$ = the IV dose; C_0 = the extrapolated plasma concentration at time zero.

For those agents that follow a two-compartment model, several V_d exist and the following formula is used to assess the *volume of the central compartment* (V_c):

$$V_c = \frac{Dose_{iv}}{A + B}$$

where A and B represent disposition constants of a two-compartment model.

In addition, the *peripheral compartment* (V_p) can be calculated as follows:

$$V_p = \frac{Dose_{iv}}{B}$$

where B is derived from the elimination or equilibrium phase of a two-compartment model.

The *total body clearance* (Cl) of a drug can be calculated as the sum of clearances by individual organs:

$$Cl = Cl_r + Cl_h + Cl_i + \ldots$$

where Cl_r = renal clearance; Cl_h = hepatic clearance; Cl_i = intestinal clearance.

B. Osmolality Formulas

To calculate *serum osmolality*, the following formula is usually applied:

Table 16.7. Osmolal Ratios of Different Alcohols

Ethanol	Ethylene glycol	Isopropanol	Methanol
4.6	6.2	6.0	3.2

Calc. Osmolality $(mOsm/kg) = 2Na + BUN/2.8 + Glucose/18$

The *osmolal gap* (*OG*) is useful in several intoxications and is calculated as follows:

OG = Measured osmolality − calculated osmolality

To calculate the contribution to measured osmolality of alcohols (also known as *osmol ratios*), the alcohol concentration (mg/dL) is divided by the numbers depicted in Table 16.7.

C. Digitalis Intoxication

To treat digitalis poisoning appropriately, it is important to assess the *digitalis body load*:

Body load (mg) = (serum digoxin concentration)

$\times 5.6 \times$ (body weight in kg) $\div 100$

The *dose of digitalis antibodies* (Digibind) is determined by dividing the body load by 0.6 mg/vial:

Dose (number of vials) = Body load (mg) $\div 0.6$ (mg/vial)

17

Trauma

Trauma is the leading cause of death in persons aged 1 to 44 years and the fourth leading cause of death overall. About 140,000 traumatic deaths occur annually. Sepsis, adult respiratory distress syndrome, and multiple organ system failure are the leading cause of death in trauma patients who survive the initial resuscitation and surgical repair of their injuries.

■ I. MULTISYSTEM TRAUMA

A. Establishment of Priorities
  1. Of highest priority in the initial evaluation are
    a. Airway maintenance
    b. Breathing and ventilation
    c. Circulation and shock management
  2. Secondary evaluation includes vital signs, complete physical (including rectal) examination. Nasogastric and urinary catheters (unless contraindicated) should generally be inserted to diagnose gastric or urinary tract hemorrhage and to allow for monitoring of urinary output.
  3. Rapid normalization of vital signs is one of the goals in trauma management.

B. Severity of Injury Scoring Systems
  1. The Glasgow coma scale (see Table 17.1) is used for assessing neurologic status in head injury.
  2. The Trauma Score (see Table 17.2) estimates physiologic severity of injury. It combines the Glasgow coma scale with other clinical indices of cardiovascular and pulmonary function.

Table 17.1. Glasgow Coma Scale

	SCORE
Eye opening	
Spontaneous	4
To verbal command	3
To pain	2
None	1
Best motor response	
Obeys verbal command	6
Localizes painful stimuli	5
Flexion withdrawal from painful stimuli	4
Decorticate (flexion) response to painful stimuli	
	3
Decerebrate (extension) response to painful stimuli	
	2
None	1
Best verbal response	
Oriented conversation	5
Disoriented conversation	4
Inappropriate words	3
Incomprehensible sounds	2
None	1
Total Score	3–15

C. Airway Management
1. Clear airway of debris or secretions
2. Avoid chin lift and neck lift/tilt if cervical spine injury is considered. Obtain cervical spine radiographs as soon as possible.

D. Oxygenation and Ventilation
1. If adequate respirations appear to be present, obtain baseline blood gases as soon as possible. Apply 100% O_2 by mask. If no spontaneous respirations, assist with bag and mask.
2. Endotracheal Intubation
   a. When necessary, intubation should usually be done by the oral route with manual in-line stabilization.
   b. Rapid-sequence induction is often indicated in patients with major trauma, head or facial injury, diminished level of consciousness, respiratory impairment: Preoxygenation, application of cricoid pressure, administration of induction agents (vecuronium 0.2 mg/kg IV, followed 3 minutes later by succinylcholine 1.0 to 1.5 mg/kg; succinylcholine is con-

Table 17.2. Trauma Score

	Points
Respiratory rate/minute	
10–24	4
25–35	3
>35	2
<10	1
0	0
Respiratory effort	
Normal	1
Shallow or retractive	0
Systolic blood pressure	
>90 mm Hg	4
70–90 mm Hg	3
50–69 mm Hg	2
<50 mm Hg	1
0	0
Capillary refill	
Normal	2
Delayed	1
None	0
Glasgow coma score	
14–15	5
11–13	4
8–10	3
5–7	2
3–4	1
Total	—

    traindicated in penetrating eye injuries, massive crush injury.), followed by intubation.

3. When a surgical airway is necessary, cricothyrotomy is the preferred procedure.
4. Most common causes for respiratory compromise: tension pneumothorax, open pneumothorax, flail chest with pulmonary contusion.

E. Circulation and Shock Management
1. Evaluation includes assessment of vital signs, level of consciousness, skin color, character of pulse, and capillary refill.
2. Shock in trauma is most commonly due to hypovolemia.
   a. Likely sites for occult hemorrhage: thorax, abdomen, pelvis, retroperitoneum, thigh.

Table 17.3. Classification of Hemorrhage

	Blood volume lost	Clinical signs
Class I	Up to 15%	Increased heart rate
Class II	15%–30%	Increased heart rate, decreased pulse pressure, minor delay in capillary refill, anxiety
Class III	30%–40%	Increased heart rate, decreased blood pressure, delayed capillary refill, clouded
Class IV	>40%	Markedly increased heart rate, sensorium decreased blood pressure, negligible urine output, markedly depressed mental status, skin cold and pale

    b. In addition, conditions producing shock that should be considered include tension pneumothorax, cardiac tamponade, myocardial contusion, spinal trauma.

3. Classification of hemorrhagic shock: see Table 17.3.
4. Treatment
    a. Class I hemorrhage: replacement of primary fluid loss with electrolyte solution.
    b. Class II hemorrhage: initial stabilization with intravenous (IV) fluids; may require blood transfusion.
    c. Class III hemorrhage: Almost always requires transfusion.
5. The patient should have at least two large-caliber (14- to 16-gauge or larger) IV lines established. Initial fluid administration should be with isotonic electrolyte solution.
    a. The administration rate should be commensurate with the clinical condition and vital signs. Fluid overload should be avoided, but adequate intravascular volume, hematocrit, and tissue perfusion must be achieved.
    b. In the hypovolemic patient, at least 2 L (20 mL/kg in a child) can be rapidly infused and the patient reassessed.
6. If shock persists despite resuscitation with IV fluids, blood replacement is indicated.
    a. Maintain a hematocrit of at least at 30%.
    b. Cross-matched blood is preferable if the patient's condition permits.

    c. If there is insufficient time for a full cross-match to be performed, type-specific (ABO and Rh compatible) blood should be administered.

    d. In patients in severe, life-threatening shock for whom type-specific blood is not available, administer type O blood (Rh negative in women of childbearing age). Subsequent cross-matching may be more difficult, however.

    e. Autotransfusion (especially administration of autologous blood from chest tube drainage) should be employed when feasible.

7. Monitor for possible complications of transfusion.

    a. Hemolytic transfusion reaction: fever, chills, and chest, back, and joint pain. Terminate transfusion, administer IV fluids and furosemide. Monitor urine output.

    b. Hypothermia may follow massive transfusion with refrigerated blood. Give blood through a warmer if possible. Monitor body temperature with a core probe.

    c. Coagulopathy may result following massive transfusion, probably on the basis of quantity and function of platelets, as well as consumption of coagulation factors. Administration of platelets is advised following rapid transfusion of each 10 U of blood. If evidence of coagulopathy exists, consider administration of fresh-frozen plasma and cryoprecipitate.

    d. Banked blood is acidemic and high in potassium, and preservative anticoagulant binds calcium. Monitor serum pH, potassium, magnesium, and calcium levels.

8. Monitor urine output: Volume replacement should produce urine output of at least 1 to 1.5 mL/kg/h.

F. Complications of Hemorrhagic Shock and Volume Resuscitation
Peripheral edema, hypothermia, cerebral edema, cardiac dysfunction (usually right ventricular failure), pneumonia, adult respiratory distress syndrome (ARDS), multisystem organ failure.

G. Cardiac Arrest

1. Perform immediate thoracotomy in patients in extremis, especially with penetrating chest trauma.

2. Therapeutic objectives include relief of cardiac tamponade, open cardiac massage, control of cardiac injuries, vascular control of major vessel or hilar injuries, and aortic occlusion for treatment of shock.

■ II. HEAD TRAUMA

Head injury is a major entity, often encountered in acute care, the head being the most frequently injured part of the body in trauma patients. Over 80,000 persons annually sustain permanent disabling injuries of the head or spinal cord.

- A. Assessment
  - 1. History
    - a. Important components are mechanism of injury and loss of consciousness. High-speed trauma (e.g., with ejection from vehicle, impact with windshield) produces a greater chance of significant injury.
    - b. Incomplete recollection by the patient of details of injury may imply a transient loss of consciousness. This symptom is not as useful if the patient is intoxicated.
  - 2. Physical Examination
    - a. Examine the scalp and face for signs of trauma, such as lacerations, ecchymoses, hemotympanum, and bleeding or clear fluid from the nostrils or ears.
    - b. Palpate the spine for tenderness or deformity. Always consider the possibility of concomitant spinal cord injury.
    - c. Focus on other injuries that affect the airway or produce respiratory or circulatory impairment.
  - 3. Neurologic Examination
    - a. This is the best tool for identifying the presence of significant intracranial injury.
      - (1) Assess the mental status (most important aspect of the neurologic examination).
      - (2) Determine focal neurologic deficit, abnormal posturing, and pathologic reflexes. Evaluate brain stem reflexes (light, corneal, gag) and ventilatory drive.
      - (3) The absence of brain stem function usually indicates the need for urgent airway intervention.
    - b. Frequent repetition of neurologic examination is necessary, especially within the first 48 hours of injury.
  - 4. Glasgow Coma Scale (GCS)
    - a. Determine the GCS score (see Table 17.1).
      - (1) Score of 13–15 = mild injury
      - (2) Score of 9–12 = moderate injury
      - (3) Score of 8 or less = severe injury
    - b. GCS is of limited usefulness in children <3 years.

B. Management
  1. Position
     When associated injuries permit, elevate the head of the bed 30 to 45 degrees, as this reduces intracranial pressure.
  2. Airway and Ventilation
     a. The highest initial priority is prevention or reduction of secondary injury due to swelling or compression of cerebral tissue by cerebral edema and raised intracranial pressure (ICP).
     b. Proper airway management reduces increased ICP. Diminished mental status (particularly a GCS score <9) is an indication for early endotracheal intubation.
     c. Chin lift and neck lift maneuvers are inappropriate if the patient with head injury is suspected of having cervical spine injury.
     d. Initial management of increased ICP includes hyperventilation.
        (1) It is often recommended to maintain arterial pCO_2 between 25 and 30 torr (mm Hg), but there is no uniform agreement on this.
        (2) Many recommend not to hyperventilate patients with $pCO_2 < 20$ torr or $pH > 7.60$.
     e. Endotracheal intubation.
        (1) Nasal intubation is relatively contraindicated; use orotracheal intubation with manual in-line stabilization.
        (2) Precede intubation with bag-valve-mask ventilation, cricoid pressure, and pharmacologic induction: lidocaine 1.5 mg/kg and succinylcholine 1.0 to 1.5 mg/kg, or vecuronium 0.1 to 0.2 mg/kg IV.
     f. When mechanical ventilation is instituted, avoid high levels (>10 cm) of positive end-expiratory pressure (PEEP), as this may increase ICP. Chest physiotherapy may also increase ICP.
  3. Osmotic Therapy and Diuresis
     a. Reduce increased ICP by reducing intracranial volume.
     b. Mannitol is the osmotic diuretic of choice. It is generally administered in rapidly deteriorating patients. It is often used to arrest neurologic deterioration when the patient is being prepared for urgent craniotomy.
        (1) Give as a 20% solution, 0.25 to 1.0 g/kg via rapid IV infusion.
        (2) ICP reduction usually occurs within 10 to 20 minutes.

    (3) Duration is limited to 2 to 6 hours following initial bolus. Continuous infusion may be required.

    (4) Monitor blood pressure, serum electrolytes, and osmolarity.

  c. Diuretics may be used alone or in combination with osmotic diuretics to reduce intracerebral fluid volume.

    (1) Furosemide is the loop diuretic of choice. Administer an IV bolus of 1 mg/kg. The onset of action is slower than mannitol, but concomitant use enhances the duration of ICP reduction by mannitol and decreases the risk of rebound ICP elevation. Repeated doses may be required.

    (2) Acetazolamide is a carbonic anhydrase inhibitor. It decreases cerebrospinal fluid (CSF) production. Administer 250 mg qid. Monitor for production of acidosis.

  d. Corticosteroids are frequently administered, but whether they diminish ICP in head trauma is controversial.

 4. Cardiovascular Support

  a. As a rule, cerebral injury does not produce hypotension (except in the agonal state).

  b. Look for an extracranial source if hypotension is present.

  c. Avoid fluid overload, but provide adequate intravascular volume and hematocrit. A pulmonary artery catheter may be required for monitoring.

C. Monitoring

 1. Intracranial Pressure

  a. Indicated in patients with severe head injury with computed tomography (CT) evidence of raised ICP. Monitoring of ICP, however, has not been proven to affect survival.

  b. Monitor by intraventricular catheter, subarachnoid bolt, or extradural pressure sensor.

  c. It is generally advised to maintain ICP at ≥ 20 mm Hg.

  d. Cerebral perfusion pressure (CPP): monitor this (CPP = mean arterial pressure [MAP] − ICP) and maintain at >60 mm Hg. If hypotension occurs, elevate arterial pressure to maintain CPP above this level, as ischemic damage may occur.

 2. Intravascular Pressure

  Arterial catheterization to allow monitoring of MAP as well as frequent blood gas determinations.

3. Head trauma may produce syndrome of inappropriate secretion of antidiuretic hormone (SIADH). This results in hyponatremia with a relatively concentrated urine (see also Chapters 9 and 14).

D. Diagnostic Studies
1. Skull Radiographs
   a. Plain skull radiographs may demonstrate skull fracture but have poor sensitivity and specificity for identifying intracranial lesions.
   b. May be useful in children <2 years of age, in whom skull fracture may identify risk of hypovolemia due to extracranial bleeding, formation of leptomeningeal cyst, and child abuse.
2. Computed Tomography
   a. CT is the diagnostic procedure of choice in assessing acute head injury. Perform CT without contrast material. CT is indicated in the patient with a decreased level of consciousness (GCS score ≤14), deteriorating mental status, focal neurologic deficit, seizures, or persistent vomiting.
   b. If the GCS score is <9, obtain CT immediately after endotracheal intubation when the patient is hemodynamically stable.
3. Magnetic Resonance Imaging (MRI)
   a. MRI is superior to CT in diffuse axonal injury.
   b. Limitations in acute injury: duration of scanning, interference of monitoring and life support equipment with magnetic field.
4. Ultrasound
   May be an option in smaller children with suspected intraventricular hemorrhage.

■ III. CRUSH INJURY

A. Traumatic Asphyxia
1. Mechanism: direct massive thoracoabdominal compression.
2. Clinical findings: blanching cyanosis of upper chest, neck and head; petechiae; edema; subconjunctival hemorrhage.
3. Associated injuries: chest wall injury, pulmonary contusion, cardiac contusion, diaphragm rupture, intra-abdominal solid and hollow viscus injury.
4. Sequelae: brachial plexus injury, spinal cord injury, transient neurologic impairment.

B. Abdominal and Pelvic Injury
   1. Crush injury accounts for 5% of pelvic fractures. May result in bladder laceration.
   2. Crush mechanism to the abdomen results in a high proportion of hollow viscus injury.

C. Skeletal Muscle Injury
   1. Results in myonecrosis. May produce rhabdomyolysis, hyperkalemia, hyperphosphatemia, hypocalcemia, and myoglobinuria.
   2. Sequelae include acute renal failure, disseminated intravascular coagulation.
   3. Follow creatine kinase (CK), electrolytes, creatinine, urine output.
   4. CK levels reach maximum 24 to 36 hours after injury. Level should decline by 50% each 48 hours thereafter. If there is an increase in CK during this time, consider recurrence of muscle necrosis.
   5. Treat acute renal failure with fluid infusion, osmotic diuresis, alkalinization (see Chapter 14).

■ IV. CHEST TRAUMA

Chest trauma is the cause of death in up to a quarter of cases of multisystem trauma. Injury may occur to the chest wall, lung, great vessels, and mediastinal viscera.

Most injuries can be initially managed with chest tube insertion and other nonoperative management.

Indications for thoracotomy include cardiac tamponade, massive hemothorax (see below); pulmonary air leak >15 to 20 L/min; aortic arch, esophageal, tracheal, or major bronchial disruption; systemic air embolism; bullet embolism; cardiac arrest.

A. Chest Wall Trauma
   1. Rib fracture is the most common chest wall injury. It is an important indicator of underlying injury.
      a. First to Third Ribs: great vessel and bronchial injury. Diminished pulse or blood pressure in arms or radiographic evidence of mediastinal hematoma (see below) are indications for arteriography.
      b. Lower Ribs: kidney, liver, spleen laceration.
   2. Flail chest occurs when three or more ribs fractured in two places or when multiple fractures are associated with sternal fracture.
      a. Clinical significance varies, depending upon the size and location of the flail segment and the extent of underlying pulmonary contusion.

    b. Obtain and follow arterial blood gases (ABGs).

    c. Splint thorax with weights, traction, or skeletal fixation.

    d. Patients with severe hypoxemia will require endotracheal intubation and positive-pressure ventilation. Observe for late development of pneumothorax, especially tension pneumothorax in the mechanically ventilated patient.

3. Sternal fracture is associated with myocardial contusion, cardiac rupture and tamponade, and pulmonary contusion. Early surgical fixation is often necessary, and urgent surgery may be indicated when costosternal dislocations produce compromise of the trachea or neurovascular structures at the thoracic inlet.

4. Analgesic methods that may be required for treatment of major chest wall injuries include parenteral opiates, epidural analgesia, and intercostal nerve block.

B. Pneumothorax

1. Usually results from penetrating trauma or blunt trauma with rib fracture. May be caused by positive-pressure ventilation (barotrauma).

2. Presence of pneumothorax requires 28–40 Fr chest tube insertion. Smaller tubes may be utilized if pneumothorax is not accompanied by hemothorax.

3. Open pneumothorax requires covering of chest wall injury with airtight dressing and insertion of chest tube.

4. Tension pneumothorax requires immediate needle decompression and chest tube insertion. Clinical findings include unilateral absence of breath sounds, severe dyspnea, tracheal shift, jugular venous distention, cyanosis.

C. Hemothorax

1. Initial treatment requires insertion of chest tube to evacuate hemothorax, reexpand lung, and monitor rate of bleeding.

2. Indications for thoracotomy include initial chest tube drainage of >1500 mL or continued bleeding of more than 300 mL/h for more than 2 to 3 hours.

D. Major Vessel Injury

1. Common cause of death in major trauma.

2. Consider when there is radiographic evidence of mediastinal hematoma: widened mediastinum, aortic knob obliteration, tracheal or nasogastric tube deviation.

3. Arteriography or CT is required for diagnosis.

E. Cardiac Tamponade

1. Most frequently occurs with penetrating injures. Suspect in chest trauma with shock and jugular venous distention.

    2. Requires thoracotomy and pericardial decompression. Pericardiocentesis may be performed if the diagnosis is uncertain or as a temporizing measure during preparation for thoracotomy.

F. Pulmonary Contusion

    Management consists of supplemental oxygen administration and mechanical ventilation with the addition of PEEP, if indicated in patients with worsening hypoxemia.

G. Myocardial Contusion

    Management consists of cardiac monitoring, echocardiography, and treatment of dysrhythmias as necessary.

■ V. ABDOMINAL TRAUMA

A. Evaluation

    1. Physical findings may be unreliable if abdominal trauma is complicated by head or other injury, or intoxication.

    2. Findings most consistently associated with internal abdominal injury are abdominal tenderness and guarding.

    3. Examine thorax for rib fractures, palpate flanks and pelvis, and perform rectal and pelvic examination.

    4. Obtain baseline hemogram, blood coagulation screen, and urinalysis.

B. Diagnostic Peritoneal Lavage (DPL)

    1. There is considerable variation in use of DPL from institution to institution.

    2. Indications may include equivocal abdominal findings, possible abdominal injury in the face of diminished sensation due to head or spinal injury, or alcohol intoxication.

    3. The major advantage is the ability to obtain a rapid indication of intraperitoneal hemorrhage.

    4. Relative contraindications: previous abdominal surgery, significant obesity, pregnancy, preexisting coagulopathy.

    5. Positive lavage consists of aspiration of >10 mL of blood, aspiration of enteric contents, or lavage fluid with red blood cell levels >100,000/mm^3, white blood cells >500/mm^3, amylase ≤20 IU/L, or bile.

C. Abdominal CT

    1. Indicated in stable patients with possible intraabdominal injury, and where DPL is being considered but is contraindicated.

    2. Advantages include ability to visualize urinary tract and retroperitoneum.

D. Penetrating Injury
   1. Antibiotics
      a. Second- or third-generation cephalosporin, e.g., cefoxitin 2 g IV q6h, or ceftazidime 1 to 2 g IV q8h, or
      b. Combination of gentamicin (1.5 to 2.0 mg/kg IV loading and 3 mg/kg/d in 3 maintenance doses) or tobramycin (1 mg/kg q8h IV) and clindamycin 600 to 900 mg q8h IV

E. Indications for Laparotomy
   1. Gunshot wounds.
   2. Stab wounds with shock, signs of peritoneal irritation, gastrointestinal bleeding, or evisceration of bowel.
   3. Blunt trauma with unstable vital signs, gastrointestinal bleeding, peritoneal irritation, pneumoperitoneum, evidence of diaphragmatic injury.
   4. There may be a role for laparoscopy in the stable patient with penetrating injury, but this method has not been used extensively in this setting.

F. Postoperative Complications
   1. Intraabdominal hemorrhage
      a. May be due to recurrent bleeding from sites not identified during surgery due to hypotension.
      b. Identify hemostasis deficiencies (thrombocytopenia, clotting dysfunction) especially if patient has had massive transfusions.
      c. If prothrombin time (PT) and partial thromboplastin time (PTT) are prolonged, administer fresh-frozen plasma.
   2. Fever: Consider wound infection, necrotizing fasciitis, peritonitis, and intraabdominal abscess.
   3. Missed intraabdominal injury: diaphragm, biliary tree, duodenum, pancreas, ureter, colon, and rectum.

G. Nonoperative Management
   1. May be suitable in patients who remain hemodynamically stable following initial resuscitation with 1 to 2 L of IV fluids. Laparoscopic repair may be another option.
      a. Normal vital signs, urine output >1.0 to 1.5 mL/h and no blood requirement.
      b. Patient must be alert.
      c. No coagulation defects.
   2. CT should establish extent of injury.
   3. Suitable injuries include
      a. Isolated splenic trauma with minor capsular tear or parenchymal injury
      b. Stab wounds without shock, peritoneal irritation, or gastrointestinal bleeding

4. Monitoring
   a. Repeat abdominal examination for signs of peritoneal irritation at least every 4 to 6 hours.
   b. Vital signs monitored every 1 to 2 hours during the first 24 hours.
   c. Serial hematocrit every 4 hours. Also monitor amylase.
   d. Repeat abdominal CT after 12 hours of observation and thereafter as indicated by clinical signs.

H. Urinary Tract Injury
   1. Evaluate with IVP or abdominal CT if gross hematuria, flank hematoma or mass, penetrating trauma with suspected urinary injury.
   2. Bladder and urethra injury: see pelvic fracture.

■ VI. MULTIPLE FRACTURES

A. General Considerations
   1. Identify fractures and dislocations, and assess distal neurocirculatory function.
   2. Complications of fractures include arterial and neural injury, hemorrhage, compartment syndrome, ARDS, fat embolization, infection, and thromboembolism.
   3. Fractures of the pelvis and femur are particularly significant because of hemorrhage potential.
   4. Dislocations of the hip and knee require prompt reduction to avoid neurovascular complications.

B. Initial Management
   1. Immobilize any injured extremity.
   2. Stabilize femur fracture in Hare or comparable traction device.

C. Arterial Injury
   1. Arterial injury may be due to transection, arterial spasm, occlusion by hematoma, external compression, arteriovenous fistula formation.
   2. Acute loss of vascular function requires emergent surgical exploration or angiography.

D. Compartment Syndrome
   1. Circulatory supply can be lost due to increased muscular compartment pressure. Most common in leg but also occurs in forearm.
   2. Earliest sign is pain with passive stretching of the extremity. Suspect if there is severe, constant pain despite reduction and immobilization.

3. Measure compartment pressure by inserting a needle connected to a manometric pressure measurement system into the soft tissue of the extremity involved; should be <30 mm Hg in the normotensive pressure.
4. Treatment is fasciotomy.

E. Infection in Open Injuries
1. Tetanus prophylaxis should be given, especially for wounds with deep tissue penetration, devitalized tissue, and burns.
2. IV antibiotics.
   a. IV first-generation cephalosporin (e.g., cefazolin 1 g IV q6h)
   b. If the wound is large or heavily contaminated, add gentamicin (1.5 to 2.0 mg/kg IV loading dose and 3 mg/kg/d in 3 maintenance doses or tobramycin (1 mg/kg q8h IV or 3 mg/kg IV single dose) if the patient has normal renal function.
3. Observe for appearance of gas gangrene (appearance of subcutaneous crepitation or soft tissue gas on radiographs).
   a. Occurs within 12 to 72 hours of injury and requires broad-spectrum antibiotics and aggressive wound debridement.
   b. Most often occurs in grossly contaminated open fractures with soft tissue damage.

F. Fat Embolism
1. Occurs most commonly in multiple fractures, especially involving femur, tibia, pelvis.
2. Onset of symptoms occurs 1 to 5 days following injury: tachypnea, hemoptysis, fever, petechiae, mental status change.
3. Hypoxemia (PaO_2 < 60 mm Hg on room air) is the most consistent finding.
4. Treatment includes correction of hypoxemia and ventilatory support with PEEP used if arterial oxygenation cannot be maintained. Management is similar to that of ARDS (see Chapter 13). Maintain a negative fluid balance. A pulmonary artery catheter may be required for management.

G. Pelvic Fracture
Pelvic fractures caused by high-energy forces have significant mortality. Hemorrhage is a major cause, as are associated injuries, sepsis, multiple organ failure, and ARDS.

Infection of pelvic hematoma may occur even in closed injuries due to hematogenous spread of bacteria.
1. Evaluation
   a. Physical Examination

   (1) Palpate pelvis to determine tenderness and instability.

   (2) Perform pelvic and rectal examination to ascertain open injury and sphincter tone.

   (3) Blood at urethral meatus or high-riding prostate on rectal examination indicates urethral tear.

  b. Radiographs

   (1) Obtain pelvic radiographs in patients suspected of sustaining pelvic fracture and in patients with multiple trauma.

   (2) CT is superior in demonstrating certain aspects of pelvic injury. Utilize in the stable patient.

 2. Hemorrhage

  a. Usually retroperitoneal, the result of venous injury to pelvic venous plexus. May be massive, exceeding several liters.

  b. Signs of persistent bleeding are an indication for external fixation of unstable pelvic fractures.

  c. Application of pneumatic antishock trousers may be helpful in temporarily controlling hemorrhage (although there is considerable controversy over efficacy). Once antishock trousers are in place, do not remove until vascular access is established and blood pressure stabilized.

  d. Consider arteriography and selective embolization for patient with continued severe hemorrhage.

 3. Associated Injuries

  a. Injuries to consider: urinary bladder perforation, vaginal or rectal laceration, posterior urethral tear.

  b. If signs of urethral injury are present, a retrograde urethrogram should be used to ascertain integrity of the urethra before urinary catheter insertion.

■ VII. SPINAL CORD INJURY

Spinal injury should be considered in any patient with multisystem injury, head or facial injury, and those who are unconscious. Maintain spinal immobilization until radiographs exclude spinal injury.

 A. Evaluation

  1. Perform a neurologic examination to determine the extent and level of injury.

   a. Examine and document motor function and sensory level.

      b. Determine if there is sacral sensory sparing or anal sphincter contraction, signs that cord injury is incomplete.

      c. Sacral reflexes (anal wink, bulbocavernosus reflex) are the first to return after spinal shock, usually within 24 hours following injury.

B. Management

   1. Endotracheal Intubation

      a. Patients may require endotracheal intubation because of paralysis of respiratory muscles.

      b. If intubation is necessary, it should be done with in-line cervical immobilization.

      c. The orotracheal approach is preferred, preceded by 100% oxygenation by mask and application of gentle cricoid pressure.

      d. Administer thiopental 25 to 200 mg and vecuronium 0.1 to 0.2 mg/kg IV or etomidate 0.3 to 0.6 µg/kg before intubation.

   2. Respiratory Care

      a. Monitor breathing with frequent vital capacity measurement. Vital capacity <10 mL/kg is an indication for ventilatory assistance.

      b. Monitor arterial blood gases for hypoxemia or hypercarbia.

   3. Corticosteroids

      a. High-dose steroid therapy is generally accepted as reducing secondary injury if started within 8 hours of injury.

      b. Administer methylprednisolone initial IV bolus 30 mg/kg followed by 5.4 mg/kg/h for the next 23 hours.

      c. Naloxone (5.4 mg/kg IV followed by infusion of 4 mg/kg/h for the following 23 hours) is frequently used in addition to corticosteroids, though its effectiveness has not been proven.

   4. Neurogenic Shock

      a. Results from injury to descending sympathetic pathways (usually in cervical and thoracic cord injuries) with loss of vasomotor tone and sympathetic cardiac innervation.

      b. Result is hypotension due to vasodilation and bradycardia, which may last for days to weeks.

      c. Administer IV fluids for initial treatment of hypotension. If hypotension persists, administer phenylephrine or dopamine.

      d. Atropine (0.5 mg) or isoproterenol may be given if heart rate <45 beats per minute.

5. Abdominal
   a. Insert a nasogastric tube for ileus and acute gastric dilatation.
   b. In patients with abdominal trauma, consider diagnostic testing (DPL or CT) to determine intraabdominal injury.
6. Urologic
   a. A bladder catheter should be in place for at least 4 days following injury, or until other injuries are stabilized and urine output is no longer being followed. After this, intermittent catheterization may be started.
   b. Tape the catheter up over the pubis to prevent urethral traction injury.
7. Traction Immobilization
   a. Traction with Garner-Wells tongs may be required to immobilize and align cervical injuries.
      (1) Weight required varies with injury.
      (2) Perform a neurologic examination, and take radiographs frequently to determine that the alignment is correct and overdistraction does not occur.
8. Autonomic Hyperreflexia
   a. Autonomic hyperreflexia is the result of increased autonomic nervous system (primarily sympathetic) activity caused by noxious stimulus from below the level of the cord lesion.
   b. Produces paroxysmal hypertension, headache, sweating, bradycardia or tachycardia, and anisocoria.
   c. Most common cause: bladder distention. Others: fecal impaction, urinary tract infection, ureterolithiasis.
   d. Treatment: Treat underlying cause (e.g., catheterize bladder). Anticholinergic drugs may be used.

■ VIII. USEFUL FACTS AND FORMULAS

A. Hemorrhage

To assess the intravascular volume resuscitation needed in a trauma patient, *normal blood volumes* according to age need to be known (see Table 17.4).

The *severity of hemorrhage* in a trauma patient can be classified as shown in Table 17.5.

To estimate how much whole blood or packed red blood cells (PRBCs) must be administered to change the hematocrit percentage to a desired amount in a trauma patient, the following formula can be utilized:

Table 17.4. Normal Blood Volumes According to Age

Normal blood volumes by age	
Newborn	85 mL/kg
Infant	80 mL/kg
Child	75 mL/kg
Adult	70 mL/kg

Table 17.5. Severity of Hemorrhage Classification Trauma Patients

Severity of hemorrhage	Blood pressure (mmHg)	Blood loss (cc)	Plasma volume (cc)
Normal	120/80	—	5000
Class I	120/80	<750	4600
Class II	115/80	1000–1250	3800
Class III	90/70	1500–1800	3200
Class IV	60/40	2000–2500	2500

$$\text{Transfusion required (mL)} = \text{Desired change in Hct} \\ \times \text{kg} \times \text{factor}$$

where Hct = hematocrit; factor = varies with the volume of blood per body weight (adults and children >2 years, a factor of 1 will achieve a Hct of 70% using PRBCs and 1.75 to achieve a Hct of 40% using whole blood).

B. Burns

Several formulas guide the initial fluid resuscitation after burn injuries. Below are the most common formulas used in clinical practice. In all these formulas, 50% of calculated volume is given during the first 8 hours, 25% of calculated volume is given during the second 8 hours, and 25% of calculated volume is given during the third 8 hours.

The *Evans formula* can be calculated as follows:

$$\text{Evans formula} = 1\,\text{mL crystalloid/kg/\% burn/24h}$$
$$1\,\text{mL crystalloid/kg/\% burn/24h}$$
$$2000\,\text{mL } D_5W/24h$$

The *Brooke formula* and the *modified Brooke formula* are calculated as follows:

$$\text{Brooke formula: } 1.5\,\text{mL crystalloid/kg/\% burn/24h}$$
$$0.5\,\text{mL colloid/kg/\% burn/24h}$$
$$2000\,\text{mL } D_5W/24h$$

Table 17.6. The Abbreviated Injury Scale

AIS score	Injury severity
1	Minor
2	Moderate
3	Serious, non-life-threatening
4	Severe, life-threatening
5	Critical
6	Maximal (correlates with death)

Modified formula = 2 mL Ringer's lactate/kg/% burn/24 h

The *Parkland formula* is calculated as

Parkland formula = 4 mL crystalloid/kg/% burn/24 h

In addition to these formulas, the evaporative water losses in patients with burns need to be calculated and replaced. *Evaporative water loss* (EWL) is calculated as

EWL(mL/h) = (25 + % BSA burned) × BSA

where BSA = body surface area.

C. Other Trauma Scoring Systems

Several trauma scoring systems are in use throughout the world. Of them, the *abbreviated injury scale* (AIS) is commonly utilized (see Table 17.6).

The *trauma score* (TS) is another commonly utilized system and is depicted in Table 17.7.

The *revised trauma score* (RTS) eliminates the assessment of capillary refill and respiratory effort and is calculated as follows:

RTS = 0.9368 GCS + 0.7326 SBP + 0.2908 RR coded values × revised score coefficient

where GCS = Glasgow coma scale; SBP = systolic blood pressure; RR = respiratory rate.

For children and infants, the *pediatric trauma score* is utilized (see Table 17.8).

D. Neurological Trauma

Within the primary survey, an early neurological trauma evaluation can be accomplished using the *AVPU method*:

A = *a*lert
V = responds to *v*erbal stimulation
P = responds to *p*ainful stimulation
U = *u*nresponsive

Table 17.7. The Trauma Score

Variable	Measurements	Score
Respiratory rate (bpm)	10–24	4
	25–35	3
	>35	2
	<10	1
	0	0
Respiratory effort	Shallow	1
	retractions	0
Systolic blood pressure (mm Hg)	>90	4
	70–90	3
	50–69	2
	<50	1
	0	0
Capillary refill	Normal	2
	Delayed	1
	Absent	0
Glasgow coma scale	14–15	5
	11–13	4
	8–10	3
	5–7	2
	3–4	1

Abbreviation: bpm, beats per minute.

Table 17.8. The Pediatric Trauma Score

Variable	+2	+1	−1
Weight (lb)	>20	10–20	<10
Airway	Normal	Maintained	Nonmaintained
Systolic BP (mm Hg)	>90	50–90	<50
CNS function	Awake	Obtunded	Coma
Open wound	None	Minor	Major
Skeletal trauma	None	Closed	Open or multiple

In those patients with severe head injuries and ICP monitoring, *cerebral perfusion pressure* (CPP) is commonly utilized in management:

CPP = MAP = ICP

where MAP = mean arterial blood pressure; ICP = intracranial pressure.

Another useful formula in neurological trauma is that of the calculation of the *pressure-volume index* (PVI), which is defined as the volume (in milliliters) necessary to raise the cerebrospinal fluid (CSF) pressure by a factor of 10:

$$PVI = \frac{\Delta V}{\log_{10}(Pp/P_0)}$$

where ΔV = volume change in the lateral ventricle using a ventricular cannula; P_0 = initial ICP; Pp = peak ICP.

18

Allergic and Immunologic Emergencies

■ I. ANAPHYLAXIS

A. Definition

Anaphylaxis is an immediate, generalized, life-threatening reaction resulting from the release of bioactive substances from mast cells and basophils.

B. Etiology

The most common causes of anaphylaxis in medical practice are depicted in Table 18.1.

C. Clinical Manifestations
1. The onset may vary from individual to individual depending on the sensitivity of the person and the route, quantity, and rate of administration of the allergen.
2. Early signs and symptoms that require a high index of suspicion may include
   a. Agitation
   b. Dizziness
   c. Headache
   d. Nausea, vomiting
3. Cutaneous involvement
   a. Generalized pruritus
   b. Flushing
   c. Urticaria
4. Upper airway obstruction as a consequence of edema of the larynx, swelling of tongue and lips (angioedema). This may result in stridor and suffocation.

Table 18.1. Common Causes of Systemic Anaphylactic Reactions

1. Drugs
    — Antibiotics (i.e., penicillins, cephalosporins, sulfonamides, vancomycin)
    — Local anesthetics (i.e., lidocaine, procaine)
    — Muscle relaxants
    — Others (i.e., insulin, protamine)

2. Foods
    — Nuts and seeds
    — Fish, shellfish
    — Milk, eggs

3. Food Additives
    — Aspartame
    — Monosodium glutamate

4. Diagnostics
    — Iodinated radiographic materials

5. Insect and snakes (stings and bites)

6. Exercise

7. Other
    — Latex gloves
    — Heterologous serum (i.e., tetanus antitoxin)

5. Respiratory failure (manifestations range from tachypnea to apnea) that may be related to the factors mentioned above as well as bronchoconstriction of the lower airways manifested by wheezing. These patients may also develop adult respiratory distress syndrome (ARDS).

6. Cardiovascular collapse: The pathophysiology is thought to be related to enhanced vascular permeability, peripheral vasodilation, and intravascular volume depletion. A heart rate increase >20 bpm from baseline and a decrease of mean arterial pressure >20 torr (mm Hg) are characteristic.

7. Dysrhythmias: Both supraventricular and ventricular rhythm disorders have been described in patients with anaphylaxis.

D. Laboratory Findings
    1. Do not wait for laboratory data to institute therapy!
    2. Patients with anaphylaxis may present with leukocytosis or leukopenia.
    3. Thrombocytopenia may appear in severe cases.

4. Immunoglobulin E (IgE) measurements may not be helpful, because many patients may manifest non-IgE-mediated anaphylaxis.

E. Management
  1. ABCs
     Secure the airway, and assist with breathing and circulation as with any other patient presenting with a potentially critical illness.
  2. The drug of choice for patients with acute anaphylaxis is epinephrine. The dosage is 0.3 to 0.5 mL of 1:1000 dilution (0.3 to 0.5 mg) subcutaneously every 10 to 20 minutes, or intravenously as described below.
  3. Antihistamines
     Traditionally, H_1-receptor antihistamines have been used; i.e., diphenhydramine (Benadryl) 25 to 50 mg intramuscularly (IM), intravenously (IV), or PO q6–8h. In theory, the combination of H_1- and H_2-receptor antihistamines might be a better chance of preventing further histamine-mediated reactions than H_1 blockers alone; i.e., cimetidine (Tagamet) 300 mg IV or PO q6h.
  4. Corticosteroids have an uncertain place in the management of acute reaction, since there is a 4- to 6-hour latent period before such agents are pharmacologically effective. The current recommended agents are hydrocortisone (Solucortef) 250 mg IV q6h or methylprednisolone (Solumedrol) 50 mg IV q6h for 2 to 4 doses.
  5. In cases of severe bronchospasm, the following drugs can be used:
     a. Metaproterenol 0.3 mL (5% solution) in 2.5 mL of saline, inhaled through a nebulizer
     b. Aminophylline loading dose of 6 mg/kg IV over 30 minutes followed by 0.3 to 0.9 mg/kg/h
  6. In patients with profound hypotension
     a. Adequate IV fluid administration (up to 1 L every 20 to 30 minutes as needed).
     b. Epinephrine 1 mL of 1:1000 dilution in 500 mL of D_5W at a rate of 0.5 to 5 μg (0.25 to 2.5 mL)/min.
     c. Norepinephrine (Levophed): 4 mg in 1 L of D_5W at a rate of 2 to 12 μg (0.5 to 3 mL)/min.
     d. Glucagon may be particularly useful in patients taking beta-adrenergic blockers. The recommended dose is 1 mg in 1 L of D_5W at a rate of 5 to 15 μg (5 to 15 mL)/min.

F. Preventive measures for patients at high risk of anaphylaxis are depicted in Table 18.2.

Table 18.2. Preventive Measures for Patients at High Risk for Anaphylaxis

1. Avoid exposure

2. Slow administration of suspected agents under medical supervision in adequate facility (i.e., ICU)

3. Optimal management of underlying disorders

4. Short- and long-term desensitization (i.e., penicillin, aspirin)

■ II. STEVENS-JOHNSON SYNDROME (ERYTHEMA MULTIFORME)

A. Definition

Erythema multiforme (EM) is an erythematous maculopapular cutaneous eruption of variable form. When EM grades into a more serious clinical state, the term Stevens-Johnson syndrome (SJS) is used.

B. Etiology

Common causes of EM and SJS are depicted in Table 18.3.

C. Clinical Manifestations

1. Prodromal symptoms may include
   a. Malaise, headache
   b. Pharyngitis, rhinorrhea
   c. Diarrhea
   d. Arthralgias
2. The earliest lesions in EM are often red, edematous papules surrounded by blanching. They enlarge to form small plaques with concentric alterations in color and morphology.
3. The so-called "Target" lesions are areas of central epidermal necrosis with or without bullae formation.
4. Patients admitted to the ICU with SJS usually present with extensive tissue necrosis and severe fluid depletion.

D. Laboratory Findings

1. Usually nondiagnostic.
2. Skin biopsy reveals a perivascular lymphocytic infiltrate in the upper dermis, subepidermal bullae formation, and endothelial cell swelling.

E. Management

1. Immediately discontinue suspected drugs or agents as well as all *nonessential* drugs.

Table 18.3. Causes of Erythema Multiforme/Stevens-Johnson Syndrome

1. Infections
   - Viral (i.e., herpes simplex, measles, hepatitis B)
   - Bacterial (i.e., streptococcus, pseudomonas)
   - Mycobacterial (i.e., tuberculosis)
   - Spirochetes (i.e., syphilis)
   - Fungal (i.e., histoplasmosis)

2. Drugs
   - Analgesics (i.e., aspirin, nonsteroidal anti-inflammatory drugs)
   - Antibiotics (i.e., sulfonamides, penicillins, tetracycline)
   - Anticonvulsants (i.e., ethosuximide)
   - Antihypertensives (i.e., minoxidil)
   - Glucocorticoids
   - H_2-blockers (i.e., cimetidine)

3. Immunizations
   - Horse serum
   - Polio vaccine
   - Pertussis vaccine

4. Neoplasms (i.e., lymphomas)

5. Connective tissue disorders (i.e., lupus erythematosus)

6. Physical agents
   - Radiation therapy
   - Sunlight

7. Others
   - Inflammatory bowel disease
   - Sarcoidosis

2. The usefulness of systemic corticosteroids in this setting is controversial. In the absence of controlled clinical trials, some authors recommend beginning therapy with prednisone 1 mg/kg/d (or IV equivalent).
3. Fluid replacement as indicated by severity of the disease.
4. Evaluate for infection, and treat appropriately.
5. Obtain consultation depending on the degree and sites of involvement (i.e., ophthalmology, plastic surgery).

■ III. ANGIONEUROTIC LARYNGEAL EDEMA

A. Definition

Angioneurotic laryngeal edema (ALE) is characterized by nonpruritic local swelling involving the face, larynx, and skin of the extremities.

B. Etiology
   1. Allergic
      Related to foods (i.e., fish), drugs (i.e., angiotensin-converting enzyme [ACE] inhibitors), inhaled substances, insect stings (i.e., bees).
   2. Hereditary
      Caused by a deficiency in C_1-esterase inhibitor. Autosomal dominant. Precipitating events may include trauma and emotional stress.

C. Clinical Manifestations
   1. Swelling of face, larynx, and skin of extremities.
   2. Depending on the progression, stridor may be a prominent feature with ensuing respiratory distress.
   3. Abdominal pain, nausea, and vomiting.

D. Laboratory Findings
   Nondiagnostic except in cases of hereditary ALE.

E. Management
   1. ABCs
      Secure the airway, and assist with breathing and circulation as with any other patient presenting with a potentially critical illness.
   2. Avoid precipitating allergens.
   3. If ALE is thought to be allergic in origin, administer parenteral epinephrine and antihistamines (as noted in "Anaphylaxis," above).
   4. Intubation is only rarely required for patients with allergic ALE, while in patients with hereditary ALE, the treatment of the acute episode may require urgent intubation or tracheostomy.

Pharmacologic Agents Commonly Used in the ICU

Acetaminophen (Tylenol):
Route: PO, PR
Dosage: 325 to 650 mg q4–6h (adults), 60 mg/kg/24h in divided doses
q4–6h (children)

Acetazolamide (Diamox):
Route: PO, IV
Dosage: Metabolic alkalosis, 250 mg q6–12h
Altitude sickness, 250 mg q6–24h

Acetylcysteine (Mucomyst):
Route: PO, IV, nebulized
Dosage: For acetaminophen toxicity
PO: Dilute to 5% with cola or other soft drink. Initial dose
140 mg/kg, then 70 mg/kg for 17 doses (do not give activated
charcoal).
IV: Load with 150 mg/kg in 200 mL D_5W over 15 minutes, then
50 mg/kg in 500 mL D_5W over 4 hours, followed by 100 mg/kg
in 100 mL D_5W over 16 hours.

Activated Charcoal (Charcoaid):
Route: PO
Dosage: For poisoning
Initial: 30 to 100 g (1 g/kg) in 250 mL water
Maintenance: 20 to 40 g q6h until drug removed from body

Adenosine (Adenocard):
Route: IV
Dosage: 3, 6, 9, 12 mg (fast IV injection)

Ammonium Chloride (generic):
Route: PO, IV
Dosage: Urine acidification, 4 to 12 g/d PO in divided doses q4–6h

Amrinone (Inocor):
Route: IV
Dosage: Bolus, 0.75 to 3 mg/kg over 2 to 3 minutes, followed by infusion of 5 to 20 μg/kg/min

Atropine (generic):
Route: PO, IV
Dosage: Bronchospasm, 1.5 to 2.0 mg by nebulizer q6h
Bradycardia, 0.5- to 1-mg IV push, repeat q5min to max. 2 mg

Bretylium (Bretylol):
Route: IV, IM
Dosage: Bolus, 5 to 10 mg/kg over 10 to 20 minutes IV, followed by a continuous infusion 1 to 5 mg/min

Carbicarb (Carbicarb):
Route: IV
Dosage: Severe acidosis, initial dose 1 mEq/kg, followed by 0.5 mEq/kg (adjust dose as indicated by clinical condition and blood pH)

Chlordiazepoxide (Librium):
Route: PO, IV, IM
Dosage: 15 to 100 mg/d in 3 to 4 divided doses

Chlorpromazine (Thorazine):
Route: PO, PR, IM
Dosage: Severe psychosis with agitation, 25 to 100 mg IM q1–4h until control is achieved

Clonidine (Catapres):
Route: PO, transdermal (In some countries IM and PR used)
Dosage: Hypertensive emergencies, 0.2 mg PO, then 0.1 mg/h to 0.7 mg or until BP is controlled

Dantrolene (Dantrium):
Route: PO, IV
Dosage: Malignant hyperthermia, initial dose 1 to 2 mg/kg IV via rapid infusion; may repeat to total 10 mg/kg if needed

dDAVP (generic):
Route: Intranasal, IV, SC
Dosage: Hemostasis, 0.3 μg/kg in NS over 15 to 30 minutes
Diabetes insipidus, 0.5 to 1 mL IV/SC bid

Diazepam (Valium):
Route: PO, IV, IM
Dosage: Status epilepticus, 5 to 10 mg IV (1 to 2 mg/min)

Diazoxide (Hyperstat):
Route: PO, IV
Dosage: Hypertensive crisis, 1 to 3 mg/kg IV (max 150 mg) q5–15min until BP is controlled

Digoxin (Lanoxin):
  Route: PO, IV, IM
  Dosage: Digitalization, 0.4 to 0.6 mg IV (may require up to 1.25 mg total); maintenance, 0.125 to 0.25 mg/d PO or IV

Dobutamine (Dobutrex):
  Route: IV
  Dosage: 2.5 to 15 µg/kg/min most commonly used

Dopamine (Inotropin):
  Route: IV
  Dosage: Dopaminergic stimulation, 0.5 to 2.0 µg/kg/min
      Alpha-, beta-dopaminergic effects, >10 µg/kg/min

Epinephrine (Epinephrine Injection):
  Route: IV, SC
  Dosage: $Beta_1$-, $beta_2$-effect, 1 to 4 µg/min
      Alpha-effects, 4 µg/min

Esmolol (Brevibloc):
  Route: IV
  Dosage: Bolus 0.5 to 1.0 mg/kg, followed by infusion at 50 µg/kg/min; maintenance 50 to 200 µg/kg/min

Fenoldopam (Corlopam):
  Route: IV
  Dosage: 0.1 to 1.0 µg/kg/min, titrate to achieve desired blood pressure

Fentanyl (Sublimaze):
  Route: IV, IM
  Dosage: Sedation/analgesia, 1 µg/kg IV/IM

Flumazenil (Romazicon):
  Route: IV
  Dosage: 0.3 mg IV

Furosemide (Lasix):
  Route: PO, IV, IM
  Dosage: 10 to 120 mg IV/IM, adjusted as necessary until desired response obtained. May use continuous infusions.

Glucagon (generic):
  Route: SC, IM, IV
  Dosage: Hypoglycemia, 0.5 to 1.0 mg SC/IM/IV, may repeat in 15 minutes
      Bradycardia, 1 to 20 mg/h

Haloperidol (Haldol):
  Route: PO, IM, IV (not FDA approved)
  Dosage: Acute psychosis, 2 to 5 mg IM q1–2h until symptoms are controlled

Heparin (Liquaenim):
Route: IV, SC
Dosage: DVT prophylaxis, 5000 U SC q8–12h
DVT/Pulmonary emboli therapy, bolus with 100 U/kg followed by a continuous infusion of 800 to 1200 U/h, titrated to maintain aPTT $1\frac{1}{2}$ to 2 times control

Hydralazine (Apresoline):
Route: PO, IV
Dosage: 5-mg IV bolus; 5- to 10-mg IV q6h maintenance

Isoproterenol (Isuprel):
Route: IV, SC, PO, inhaled
Dosage: Infusion 1 to 10 μg/min

Ketorolac Tromethamine (Toradol):
Route: PO, IM
Dosage: Initial dose 30 to 60 mg IM, then 15 to 30 mg q6h

Labetalol (Normodyne):
Route: PO, IV
Dosage: Rapid BP control, IV bolus 5 to 20 mg (slowly); repeat after 5 minutes if needed. Continuous infusion of 1 mg/mL started at 1 to 2 mg/min, and titrated to effect.

Lidocaine (Xylocaine):
Route: IV, IM, SC
Dosage: Bolus 1.0 to 1.5 mg/kg followed by 1 to 4 mg/min

Lorazepam (Ativan):
Route: PO, IV, IM
Dosage: 2 to 10 mg/d in divided doses PO/IV/IM (some patients may require continuous infusions).

Mannitol (Osmitrol):
Route: IV
Dosage: For cerebral edema, IV infusion 0.15 to 2.0 g/kg as 15% to 25% solution over 30 to 60 minutes; max. dose is up to 6 g/kg/24h.

Meperidine (Demerol):
Route: PO, IM, IV, SC
Dosage: 50 to 150 mg q3–4h

Midazolam (Versed):
Route: IV, IM
Dosage: 1 to 4 mg q2–6h

Morphine (Duramorph):
Route: IM, IV, PO, PR
Dosage: 5 to 10 mg q4–6h (some patients may require continuous infusions).

Naloxone (Narcan):
  Route: IV, IM, SC
  Dosage: 0.4 to 2.0 mg IV; may repeat up to 10 mg. Continuous IV
  infusion at 4 to 5 µg/kg/min.

Nitroglycerin (Nitroglycerin):
  Route: PO, IV, SL, topical
  Dosage: 10 to 400 µg/min IV

Norepinephrine (Levophed):
  Route: IV
  Dosage: 4 to 10 µg/min

Phenobarbital (Barbita):
  Route: PO, PR, IM, IV
  Dosage: Status epilepticus, 10 mg/kg IV at 50 mg/min; up to 20 mg/kg
  total (adults)

Phentolamine (Regitine):
  Route: IV, IM
  Dosage: 5 mg IV/IM prn, taper to effect (adult); 0.1 mg/kg IV prn
  (pediatric).

Phenylephrine (Neo-Synephrine):
  Route: IV
  Dosage: 15 mg dissolved in 250 mL D_5W (60 µg/mL); start at 20 to
  30 µg/min, titrate to desired BP

Procainamide (Procainamide):
  Route: PO, IV
  Dosage: 100 mg/min IV to effect or to total dose of 1000 mg,
  followed by infusion 2 to 6 mg/min

Prochlorperazine (Compazine):
  Route: PO, IM, IV, PR
  Dosage: 5 to 10 mg PO tid/qid; 5 to 10 mg IV q3–4h; 25 mg PR bid

Propofol (Diprivan):
  Route: IV
  Dosage: 2 to 15 cc/h by continuous infusion to achieve the desired
  level of sedation

Propranolol (Inderal):
  Route: PO, IV
  Dosage: Titrate 0.5 to 1.0 mg IV q5min to effect.

Protamine (Protamine sulfate):
  Route: IV
  Dosage: 1 mg for each 90 U of lung heparin or 1 mg for each 115 U
  intestinal heparin, by slow injection over 1 to 3 minutes; max.
  dose 50 mg in 10 minutes.

Sodium Bicarbonate (Sodium Bicarbonate Injection):
  Route: IV, PO
  Dosage: Severe acidosis, initial dose 1 mEq/kg, followed by 0.5 mEq/kg; adjust dosage as indicated by clinical condition and blood pH.

Sodium Nitroprusside (Nipride):
  Route: IV
  Dosage: Mix 50 mg in 250 mL D_5W. Start at 0.5 µg/kg/min and titrate to effect.

Sodium Polystyrene Sulfonate (Kayexelate):
  Route: PO, PR
  Dosage: 15 g, PO q6–24h

Succinylcholine (Anectine):
  Route: IV, IM
  Dosage: 1 to 1.5 mg/kg IV; 2 to 4 mg/kg IM (pediatric use only)

Thiopental (Pentothal sodium):
  Route: IV, PR
  Dosage: General anesthetic, 2 to 3 mL 2.5% solution (50 to 75 mg) IV q20–40s until desired effect reached
  Seizures, 75 to 125 mg IV

Trimethaphan (Arfonad):
  Route: IV
  Dosage: Start at 0.3 mg/min and titrate to effect.

Abbreviations: aPTT, activated partial thromboplastin time; BP, blood pressure; IM, intramuscular; IV, intravenous; NS, normal saline; PO, by mouth; PR, by rectum; SL, sublingual.

Common Laboratory Values in the ICU

The most common laboratory values used in the assessment of critically ill patients are presented in this chapter. They have been organized in alphabetical order and according to biologic source where; (P) represents plasma, (B) blood, (S) serum, (U) urine, (CSF) cerebrospinal fluid, (RBCs) red blood cells and (WBCs) white blood cells. These values are not intended to be definitive, since normal ranges vary from hospital to hospital. Both traditional units and system international (SI) units are presented.

α1-Antitrypsin (S)
150 to 350 mg/dL (dual report) (SI: 1.5 to 3.5 g/L)

17-Ketogenic steroids (as dehydroepiandrosterone) (U)
Female: 7 to 12 mg/24 h (SI: 25 to 40 μmol/d)
Male: 9 to 17 mg/24 h (SI: 30 to 60 μmol/d)

17-Ketosteroids (as dehydroepiandrosterone) (U)
Female: 6 to 17 mg/24 h (SI: 20 to 60 μmol/d)
Male: 6 to 20 mg/24 h (SI: 20 to 70 μmol/d)

Alanine aminotransferase (ALT) (S)
0 to 35 (35°C) U/L (SI: 0 to 35 U/L)

Albumin (S)
4.0 to 6.0 g/dL (SI: 40 to 60 g/L)

Ammonia (P)
As ammonia (NH_3): 10 to 80 μg/dL (dual report) (SI: 5 to 50 μmol/L)
As ammonium (NH_4): 10 to 85 μg/dL (dual report) (SI: 5 to 50 μmol/L)
As nitrogen (N): 10 to 65 μg/dL (dual report) (SI: 5 to 50 μmol/L)

Amylase (S):
  0 to 130 (37°C) U/L (SI: 0 to 130 U/L)
  50 to 150 Somogyi units/dL (SI: 100 to 300 U/L)

Aspartate aminotransferase (AST) (S)
  0 to 35 (37°C) U/L (SI: 0 to 35 U/L)

Bilirubin (S)
  Total: 0.1 to 1.0 mg/dL (dual report) (SI: 2 to 18 μmol/L)
  Conjugated: 0 to 0.2 mg/dL (dual report) (SI: 0 to 4 μmol/L)

Calcium (S)
  Male: 8.8 to 10.3 mg/dL (dual report) (SI: 2.20 to 2.58 mmol/L)
  Female: <50 years, 8.8 to 10.3 mg/dL (dual report) (SI: 2.20 to 2.58 mmol/L)

Calcium, normal diet (U)
  <250 mg/24 h (SI: <6.2 mmol/d)

Carbon dioxide content (CO_2 + HCO_3) (B, P, S)
  22 to 28 mEq/L (SI: 22 to 28 mmol/L)

Chloride (S)
  95 to 105 mEq/L (SI: 95 to 105 mmol/L)

Cholesterol esters, as a fraction of total cholesterol (P)
  60% to 75% (SI: 0.60 to 0.75)

Complement, C3 (S)
  70 to 160 mg/dL (SI: 0.7 to 1.6 g/L)

Copper (S)
  70 to 140 μg/dL (SI: 11.0 to 22.0 μmol/L)

Cholesterol (P)
  <200 mg/dL (dual report) (SI: <5.20 mmol/L)

Copper (U)
  <40 μg/24 h (SI: <0.6 μmol/d)

Corticotropin (ACTH) (P)
  20 to 100 pg/mL (SI: 4 to 22 pmol/L)

Creatine kinase (CK) (S)
  0 to 130 (37°C) U/L (SI: 0 to 130 U/L)

Creatine kinase isoenzymes, MB fraction (S)
  >5% in myocardial infarction (SI: >0.05)

Creatine (U)
  Male: 0 to 40 mg/24 h (SI: 0 to 300 μmol/d)
  Female: 0 to 80 mg/24 h (SI: 0 to 600 μmol/d)

Creatine (S)
  Male: 0.17 to 0.50 mg/dL (SI: 10 to 40 μmol/L)
  Female: 0.35 to 0.93 mg/dL (SI: 30 to 70 μmol/L)

Creatinine (U)
Variable g/24h (Dual report) (SI: variable mmol/d)

Creatinine (S)
0.6 to 1.2mg/dL (dual report) (SI: 50 to 110μmol/L)

Creatinine clearance (S, U)
75 to 125mL/min (dual report) (SI: 1.24 to 2.08mL/s)

Cystine (U)
10 to 100mg/24h (SI: 40 to 420μmol/d)

Dehydroepiandrosterone (U)
Female: 0.2 to 1.8mg/24h (SI: 1 to 6μmol/d)
Male: 0.2 to 2.0mg/24h (SI: 1 to 7μmol/d)

Digoxin, therapeutic (P)
0.5 to 2.2ng/mL (dual report) (SI: 0.6 to 2.8mmol/L)
0.5 to 2.2μg/L (dual report) (SI: 0.6 to 2.8mmol/L)

Erythrocyte sedimentation rate (B)
Female: 0 to 30mm/h (SI: 0 to 30mm/h)
Male: 0 to 20mm/h (SI: 0 to 20mm/h)

Estradiol, male > 18 years (S)
15 to 40pg/mL (dual report) (SI: 55 to 150pmol/L)

Ethyl alcohol (P)
<100mg/dL (SI: <22mmol/L)

Etiocholanolone
Female: 0.8 to 4.0mg/24h (SI: 2 to 14μmol/d)
Male: 1.4 to 5.0mg/14h (SI: 4 to 17μmol/d)

Testosterone (P)
Female: <0.6ng/mL (dual report) (SI: <2.0nmol/L)
Male: 4.0 to 8.0ng/mL (dual report) (SI: 14.0 to 28.0nmol/L)

Fibrinogen (P)
200 to 4300mg/dL (SI: 2.0 to 4.0g/L)

Follicle-stimulating hormone (FSH) (P)
Female: 2.0 to 15.0mIU/mL (SI: 2 to 15IU/L)
Peak production: 20 to 50mIU/mL (SI: 20 to 50IU/L)
Male: 1.0 to 10.0mIU/mL (SI: 1 to 10IU/L)

Follicle-stimulating hormone (FSH) (U)
Follicular phase: 2 to 15IU/24h (SI: 2 to 15IU/d)
Midcycle: 8 to 40IU/24h (SI: 8 to 40IU/d)
Luteal phase: 2 to 10IU/24h (SI: 2 to 10IU/d)
Menopausal women: 35 to 100IU/24h (SI: 35 to 100IU/d)
Male: 2 to 15IU/24h (SI: 2 to 15IU/d)

Gamma-glutamyltransferase (GGT) (S)
0 to 30 (30°C) U/L (SI: 0 to 30 U/L)

Glucose (P)
70 to 110 mg/dL (dual report) (SI: 3.9 to 6.1 mmol/L)

Hematocrit (B)
Female: 33% to 43% (SI: 0.33 to 0.43)
Male: 39% to 49% (SI: 0.39 to 0.49)

Hemoglobin (B)
Male: 14.0 to 18.0 g/dL (SI: 140 to 180 g/L)
Female: 11.5 to 15.5 g/dL (SI: 115 to 155 g/L)

Hemoglobin (B)
Female: 12.0 to 15.0 g/dL (SI: 120 to 150 g/L)
Male: 13.6 to 17.2 g/dL (SI: 136 to 172 g/L)

Immunoglobulins (S)
IgG: 500 to 1200 mg/dL (SI: 5.00 to 12.00 g/L)
IgA: 50 to 350 mg/dL (SI: 0.50 to 3.50 g/L)
IgM: 30 to 230 mg/dL (SI: 0.30 to 2.30 g/L)
IgD: <6 mg/dL (SI: <60 mg/L)
IgE:
   0 to 3 years: 0.5 to 1.0 U/mL (SI: 1 to 24 µg/L)
   3 to 80 years: 5 to 100 U/mL (SI: 12 to 240 µg/L)

Iron (S)
Male: 80 to 180 µg/dL (dual report) (SI: 14 to 32 µmol/L)
Female: 60 to 160 µg/dL (dual report) (SI: 11 to 29 µmol/L)

Iron-binding capacity (S)
250 to 460 µg/dL (dual report) (SI: 45 to 82 µmol/L)

Ketosteroid fractions (U)
Androsterone:
   Female: 0.5 to 3.0 mg/24 h (SI: 1 to 10 µmol/d)
   Male: 2.0 to 5.0 mg/24 h (SI: 7 to 17 µmol/d)

Lactate dehydrogenase (S)
50 to 150 (37°C) U/L (SI: 50 to 150 U/L)

Lactate dehydrogenase isoenzymes (S)
LD_1: 15% to 40% (SI: 0.15 to 0.40)
LD_2: 20% to 45% (SI: 0.20 to 0.45)
LD_3: 15% to 30% (SI: 0.15 to 0.30)
LD_4 and LD_5: 5% to 20% (SI: 0.05 to 0.20)
LD_1: 10 to 60 U/L (SI: 10 to 60 U/L)
LD_2: 20 to 70 U/L (SI: 20 to 70 U/L)
LD_3: 10 to 45 U/L (SI: 10 to 45 U/L)
LD_4 and LD_5: 5 to 30 U/L (SI: 5 to 30 U/L)

Lead, toxic (B)
>60 µg/dL (dual report) (SI: >2.90 µmol/L)

Lead, toxic (U)
>80 µg/24 h (dual report) (SI: >0.40 µmol/d)

Lipids, total (P)
400 to 850 mg/dL (dual report) (SI: 4.0 to 8.5 g/L)

Lipoproteins (P)
Low-density (LDL), as cholesterol: 50 to 190 mg/dL (dual report)
(SI: 1.30 to 4.90 mmol/L)
High-density (HDL), as cholesterol:
Male: 30 to 70 mg/dL (dual report) (SI: 0.80 to 1.80 mmol/L)
Female: 30 to 90 mg/dL (dual report) (SI: 0.80 to 2.35 mmol/L)

Magnesium (S)
1.8 to 3.0 mg/dL (dual report) (SI: 0.80 to 1.20 mmol/L)

Mean corpuscular hemoglobin concentration (B)
Mass concentration: 33 to 37 g/dL (SI: 330 to 370 g/L)
Substance concentration (Hb[Fe]): 33 to 37 g/dL (SI: 20 to 23 mmol/L)

Mean corpuscular hemoglobin (B)
Mass concentration: 27 to 33 pg (SI: 27 to 33 pg)
Substance concentration (Hb[Fe]): 27 to 33 pg (SI: 1.68 to 2.05 fmol)

Mean corpuscular volume (B)
Erythrocyte volume: 76 to 100 µm³ (SI: 76 to 100 fL)

Phenytoin, therapeutic (P)
10 to 20 mg/L (SI: 40 to 80 µmol/L)

Phosphatase, acid (prostatic) (P)
0 to 3 King-Armstrong U/dL (SI: 0 to 5.5 U/L)

Phosphatase, alkaline (S)
30 to 120 U/L (SI: 30 to 120 U/L)

Phosphate (as phosphorus) (S)
2.5 to 5.0 mg/dL (dual report) (SI: 0.80 to 1.60 mmol/L)

Platelets (B)
150 to 450 10³/mm³ (SI: 150 to 450 10⁹/L)

Potassium (S)
3.5 to 5.0 mEq/L (SI: 3.5 to 5.0 mmol/L)

Progesterone (P)
Follicular phase: <2 ng/mL (SI: <6 nmol/L)
Luteal phase: 2 to 20 ng/mL (SI: 6 to 64 nmol/L)

Protein, total (U)
<150 mg/24 h (SI: <0.15 g/d)

Protein, total (S)
6 to 8g/dL (SI: 60 to 80g/L)

Protein, total (CSF)
<40mg/dL (SI: <0.40g/L)

Red blood cell count (erythrocytes) (B)
Female: 3.5 to 5.0 10^6/mm³ (SI: 3.5 to 5.0 10^{12}/L)
Male: 4.3 to 5.9 10^6/mm³ (SI: 4.3 to 5.1 10^{12}/L)

Red blood cell count (CSF)
0/cu mm (SI: 0 10^6/L)

Reticulocyte count (adult) (B)
10,000 to 75,000/cu mm (dual report) (SI: 10 to 75 10^6/L)
Number fraction: 1 to 24 0/00 (No. per 1000 erythrocytes) (SI: 1 to 24 10^{-3})
0.1% to 2.4% (SI: 1 to 24 10^{-3})

Sodium (S)
135 to 147mEq/L (SI: 135 to 147mmol/L)

Sodium ion (S)
135 to 147mEq/L (SI: 135 to 147mmol/L)

Sodium ion (U)
Diet-dependent mEq/24h (SI: 5 to 25mmol/d)

Steroids (U)
Hydroxycorticosteroids (as cortisol):
Female: 2 to 8mg/24h (SI: 5 to 25µmol/d)
Male: 3 to 10mg/24h (SI: 10 to 30µmol/d)

Thyroxine (T_4) (S)
4 to 11µg/dL (dual report) (SI: 51 to 142nmol/L)

Thyroxine-binding globulin (TBG) (S)
12 to 28µg/dL (dual report) (SI: 150 to 360nmol/L)

Thyroxine, free (S)
0.8 to 2.8ng/dL (dual report) (SI: 10 to 36pmol/L)

Triodothyronine (T_3) (S)
75 to 220ng/dL (SI: 1.2 to 3.4nmol/L)

Urate (as uric acid) (S)
2.0 to 7.0mg/dL (SI: 120 to 140µmol/L)

Urate (as uric acid) (U)
Diet-dependent g/24h (SI: diet-dependent mmol/d)

Urea nitrogen (S)
8 to 18mg/dL (dual report) (SI: 3.0 to 6.5mmol/L of urea)

Urea nitrogen (U)
 12 to 20 g/24 h (dual report) (SI: 430 to 700 mmol/d of urea)

Urobilinogen (U)
 0 to 4.0 mg/24 h (SI: 0.0 to 6.8 µmol/d)

White blood cell count (B)
 3200 to 9800/mm^3 (SI: 3.2 to 9.8 10^9/L)

White blood cell count (CSF)
 0 to 5/cu mm (SI: 0 to 5 10^6/L)

Zinc (S)
 75 to 120 µg/dL (SI: 11.5 to 18.5 µmol/L)

Zinc (U)
 150 to 1200 µg/24 h (SI: 2.3 to 18.3 µmol/d)

Index